DANGERS

of

Excessive
Antioxidants

IN CANCER PATIENTS

A Health Impact Statement and Selective Review for the Medical Professional and Educated Consumer

BY

PROF. HON. RANDOLPH M. HOWES, M.D., Ph.D.

Physician, Surgeon and Scientist (Biochemist)

DANGERS
of
Excessive
Antioxidants
IN CANCER PATIENTS

BY
PROF. HON. RANDOLPH M. HOWES, M.D., Ph.D.
Physician, Surgeon and Scientist (Biochemist)

Adjunct Assistant Professor of Plastic Surgery,
The Johns Hopkins Hospital, Baltimore, MD USA

Espaldon Professor of Plastic and Reconstructive Surgery,
University of Santo Tomas, Manila, Philippines

Adjunct Professor of Biological Sciences,
Southeastern Louisiana University

Founder, Director and Chairman of the Scientific Advisory Board;
U.S. Medical Scientific Research Foundation, Inc.

Acknowledgements

Special thanks Don Neale Piatt, Sr. for expert proof reading.
Also, special thanks to Michael R. Root, M.S. for his unwavering encouragement.

I despise precious time wasted,
for it alone, is the unfinished canvas
displaying the portrait of my life.

R. M. Howes, M.D., Ph.D.
9/7/09

Notice to users:

Disclaimers:

Please note: only your personal physician or other health professional you consult can best advise you on matters of your health based on your medical history, your family medical history, your medication history, and how information from any of these databases may apply to you. Neither Dr. Howes nor any party involved in creating, producing or delivering this web site shall be liable for any damages arising out of access to or use of this material or web site, or any errors or omissions in the content thereof.

The information given herein is not intended as medical advice. Always consult with your doctor for underlying illness. Before beginning dietary investigation, consult a dietician or a physician with an interest in nutrition. Information is drawn from the scientific literature, web research, and personal enquiry; while all care is taken, information is not warranted as accurate and the author cannot be held liable for any errors and omissions.

Financial disclosure:

Dr. Howes has no financial conflicts of interest and is not involved in the sale of dietary supplements or fitness equipment. The author holds no stocks or interests in companies in the food additive or antioxidant supplement business.

ABOUT THE AUTHOR
RMH Biographical sketch:

Dr. Howes was the first in the history of Tulane School of Medicine to be awarded a Doctorate of Medicine degree and a Ph.D. in Biochemistry at the same time. He was trained as a General surgeon and a Plastic surgeon at the prestigious Johns Hopkins Hospital, in Baltimore, Maryland. He was the first in the history of Johns Hopkins Hospital to obtain board eligibility in both general and plastic surgery in a six year period.

Dr. Howes invented the triple lumen venous catheter, which has been credited with helping save the lives of over 20 million critically ill patients worldwide. His catheter is the number one venous catheter in the world today and his name is well recognized in over 100 countries. He has been recognized as a humanitarian, visionary, entrepreneur, singer, songwriter, inventor and author.

He received the Harper Award for innovative research from the American College for Advancement in Medicine, served as their keynote speaker and his peers refer to him as "a walking encyclopedia on oxygen metabolism."

He is a Dr. Norman Vincent Peale Unsung Hero award winner, which recognized his awesome versatility. Additionally, even though he does not like talking about it, he is a self made multi-millionaire.

He is currently doing extensive research on cures for cancer and heart disease and development of revolutionary treatment modalities. He has written 16 books over the past 8 years on the subject of oxygen metabolism, as it relates to protection from cancer, heart disease, diabetes, malaria, HIV/AIDS, Alzheimer's disease, aging and arthritis. He has written many scientific and medical papers and has lectured nationally and internationally.

His research has shown that currently popular antioxidant vitamins, such as vitamins A & E, (and vitamin C to a lesser extent) can be harmful and that oxygen free radicals protect us from bacterial, fungal and viral infections and they help to control cancer growth. He has developed an effective, inexpensive singlet oxygen generating system, from orthomolecular agents, for the treatment of cancer and heart disease. He is passionate about his research and hopes to have his discoveries at the patient's bedside in his lifetime.

There are over 6,000 pages in his magnum opus and at the Howes World Selective Library on Oxygen Metabolism.

Over 3,000 pages of his opus are available online in a searchable format
www.iwillfindthecure.org

To put one's faith in people
is to seek disappointment.
To put one's faith in ideas of discovery
is to be pestered by never-ending curiosity.

R. M. Howes, M.D., Ph.D.
9/7/09

Companion Papers:

Citation: R. Howes: Mythology of Antioxidant Vitamins?. The Journal of Evidence-Based Alternative and Complimentary Medicine. April, 2011. 16(2): 149-189.

Citation: R. Howes: Cancer Therapy: A Review with Scientific Validation for the Role of Electronically Modified Oxygen Derivatives in Oncologic Treatment Modalities. The Internet Journal of Alternative Medicine. 2010 Volume 8 Number 1.

Citation: R. Howes: Hydrogen Peroxide: A review of a scientifically verifiable omnipresent ubiquitous essentiality of obligate, aerobic, carbon-based life forms. The Internet Journal of Plastic Surgery. 2010 Volume 7 Number 1.

Howes M.D., PhD., R. (2009). Dangers of Antioxidants in Cancer Patients: A Review. PHILICA.COM Article number 153. Published 7th February, 2009. (20 pages)

Howes M.D., PhD., R. (2008). Aging and anti-aging claims: a review on antioxidant vitamins A, C & E. PHILICA.COM Article number 116. Published on 12th January, 2008. (16 pages)

Howes M.D., PhD., R. (2007). Sleep: An original "radical" proposal. PHILICA.COM Observation number 42. Published on 5th October, 2007. (1 page)

Howes M.D., PhD., R. (2007). Antioxidant Vitamins A, C & E; Death in Small Doses and Legal Liability? PHILICA.COM Article number 89. Published on 5th April, 2007. (23 pages)

Howes M.D., PhD., R. (2007). Cancer, Apoptosis and Reactive Oxygen Species: A New Paradigm. PHILICA.COM Article number 86. Published on 26th February, 2007. (11 pages)

Howes M.D., PhD., R. (2007). Antioxidant Vitamins A, C and E: Assessing Potential for Harm. PHILICA.COM Article number 83. Published on 15th February, 2007. (14 pages)

Howes M.D., PhD., R. (2007). The Consequent Downfall of the Free Radical Theory. PHILICA.COM Article number 75. Published on 22nd January, 2007. (9 pages)

Howes, R.M.: "The Free Radical Fantasy," The Annals of New York Academy of Sciences, 2006, Vol. 1067, pp. 22-26.

Available at:

www.philica.com
www.medi.philica.com
www.iwillfindthecure.org

Experience is the primo teacher,
enlightening us as to how little we really know.

R. M. Howes, M.D., Ph.D.
9/7/09

Prof Randolph M. Howes MD, PhD

OTHER BOOKS PUBLISHED:

#1 The Fire Eaters, Molding your own destiny more easily, Carnivore Press, © 1982

#2 Uplift, The Answer Book to your plastic and cosmetic surgery questions, Carnivore Press, © 1986

#3 The Pundit Speaks, An Anthology of Neoclassical Poetic Philosophy, Carnivore Press, © 1990

#4 The Pundit Speaks, Volume II, An Anthology of Neoclassical Poetic Philosophy, Free Radical Press, © 1994

#5 The Pundit Speaks, Volume III, An Anthology of Neoclassical Poetic Philosophy, Free Radical Press, © 1996

#6 The Fable of the Chocolate Covered Strawberry Coloring Book, Free Radical Press, © 2001

#7 The Pundit Speaks, Volume IV, An Anthology of Neoclassical Poetic Philosophy, Free Radical Press, © 2003

#8 The Pundit Speaks, Volume V, An Anthology of Neoclassical Poetic Philosophy, Trafford Publishing, © 2009

#9 Death In Small Doses? Trafford Publishing, © 2010

#10 Antioxidant Overkill, Free Radical Publishing, © 2011

DEDICATION

To any and all who fanned the flames
of enthusiasm within me, who taught me humility and
who loved me, even if it was just a little.

TABLE OF CONTENTS:

The U.T.O.P.I.A. Institute and Free Radical Publishing Co.

Truly passionate writers,
both scientific and otherwise,
will not quit,
'till they keel over on their keyboards,
never having finished their perceived tasks.

R. M. Howes, M.D., Ph.D.
4/10/11

THE LITTLE PICTURE
THE BIG PICTURE
HOWES NEW RULES
Summary of things that I know

- The role of heme and the mitochondrion in the chemical and molecular mechanisms of mammalian cell death induced by the artemisinin anti-malarials
- Confusing data: antioxidants cure cancer and peroxide blocks apoptosis

THE SCIENTIFIC VOYAGER

The vast immensity of the data ocean surrounds and engulfs you.
At first, you glimpse something foggy on the far away research horizon.
You diligently pursue, in that direction, to get a better look.
A distant shape is then suggested, but needs considerable clarification.
You move in, study it intensely - all possibilities, intensively.
An image of enlightenment begins to form.
It has a pattern and design….but is it real or just another illusion?
More study, more study, more study and
now it congeals into focus. Your mind's eye can see it ever so clearly.
It is a magnificent island of discovery
jutting out of a raging sea of unknowns.
Now, you must step out onto its slippery rock surface
to be scientifically satiated.
There….you feel it solidly under your feet. Eureka!
But how do you inform others of your discovery?
How do you bring them onshore with you?
Carefully, very, very carefully
for many are still blind,
still uninformed, still misinformed, still lost at sea!
Yet, for you, the tumultuous journey is at an end.
You are scientifically satisfied….
'till you launch the next inquiry.

R. M. Howes, M.D., Ph.D.
4/1/11

Preliminary warning:
IN GENERAL,
STUDIES HAVE SHOWN THAT
ANTIOXIDANTS ARE NEITHER TOTALLY SAFE
NOR PREDICTABLY EFFECTIVE.

R. M. Howes, M.D., Ph.D.

4/18/11

(EMODs, electronically modified oxygen derivatives) (apoptosis, cellular suicide)

There are twenty seven (27) types of human cancer cell types and nine (9) murine cancer cell types that can be killed by EMODs and in which the killing can be blocked by antioxidants, thereby providing antioxidant protection and shielding of the cancer cells. Published data has shown that antioxidants blocked the killing of the following human and murine cancer cell types by EMODs:

human breast cancer (J. Nutr. 134, 2004) (Gundimeda et al, 1996) (Peralta et al, 2006) (Aykin-Burns et al, 2009) (Xiao et al, Mol Cancer Ther. 2006)

human prostate carcinoma (Xiao et al, 2006) (Wu et al, 2005) (Singh et al, 2005) (Cho et al, 2005) (Milanesa et al, 2000)

human non-small cell lung cancer (Ling et al, 2003) (Wu et al, 2006)

human colon adenocarcinoma (Wenzel et al, 2005)

human colon cancer (Wenzel et al, 2004) (Aykin-Burns et al, 2009)

human colorectal carcinoma (Chen et al, 2004) (**Gali-Muhtasib** et al, 2008)

human ovarian cancer cells (Pak et al, 2011)

human melanoma (Marcin et al, 2005) (Okroj et al, 2006) (Nishikawa et al, 2004) (Grimm et al, 2011)

human metastatic melanoma (Kirshner et al, 2008)

human head and neck cancer (Mattson et al, 2009)

human lymphoma (J. Nutr. 134, 2004) (Mansat-De Mas et al, 1999)

human leukemia (Hileman et al, 2004) (McKallip et al, 2006) (Hou et al, 2005) (Feng et al, 2007) (Yedjou et al, 2008) (Hiraoka et al, 1998)

human hepatoma (Wu et al, 2004) (Wu, Ng, Lin, 2004)

human hepatocellular liver carcinoma (Shimoda et al, 2003)

human pancreatic cancer (Maehara et al, 2004)

human multiple myeloma (Grad et al, 2001) (Ahmad et al, 1997) (Gupta et al, 2000) (Nakazato et al, 2005) (Isham et al, 2007)

Burkitt's lymphoma (Ahmad et al, 1997) (Gupta et al, 2000) (Nakazato et al, 2005) (Ahmad et al, 1997)

human chronic lymphocytic leukemia (Kay, 2006) **(Chandra et al, 2003)** (Shanafelt et al, 2005) (Mow et al, 2002) (Biswas S, et al, 2010)

human acute myeloid leukemia (Kay, 2006) **(Chandra et al, 2003)** (Shanafelt et al, 2005) (Mow et al, 2002)

human promyelocytic leukemia (Hou et al, 2005)

human erythromyeloid leukemia (Wagner et al, 2000)

human epithelial cancer cells (breast and colon) (Aykin-Burns et al, 2009)

human endometrial cancer (Llobet et al, 2008)

human bladder cancer cells (Miyajima et al, 1999)

human invasive bladder cancer (Miyajima et al, 1999 - human bladder cancer KU-1 cell line)

human glioblastoma cells (Lee et al, 2004)

human osteosarcoma (Ahmad et al, 2005)

murine pheochromocytoma (Jang, Surh, 2001)

murine retinoblastoma (Salganik et al, 2000)

murine thymoma (Tome et al, 2001)

murine lymphoma- six cell types (Nathan et al, vol 153, 1981)

murine leukemia (Wagner et al, 1996)

murine fibrosarcoma (Teicher et al, 1994)

murine neuroblastoma (Prasad et al, PNAS. 1979)

murine mammary cancer (Bracke et al, 1999)

murine brain cancer (Zeisel (2), 2004)

Part of this list was compiled in 2009 and has been updated for this book. (Howes, Philica. Feb 7, 2009).

It is evident to many investigators that the in vitro apoptogenic agents function as prooxidants.

(Hail et al, 2008).

27 SPECIFIC HUMAN CANCER CELL TYPES SHIELDED BY ANTIOXIDANTS: This expanded section includes identification of cell types with references.

HUMAN _BREAST_ CANCER CELLS: T47D human mammary carcinoma, human breast cancer cells (**MDA-MB-231** and **MCF-7**), human breast cancer cells - **MCF-7** human breast cancer cells (Doroshow, 1986) (J. Nutr. 134, 2004)

(Gundimeda et al, 1996) (Peralta et al, 2006) (Aykin-Burns et al, 2009) (Xiao et al, Mol Cancer Ther. 2006)

HUMAN _PROSTATE_ CANCER CELLS: androgen-independent human prostate cancer **PC-3** cells, (Xiao et al, 2006) (Wu et al, 2005) **PC-3** and **DU145** human prostate cancer cells (Singh et al, 2005), **DU145** prostate cancer cells (Cho et al, 2005) (Milanesa et al, 2000)

HUMAN _NON-SMALL CELL LUNG_ CANCER CELLS: human **H460** non-small cell lung cancer Cells (Ling et al, 2003) (Wu et al, 2006)

HUMAN _COLON ADENOCARCINOMA_ CELLS: **HT-29** human colon cancer cells (Wenzel et al, 2005), **SW480** human colon adenocarcinoma cell line (Aykin-Burns et al, 2009)

HUMAN _COLON_ CANCER CELLS: **HT-29** human colon cancer cells (Wenzel et al, 2004), human colon and breast cancer cells (**HT29** human colon cancer cells, **HCT116** human colon cancer cells, **SW480** human colon adenocarcinoma cells and **MB231** human breast cancer cells) (Aykin-Burns et al, 2009)

HUMAN _COLORECTAL_ CARCINOMA CELLS: colon cancer cells **HCT116** (**Gali-Muhtasib** et al, 2008), colorectal carcinoma cells (**HT29, COLO205, COLO320-HSR**) (Chen et al, 2004)

HUMAN _OVARIAN_ CANCER CELLS: SKOV-3 human ovarian carcinoma cells (Pak et al, 2011)

HUMAN _MELANOMA_ CELLS: (Marcin et al, 2005) (Okroj et al, 2006), **MDA-MB-435S** cells (originally a model for metastatic human breast cancer but now genetically tests more closely to human melanoma cell lines) (Nishikawa et al, 2004) (Grimm et al, 2011)

HUMAN _METASTATIC MELANOMA_: actual human patients were used - not cell cultures (Kirshner et al, 2008)

HUMAN _HEAD AND NECK_ CANCER CELLS: FaDu, Cal-27, and **SQ20B** head and neck cancer cells (Mattson et al, 2009)

HUMAN _LYMPHOMA_ CELLS: U937 histiocytic lymphoma cells (Mansat-De Mas et al, 1999) (J. Nutr. 134, 2004)

HUMAN _LEUKEMIA_ CELLS: (Hileman et al, 2004) (McKallip et al, 2006) (Hou et al, 2005), **HL-60** human leukemia cells (Feng et al, 2007) (Yedjou et al, 2008), **PLB-985** human myeloid leukemia cells (Hiraoka et al, 1998)

HUMAN _HEPATOMA_ CELLS: PLC/PRF/5 human hepatoma cells (Wu et al, 2004), **PLC/PRF/5** human hepatoma cells (Wu, Ng, Lin, 2004)

HUMAN _HEPATOCELLULAR LIVER_ CARCINOMA CELLS: human hepato-cellular carcinoma (HCC) cell clone **P1(0.5),** derived from the **PLC/PRF/5** cell line (P5) (Shimoda et al, 2003)

HUMAN _PANCREATIC_ CANCER CELLS: pancreatic **PC-12** cancer cells (Maehara et al, 2004)

HUMAN _MULTIPLE MYELOMA_ CELLS: 4 human MM cell lines: 8226/S, 8226/Dox40, U266, and U266/Bcl-x(L) (Grad et al, 2001), (Ahmad et al, 1997) (Gupta et al, 2000) (Nakazato et al, 2005), **CD138⁺** myeloma cells (Isham et al, 2007)

BURKITT'S _LYMPHOMA_ CELLS: (Ahmad et al, 1997) (Gupta et al, 2000), Human malignant B-cell lines including myeloma cells (**IM9, RPMI8226, and U266**) and Burkitt's lymphoma cells (**HS-sultan**) (Nakazato et al, 2005), (Ahmad et al, 1997)

HUMAN _CHRONIC LYMPHOCYTIC LEUKEMIA_ CELLS: (Kay, 2006), **CLL B-cells, K562 cells** (Chandra et al, 2003) (Shanafelt et al, 2005) (Mow et al, 2002), **HuID10** chronic lymphocytic leukemia cells (Biswas S, et al, 2010)

HUMAN _ACUTE MYELOID LEUKEMIA_ CELLS: (Kay, 2006) (Chandra et al, 2003) (Shanafelt et al, 2005), **K562** cells and **bcr/abl-transduced FDC-P1** cells and **myeloid progenitors** (Mow et al, 2002)

HUMAN _PROMYELOCYTIC LEUKEMIA_ CANCER CELLS: HL-60 human leukemia cells (Hou et al, 2005)

HUMAN _ERYTHROMYELOID LEUKEMIA_ CELLS: K562 human erythro-leukemia cell line (Wagner et al, 2000) (acute nonlymphocytic leukemia cell line)

HUMAN _EPITHELIAL_ CANCER CELLS: (breast and colon): human colon and breast cancer cells (**HT29** human colon cancer cells, **HCT116** human colon cancer cells, **SW480** human colon adenocarcinoma cells and **MB231** human breast cancer cells) (Aykin-Burns et al, 2009)

HUMAN _ENDOMETRIAL_ CANCER CELLS: cell line not available unless purchase article (Llobet et al, 2008)

HUMAN _BLADDER_ CANCER CELLS: human bladder cancer **KU-1 cell line** (Miyajima et al, 1999)

HUMAN _INVASIVE BLADDER_ CANCER CELLS: (Miyajima et al, 1999 - human bladder cancer **KU-1** cell line)

HUMAN _GLIOBLASTOMA_ CELLS: human glioblastoma cell line **U251** (Lee et al, 2004)

HUMAN _OSTEOSARCOMA_ CELLS: several different human cancer cell lines, i.e., **PC-3, DU145, MDA-MB231, and HT-29** and **human osteosarcoma** cells lacking functional mitochondrial electron transport chains (rho0) (Ahmad et al, 2005)

9 SPECIFIC MURINE (mouse and rat family) CANCER and CELL LINES SHIELDED BY ANTIOXIDANTS

MURINE _PHEOCHROMOCYTOMA_ CELLS: rat pheochromocytoma **(PC12)** cells (Jang, Surh, 2001)

MURINE _RETINOBLASTOMA_: The **TgT**$_{121}$ transgenic line was previously referred to as LST1137-5 (Salganik et al, 2000)

MURINE _THYMOMA_ CELLS: mouse thymoma cells **WEHI7.2** (Tome et al, 2001)

MURINE _LYMPHOMA_ - SIX CELL TYPES: L5178Y mouse lymphoma cells (Agarwal et al, 1991), (Nathan et al, vol 153, 1981)

MURINE _LEUKEMIA_ CELLS: murine leukemia cells **L1210** (Wagner et al, 1996)

MURINE _FIBROSARCOMA_ CELLS: murine fibrosarcoma cells **FSaII** (Teicher et al, 1994)

MURINE _NEUROBLASTOMA_ CELLS: mouse neuroblastoma cells **NBP$_2$** cells (Prasad et al, PNAS. 1979)

MURINE _MAMMARY_ CANCER: female nude mice inoculated with human **MCF-7/6** mammary adenocarcinoma cells. (Bracke et al, 1999)

MURINE _BRAIN_ CANCER:TgT$_{121}$ transgenic mouse model, which spontaneously develops brain cancer (Zeisel (2), 2004)

OTHER known human cancer cell types killed by EMODs

- **human prostate cancer cells:** androgen-independent human prostate cancer **PC-3 (Wt)** cells (Venkataraman et al, 2004), (Venkataraman et al, 2005),

- **human diploid leukemia cells: PLB-985** myeloid leukemia cells (Hiraoka et al, 1998)

- **human leukemia cells isolated from patients:** human monoblastic **ML-1 and lymphoblastoid T-cell Jurkat** lines (Pelicano et al, 2003) (McKallip et al, 2006) (Ahmad et al, 2003)

- **human colon cancer cells: HT-29** colon cancer cells (Malik et al, 2003)

INTRODUCTION

This book is drawn from scientific evidence and not from "overly speculative guessing." I have found striking commonalities between the interactions of EMODs (electronically modified oxygen derivatives, formerly known as ROS, reactive oxygen species) and pathogens and cancer. These shared mechanisms of action are seen within chemotherapy, radiation therapy, photodynamic therapy, apoptosis and pathogen kill by certain antibiotics, all of which substantially involve a central and critical role for EMODs.

It is my belief that the magnitude of these underlying biochemical facts and theoretical projections have been overlooked or denied by those recommending antioxidants to cancer patients or cancer survivors. **There can be no doubt that EMODs are at the very heart of naturally-occurring and/or therapeutically induced apoptosis.** Thus, theoretically, excessive antioxidant activity can be seen as being counter to the very intent of the anti-cancer therapeutic modalities and opposed to natural apoptotic cellular control and turn over, especially as it relates to limiting cancer development, growth and propagation.

Scientific inquiry can never be completed,
only extended.

R. M. Howes, M.D., Ph.D.
9/7/09

Perpetually repeated false impressions and exaggerated inaccuracies have led to the acceptance of flawed theories and disproved hypotheses. Yet, the inaccuracies and the theories, relative to oxygen free radicals, appear to live on and they are now, more than ever, erroneously referred to in the scientific literature as proven facts.

I have become increasingly skeptical and weary of overly exaggerated interpretations of in vitro studies and at epidemiological associations which are presented and touted as cause and effect relationships. By definition, a cause invariably leads to its effect. A cause and effect relationship has been erroneously inferred between electronically modified oxygen derivatives, EMODs (reactive oxygen species, ROS) and exaggerated disease estimates (exceeding 100 diseases, including aging).

Yet, there is not one proven case of a cause and effect relationship between any disease and electronically modified oxygen derivatives (EMODs). To the contrary, there is increasingly convincing evidence that the injudicious use of antioxidants can lead to increased risk of cancer, stroke, heart disease and overall mortality. Further, there is overwhelming evidence that a deficiency level of EMODs is directly linked to repeated infections and tumorigenesis in chronic granulomatous disease, HIV/ AIDS patients and those who are immunosuppressed.

In actuallity, free radicals perform a crucial role in normal, healthy physiological process-es like our immune system and promote (prooxidative reactions) beneficial oxidation. It is important to realize that many vitamins and supplements classified as antioxidants (or so-called antioxidants) are actually redox agents, meaning they act as antioxidants in some instances and prooxidants in others. This markedly increases the difficulty of intrepreting redox data and is seldom addressed in the literature.

A major paradigm-shift is in order as regards the old and predominately accepted free radical theory. EMODs naturally surround us externally in the atmosphere and on the skin, secondary to reactions of O_2 with UV light. We inhale and exhale EMODs, we drink them, we eat them in raw and cooked foods, we generate them in the digestion of foods and we find them present in the excretory organs of the gastrointestinal tract and the urinary system.

> The only oxygen we need is
> one pint per breath at the rate of
> only a minimum of 21,600 times per day.
> Other than that….
>
> R. M. Howes, M.D., Ph.D.
> 9/12/09

In fact, superoxide and hydrogen peroxide are ubiquitous and omnipresent in steady state levels in all aerobic cells, especially in post mitotic cells with high oxygen consumption, such as the brain and the heart. Thus, I ask, "How toxic can EMODs really be?"

The currently accepted tortured logic of the free radical theory teaches that oxygen and its radicals are highly toxic, even lethal. I believe that my review of the overall literature shows that they are wrong. I believe that these EMODs are primarily "protective prooxidants." Further, I believe that they are of low toxicity, considering the fact that all of our aerobic cells are continually bathed in steady state levels of EMODs, throughout our entire lifetime.

In the 1960's and the 1970's, a group at Baylor University Medical Center found that intra-arterial and intravenous administration of hydrogen peroxide would aid in killing cancer and pathogens and aid in the regression of arteriosclerotic plaque. I believe that hydrogen peroxide is the most prevalent, and perhaps the most significant EMOD in the body, even exceeding the well recognized importance of nitric oxide.

Followers of the free radical theory and the mitochondrial theory of aging say that aging is a stochastic (random) disease of accumulation of damaged products of oxidation and I say that aging and disease are, at least in part, the result of deficiency states, especially of EMODs. Contrary to the expectations of the free radical theory, those who seem to have the best health are the individuals who exercise and who metabolize the highest levels of oxygen and generate the highest levels of EMODs.

Oxygen consumption increases up to 20 times greater with exercise than the resting level, resulting in an elevated flow of oxygen through the mitochondrial electron-transport chain and a nigh stoichiometric increase in EMOD production. I believe that we should "consider exercise to be a medicine" and that each episode of exercise is equivalent to a substantial dose of EMODs. According to the free radical theory, the presence of the alleged damaging EMODs, secondary to exercise, would promote increases in diseases and aging but, that does not happen.

Conversely, hypoxia allows cancer cells to be more aggressive, to metastasize and impairs the effect of radiation, which is based on the generation of tumoricidal EMODs.

Conditions which substantially decrease the amount of oxygen available to the cell, at the EMOD production level in the electron transport chain and oxidative phosphorylation, will predictably cause or result in the manifestation of disease and/or cell death. Twice Nobel Laureate, Otto Warburg has said that disease is a problem of oxygenation but I say that it is, specifically and in particular, a problem of oxidation. This oxidation is based on relative levels of EMODs.

We have been "radically" misled by the teachings of the free radical theory. In 2004, I published a 767 page e-book entitled, "U.T.O.P.I.A. Unified Theory of

Oxygen Participation In Aerobiosis," which outlined a unique, new "radical" paradigm to explain EMODs and their association with cellular redox status, homeostatic self healing and prooxidant protection against pathogens and neoplasia. I concluded that deficient EMOD levels "allow" for the development of pathogens, cancer and, in part, aging. Normal EMOD levels maintain homeostasis and the redox status of the cell and high EMOD levels kill pathogens and cancer. Our body protects us with the primary way that it has available to it, which is by utilizing oxidative biochemistry.

There is not one major medical breakthrough based on the free radical theory (i.e., EMODs are harmful and deleterious agents)....NONE!

The flow of electrons and protons, via oxygen and the EMODs, is essential for energizing our state of being alive, as evidenced by Peter Mitchell's Nobel winning chemiosmotic theory. Oxygen free radicals are designed to provide for the flow of electrons and I believe that some antioxidants are designed as possible co-oxidants or pre-oxidants (not oxidant scavengers or quenchers) in promotion of this electron/proton flow. Otherwise, one can not explain the prooxidant activity of antioxidants.

By design, the shift back and forth between two alternating oxidation states, via single-electron-transfer reactions, is the property that makes iron and copper such essential components of the hemeproteins and enzyme complexes in the endoplasmic reticulum and the mitochondrial electron transport system. Transition metals are designed to exist in several alternating spin-states and are able to relieve the π-electron spin restrictions of ground state dioxygen. The coordination of biomolecules by transition metals almost always involves the d-orbitals of the metal.

Iron and copper can serve as prooxidants and deficiency states of both are associated with an increased incidence of cancer, infections and arthritis. As with oxygen, many atoms and molecules are designed to promote vital electron/proton flow and to metabolically proceed via free radical species.

In 2005, I published a 931 page e-book, a companion to U.T.O.P.I.A., entitled, "The Medical and Scientific Significance of Oxygen Free Radical Metabolism," which solidified my Unified Theory, based on an extensive review of the world's literature on oxygen metabolism. In this book, I further developed my theory that EMODs are the fundamental basic elements for prooxidant protection from pathogens and neoplasia and that they are responsible for oxidative self-healing and for staving off death. They keep countless pathogens and neoplastic cells continually in check and they respond to bodily injury, such that they can assist in collagen synthesis and wound healing.

At least 200 genes and signal transducing proteins have been reported to be sensitive to reductive and oxidative (redox) states within the cell. Just as the body has the fibrinolytic system which continually keeps blood from clotting intravascularly, the body has oxidative systems which keep cancer from growing, plaques from forming, herpetic lesions from developing and cataracts from coalescing.

My review of the literature revealed that spontaneous regression is seen in cancers, arteriosclerosis, cataract formation, HIV/AIDS, arthritis, etc. This gives strong support to the position that we must have in place an intrinsic system to hold in abeyance or reverse these conditions or they would remain or progressively get worse.

In 2006, I published a 274 page e-book entitled, "Hydrogen Peroxide: Monograph 1: Scientific, Medical and Biochemical Overview and Monograph 2: Antioxidant Vitamins: A, C & E: Equivocal Scientific Studies." We need to change directions from the library to laboratory and to move on to the patient's bedside.

During 2004 and 2005 I lectured both nationally and internationally to present my Unified Theory to qualified scientists and physicians for their critique and/or acceptance. I lectured to the graduating medical class at the University of Santo Tomas and to the Philippine Association of Plastic and Reconstructive Surgeons in Manila as the Espaldon Professor of Plastic Surgery; at the 40th Annual Meeting of American Academy of Environmental Medicine (AAEM) for a requested two lectures; at the Orthomolecular Health Medicine Society (OHMS) for a requested two lectures; as the Keynote Speaker and recipient of the 2005 Harold Harper Award at the 64th Regional Education Conference of the American College for Advancement in Medicine (ACAM); as the Visiting Professor at the Johns Hopkins Plastic Surgery Division; at the International College of Integrative Medicine (ICIM); and at the 11th Congress of the International Association of Biomedical Gerontology in Denmark, following the opening lecture of Dr. Denham Harman (father of the free radical theory). I am currently trying to find funding and to set up investigational cancer studies at the University of Santo Tomas, utilizing my singlet oxygen delivery system and to set up a wide array of oxidative clinical and laboratory studies needing funding at the Johns Hopkins Hospital.

Passion for my work is obvious in my lectures and this was reflected by the fact that I was the only lecturer who was asked to present two lectures at two of the above conferences (AAEM and OHMS). Dr. John Wilson, program coordinator of the AAEM, told the attendees that my first talk had created a "firestorm" of discussion and thus, I was asked to speak a second time. At the IABG-Denmark meeting, I directly and respectively challenged Dr. Harman's free radical paradigm. Further, the American College for Advancement in Medicine presented me with their 2005 Harold Harper Award, recognizing a "visionary in the field of preventive medicine, which transmits new medical thinking to new physicians in a clear and forceful manner." The cost of the above activities have been covered by utilizing my personal funds, exclusive of some honoraria.

I have had the opportunity to work closely with many of the great minds of medical science. My biochemistry mentor at Tulane was Dr. Richard Steele, whose mentor was Nobel Laureate, Dr. Albert Szent Gyorgii. While at Tulane, I worked as a technician with Nobel Laureate, Dr. Andrew V. Schally, co-isolator of thyrotropin releasing factor. At Tulane, I had the privilege of meeting and speaking with Nobel Laureate, Dr. Linus Pauling, and Dr. Wald, who was interested in the fact that I was the first in the history of Tulane to complete a doctorate of medicine and a doctorate in biochemistry simultaneously, which they felt could help bridge the chiasm between physicians and scientists.

While completing my general surgery and plastic surgery training at the Johns Hopkins Hospital, I had the opportunity to work with the late Dr. Albert L. Lehninger, who contributed so much to the study of the mitochondrion and I was able to conduct research on oxygen free radicals throughout my general and plastic surgery residencies. In later years, I had many fascinating conversations with Nobel Laureate, Dr. Fritz Lipmann, discoverer of co-enzyme-A and its importance in intermediary metabolism. While at a meeting at Johns Hopkins, I presented an original poem entitled, "Nitric Oxide: Radical Thoughts in vein," to Nobel Laureate, Dr. Louis Ignarro. I feel that exposure to these great minds has been influential in helping me envision new landmark paradigms in the formulation of my innovative research.

In 2003, following two presentations to the board of directors of Arrow International, Inc., I convinced them to fund a pilot study for my singlet oxygen cancer therapy system. We jointly agreed to hire a lab at Tuft's Medical School to conduct my studies. It was agreed by all involved that I would be the first author of any and all papers produced by this research. However, after my singlet oxygen system produced successful results with a 22% kill of human squamous cell carcinoma, which had been transplanted into athymic mice, the head of the lab insisted that he should be the first author because his lab had physically run the study (which Arrow and I had specifically hired and paid him to do).

I steadfastly stood my ground and refused to allow him to usurp undue credit for my innovative ideas and to try to take credit for my Unified Theory paradigm.

Consequently, I missed out on a major publication and had to settle for including it in my second book. I am persistence personified, as I pointed out in my 1982 book entitled, "The Fire Eaters: Molding your own destiny more easily." More and more physicians are being attracted to my Unified Theory paradigm and are seeking to utilize combinatorial oxidative therapies for their patients.

Basic energy-producing metabolism for aerobic organisms starts with $^3sgO_2$ (ground state oxygen) and ends with H_2O (water). The primary intermediate oxygen derivatives are O_2^- (superoxide anion radical), H_2O_2 (hydrogen peroxide), the hydroxyl radical (.OH) and its primary electronic excitation state, $^1d_gO_2$ (metastable singlet delta oxygen).

Both O_2^- and H_2O_2 are essential steps in the mitochondrial electron transport chain and its coupling to oxidative phosphorylation for ATP (adenosine triphosphate) energy production. All other EMODs are formed by secondary mechanisms.

Nothing is more disturbing than the claims by thousands of researchers that O_2 is a toxic killer, contrasted with the claims of thousands of alternative practitioners that O_2 therapy is a miracle cure. In considering the incredible range of results seen with varying qualified laboratory investigators and in view of the diametrically opposed clinical results, seen with clinicians versus practitioners of alternative medicine, there is an eminent need for a view towards innovative unification. However, acceptance of my Unified Theory will require studies performed in strict accordance with the scientific method and conducted at a well recognized academic institution.

Presently, our methods for treating cancer, atherosclerosis, diabetes, HIV/AIDS, arthritis and malaria lack a high degree of effectiveness and we have poor models for prevention of these diseases. The Howes Singlet Oxygen Delivery System is a quantitative, highly reproducible, reliable, nonradicallic, single-step method, which is completely made of crucial physiological compounds and which breaks down into needed end products. My system utilizes the principles of the Foote reaction, which combines hydrogen peroxide with sodium hypochlorite to yield electronically excited singlet molecular oxygen, sodium chloride and water.

The Howes Singlet Oxygen Delivery System produces rapid cancer cell kill, with minimal damage, if any, to normal cells because normal cells have the biochemical requirements to deal with a steady state of singlet oxygen and EMODs on an ongoing basis. Biochemically, it does not get any better than this.

Once the simplicity of my singlet oxygen delivery system is understood and its potential bactericidal, virucidal, fungicidal, parasiticidal and tumoricidal properties are appreciated, we should have the ability to successfully treat a vast variety of bacterial diseases, such as sepsis and methicillin resistant infections; fungal infections; parasitic infestations such as malaria; viral infections such as HIV/AIDS, Epstein Barr and rotaviruses and any virus with a lipid coat; and all cell types of neoplastic diseases, including metastatic lesions.

The ability to stack or use oxidative therapies in a combinatorial manner offers unbelievable possibilities for selectively targeting pathogens and neoplasia, while not producing significant damage to normal cells (Please refer to my book entitled, *Antioxidant Overkill,* published 2011). This aspect alone could help us avoid some of the 100,000 annual deaths attributed to adverse drug reactions and could represent a paradigm shift from reliance on harmful pharmaceuticals to a system which duplicates the body's natural oxidative healing and protective mechanisms.

I have been involved with studies in oxidative metabolism and electronic excitation states since the mid 1960s, when I worked with Dr. Richard H. Steele in the Department of Biochemistry at Tulane School of Medicine. Pioneering work by Dr. Steele and I, in the 1970s on microsomal lipid peroxidation and aryl-hydroxylations, demonstrated evidence for the generation and participation of electronic excitation states, namely singlet oxygen. We were the first to demonstrate the functional generation of an electronic excitation state, exclusive of vision, in mammalian systems. Our work was supported in 2002 by the work of Yasui et al who presented evidence for singlet oxygen involvement in rat and human cytochrome P450-dependent substrate oxidations.

While studying widely divergent biological electronic excitation generating systems, such as the microsomal mixed function oxidases, the neutrophil respiratory burst, and proline hydroxylation for collagen biosynthesis, I believed that these oxidative systems shared a point of convergence, expressed in the Howes Excytomer Pathway, involving superoxide anion and electronically excited singlet oxygen, which was published in Perspectives in Biology and Medicine in 1977.

Photodynamic therapy (PDT) is used to treat diseases ranging from cancer to psoriasis and utilizes injectables or ointments, which are light-activated to produce singlet oxygen. PDT will also dissolve arteriosclerotic plaque and kill cancer cells. Furthermore, I saw an additional commonality with generation of singlet oxygen produced by the steady-state physiological oxidative reagents containing an organic peroxide and the salt of hypohalous acid. Subsequently, I reasoned that the peroxide/hypochlorite oxidative system may represent an ideal method of singlet oxygen delivery for effectively treating premalignant and malignant lesions, while simultane-ously eliminating many of the drawbacks associated, not only with photodynamic therapy (PDT), but with all other conventional methods of cancer therapy. It has been shown that phagocytic cells can kill cancer cells with the respiratory burst, when there is a sufficiency of EMODs. This work begs to be investigated.

I fully realize that I am swimming upstream, against a downward tide of established oxygen free radical articles and authors but their paradigm has proven to be a highly unreliable predictor of clinical results in humans. I have developed a new paradigm of predictability to more correctly explain current scientific and clinical observations.

Traditional grants are presented to projects which follow the beaten path of ac-cepted scientific dogma. Usually, there is little tolerance for or financial support given to new paradigms and innovative approaches. In my case, since I am working with non-patentable agents, such as hydrogen peroxide and sodium hypochlorite, the standard "pharmaceutical pot of gold for funding" has no interest in support-ing such ground breaking paradigms. They have no profit motive to pursue any of these studies.

Yet, my work could promote research which could yield effective, inexpensive and readily available treatment modalities for all countries of the world. The potential to relieve pain and suffering for all the people of the world fuels the fire of innova-tion and discovery, which burns so brightly within my heart.

Unfortunately, traditional oxidative therapies, as practiced by alternative practitio-ners, have been considered to be on the fringe of orthodox allopathic medicine. Thus, many oxidative therapies of the past, such as ozone therapy, intravenous hy-drogen peroxide treatments, ultraviolet irradiation of blood and hyperbaric oxygen treatments have not received funding for in depth scientific study and scrutiny. The time to investigate oxidative studies, which mimic the body's prooxidant protective mechanisms, utilizing hydrogen peroxide, hypochlorite and singlet oxygen is now.

Nonetheless, my life has been dedicated to the fields of medicine and science and my passion for discovery is greater than ever. My dream is to have oxidative therapies at the patient's bedside in my lifetime. Please help me make this hap-pen. I deeply appreciate your interest and support. Getting these oxidative studies started, will mean that they will be carried on when I am gone. In the name of all patients, I can not ask for more. Thank you.

According to the American Cancer Society, in 2011 there are almost 12 million cancer survivors in the United States of America. If these individuals are taking antioxidants, this theoretically represents a huge potential public health problem, whereby these survivors are endangering their current and future well being, by unintentionally sheltering cancer cells secondary to excessive antioxidant use.

This prediction is verified by the studies showing increased risk of cancer development in individuals receiving antioxidant supplements (please see my books, *Death In Small Doses?* and *Antioxidant Overkill*).

Should patients be counseled against using antioxidant supplements to prevent or treat cancer? You bet they should!

I present approximately 106 studies showing EMODs are responsible for cancer cell killing (induction of apoptosis).

I present approximately 50 studies showing that antioxidants can block EMOD induced apoptosis.

I present one hundred eighteen (118) human studies showing antioxidant ineffectiveness in cancer treatment or prevention and of this thirty nine (39) studies showing harmful antioxidant effects (added to and taken from book Two, *Death in small doses?* and from *Antioxidant Overkill*).

THE LITTLE PICTURE

Provision of excess antioxidants to individuals who do not need them is unwise and can be harmful. Please read my books, *Death In Small Doses?*, and *Antioxidant Overkill*. Only ingest specific naturally occurring antioxidants if there is a proven antioxidant deficiency. Otherwise, there is a likelihood that you may be interfering with the intent to your tumoricidal therapy and of your overall health.

According to the Centers for Disease Control and Prevention, one in 20 adults in America is a cancer survivor. In 2007, there were about 11.7 million Americans with a history of cancer and that number in 2011 is about 12 million.

It is said that cancer is a big business, about $200 billion a year and it claims more than 1,500 Americans each day.

In addition to educating cancer survivors, we must endeavor to educate the general public and medical personnel, especially doctors and nurses about the potential dangers of excessive antioxidant ingestion.

None of the dietary supplements have been evaluated by the U.S. Food and Drug Administration for either safety or effectiveness….NONE! None of the dietary supplements can claim to diagnose, prevent, treat or cure any disease….NOT ONE SINGLE DISEASE! What else do you need to know?

We need a certain level of antioxidants to supply electrons to oxygen. Naturally occurring antioxidants from fruits and vegetables are the best source. Synthetic chemically concocted antioxidants are the worst. Synthetics do not work like the natural antioxidants and vitamins present in fruits and vegetables.

Antioxidant stacking (overloading) leads to an EMOD insufficiency, which allows for disease manifestation and coexistence of various common pathological conditions, such as cancer, strokes and heart disease. Again, please read both of my previous books, *Death In Small Doses?* and *Antioxidant Overkill.*

THE BIG PICTURE

(EMODs, electronically modified oxygen derivatives) (apoptosis, cellular suicide)

Nutritional and genetic interventions to boost anti-oxidants have generally failed to increase life-span (or cure common diseases). Furthermore, the free radical theory fails to explain why exercise causes higher levels of so-called EMOD (oxyradical) damage, but generally promotes healthy aging. Antioxidants have been a miserable failure in the prevention of diseases (especially cancer) or aging. (Brewer, 2010).

Radiation kills cancer cells by concentrating massive amounts of oxygen free radicals (EMODs, ROS) directly into tumors. Radiation works because it generates oxygen derivatives (EMODs), which then kill the cancer. (Little et al, 1993).

Approximately 60% of cancer patients in the United States receive radiotherapy. (Borek, 2004).

Chemotherapeutics can generate purposeful cancer killing prooxidants (EMODs) by exogenous drug administration. Like radiation, Chemotherapy frequently works because it produces oxygen derivatives (EMODs), which then kill the cancer. (Conklin, 2000).

Reduction in EMOD levels generated by chemotherapeutic agents has the same effect as a reduction in dose. In short, antioxidants can reduce the effectiveness of chemotherapeutic drugs. (Erhola et al, 1996).

In most forms of cellular suicide, the death signaling cascade utilizes reactive oxygen species (EMODs) as essential intermediate messenger molecules. In other words, EMODs are a primary means of killing cancer cells. (Albright et al, 2003) (Vrablic et al, 2001) (Slater et al, 1995) (Johnson et al, 1996) (Sugiyama et al, 1996).

The prevalence of antioxidant dietary supplement use is higher among cancer survivors (and medical personnel) than among the general population, and the supplements being used are increasingly complex mixtures of ingredients. More cancer survivors use antioxidants than does the normal population. (Rock et al, 2004).

Six in ten women (60.5 %) reported using antioxidants during breast cancer treatment, which included chemotherapy, radiation, and tamoxifen (anti-estrogen) therapy. (Greenlee et al, 2009). Antioxidant use is very common in breast cancer patients.

About seven in ten antioxidant users (69.3 percent) used high doses, defined as higher than the dose contained in a Centrum multivitamin. That is, excessive antioxidant use is rampant in cancer survivors. (Greenlee et al, 2009).

Patients are increasingly self-prescribing antioxidant therapy during chemotherapy and radiation therapy as a result of market forces and aggressive advertising by antioxidant manufacturers. Cancer survivors have been misled to believe that antioxidants are good for them and consequently they buy them and take them. (De Maria et al, 1992).

Results from three large randomized controlled trials (ATBC study, the CARET study and the SELECT study), indicated that the use of beta-carotene and vitamin E (and perhaps selenium) supplements in conjunction with radiation therapy is contraindicated and should be avoided. These three studies had a total of 82,980 human participants and were all shut down about 21 months early due to the fact that the supervisory physicians detected obvious harmful effects of the antioxidants and felt it unethical to continue these studies. To me, this speaks volumes about the dangers of excessive antioxidant consumption!

The mechanisms of action of chemotherapeutic drugs (and PDT and radiotherapy) and antioxidants are chemically understood well enough to predict their apparent interactions and to suggest that considerable care should be exercised with respect to both clinical decisions and study interpretation. In short, we know that antioxidants can block the intended therapeutic effects of chemo, radiation and PDT. (Chabner et al, 1990). Note: They can also block the effects of antibiotics, many of which are dependent upon EMODs.

Ergo, **anything (specifically, antioxidants) that significantly interferes with EMOD production or activity (i.e., EMOD-induced apoptosis) must, to some degree, interfere with the efficacy and purpose of the primary cancer treatment.**

Logically, for utmost patient safety, antioxidants should be avoided during chemo, PDT or radiation therapy, unless there is unequivocal proof that their benefits outweigh their potential risk. I show that the potential harmful risk of antioxidants in cancer patients is evident by the magnitude of the accumulated scientific data.

A 2005 report concluded that cancer patients should avoid antioxidant supplements while receiving chemotherapy or radiation treatment. (D'Andrea, 2005).

Also, **a Wall Street Journal article argued that antioxidants could block the beneficial effects of standard cancer therapy.** (Parker-Pope, 2005).

A 2008 article, in the ***Journal of the National Cancer Institute,*** published a review of randomized trial data, which suggested that **cancer patients should avoid the routine use of antioxidant supplements because they may potentially decrease the efficacy of radiation therapy by protecting the tumor and reducing overall survival.** (Lawenda et al, 2008).

Actually, the relevant concept is quite simple: increased antioxidants (which decrease cancer cellular killing) decrease EMODs and apoptosis; whereas, decreased antioxidants increase EMOD affectivity and increase cancer cellular killing. It can be intentionally confused but it is basically that straight forward in systems relying on EMOD cytotoxicity and subsequent tumor apoptosis.

The *Harvard Science Review*, Spring 2010, published an article entitled, "**Antioxidants not heaven-sent.**" They cited my 2006 paper on the Free Radical Fantasy and stated, "It may come as a surprise that the current scientific consensus is that there is no health benefit to taking antioxidant supplements."

In February 2011, *Newsweek* magazine published an article entitled, "**Antioxidants Fall From Grace.**" Also saying, "The popular dietary components may not do any good, and may actually harm."

HOWES' NEW RULES

Following my exhaustive studies of the world literature and my selective reviews on oxygen metabolism, I have compiled these new rules for cancer patients.

Howes' Rules For Antioxidant Use In Cancer Patients Or Patients With Premalignant Conditions:

Howes Rule One: Any medicine or supplement that is taken during cancer radiotherapy, chemotherapy or photodynamic therapy should have been tested to prove that it does not protect or promote neoplastic cells, because safeguarding tumor cells would defeat or negate the explicit intended effect and purpose of the anti-cancer (tumoricidal) treatment or therapy.

Howes Rule Two: Any reduction in a therapy's cancer-killing ability is in direct conflict with the overall medical treatment objective and the patients' ultimate well being and should therefore be avoided.

Howes Rule Three: Based on significant prior data, excessive antioxidant levels theoretically, and in fact, promote an environment that is beneficial to tumor cell growth and survival. Condiderable scientific evidence has shown that antioxidants can serve as shields for tumorous cells. Patients with known premalignant conditions or cancer (including survivors) should avoid antioxidant over use until further research shows otherwise.

Howes Rule Four: Even if an antioxidant is shown to reduce adverse effects of primary cancer treatments, it must be proven not to diminish the tumoricidal activity of the anti-cancer therapy. If it decreases the tumoricidal intent, in any way, it must be used with extreme caution, if at all, and the patient must be informed of its possible harmful effect.

Summary of things that I know: (EMODs, electronically modified oxygen derivatives) (apoptosis, cellular suicide)

- EMODs are major players for inducing apoptosis and killing pathogens

- Cancer cells are killed primarily by apoptosis (and necrosis)

- Thus, EMODs are major participants (activators) in cancer cell death

- Antioxidants can block the activity (and signaling) of EMODs

- Antioxidants can block cancer cell kill

- Thus, it is theoretically counterintuitive and likely counter productive for cancer patients or patients with premalignant conditions to take antioxidants, either before, during or after treatment, even though some antioxidants are claimed to slightly reduce adverse effects of chemo or radiation therapy.

Even though it is true that chemo and radiotherapy can cause harmful and painful adverse side effects, excessive antioxidants will theoretically interfere or negate the intent of the treatments.

I strongly recommend against the use of unneeded antioxidants by cancer survivors, until further research yields a clear and unequivocal conclusion. After all, **"Why risk defeating the purpose of your cancer treatment, even by a small amount, by ingesting unnecessary antioxidants?"** The occurrence of adverse events could negate any potential benefits of treatments.

Acceptance of things as they are,

rings the death knoll

for excitement or discovery.

R. M. Howes, M.D., Ph.D.

9/27/09

SECTION ONE:

An overall view

Prof Randolph M. Howes MD, PhD

The World Cancer Research Fund (WCRF) conducted a landmark study on cancer prevention that Professor Martin Wiseman, project director, said "represents the most definitive advice on preventing cancer that has ever been available anywhere in the world." The 10/31/07 report, which selected 7,000 studies from a world-wide pool of 500,000 written since records began in the 1960s, produced five key findings. One of those findings, that is particularly important and relevant, is that, "*It did not recommend dietary supplements as (cancer) prevention.*" The production of the second expert report was a huge undertaking for the WCRF global network, in-volving over 100 scientists from 30 different countries. WCRF/AICR commissioned and funded the report, but the content has been driven by an independent panel of 21 world renowned scientists. The Expert Panel worked for five years to assess the research and their conclusions and recommendations are firmly based on the scientific evidence.

This was a blow to those pushing antioxidants as a means of cancer prevention but this is just a glimpse of the nonsense/nonscience surrounding the injudicious use of antioxidants.

Are antioxidants a boon or a bust?

"Are antioxidants a boon or a bust?" The "jury is no longer out." Although antioxi-dants have benefits in normal amounts, it is currently recommended to take them only if you have a known deficiency. It is especially important not to take superflu-ous amounts. If they are not needed, do not take them.

Yet, people are encouraged by strong marketing forces to buy antioxidants and be exposed to their harmful potential and to their unnecessary costs. These unfortu-nate circumstances are sad for those who pay the bills — and sadder for patients who did not need them to start with.

My past two books, *Death In Small Doses?* and *Antioxidant Overkill*, emphasized the negative studies regarding antioxidants and of their potential harm. But, it is well known that studies with significant positive results are easier to find than those with 'negative' results.

This so called **publication bias** can arise from the tendency of authors to sub-mit or journals to accept manuscripts that have a positive rather than a negative or neutral result. It can also be the consequence of deliberately overemphasizing positive results or even worse: the results can be *"embellished"*, (partly) faked or negative results can be manipulated, hidden or completely undisclosed. This must always be kept in mind when reading about antioxidants or medications.

**In my editorials regarding out-of-control Big Pharma,
I merely represent an annoying chigger attacking
the dangling, sweaty scrotum of a gargantuan elephant.
I can't really hurt the beast but
assuredly, I can irritate the hell out of it.**
R. M. Howes, M.D., Ph.D.
9/20/09

My books contain extensive bibliographic, peer-reviewed references and abstracts summarizing original articles from the best primary research and most respected clinical journals. I have carefully selected articles from thousands of journals and from all countries around the world, which makes my books especially comprehensive and exceptionally representative of the current state of scientific evidence based data, as it relates to the biochemistry of oxygen metabolism, antioxidants and redox chemistry.

Yet, the literature is filled with "may" articles. This means that no one can prove it true or disprove it, just like the "possibly, could, should, might or could be or thought to be" articles. Combine this with "fuzzy math" (contrived statistics) and we have a major problem in sorting out truth in today's so-called scientific articles.

SUMMARY: Points *against* the use of antioxidants with chemo or radiation therapy

(STUDIES AGAINST EXCESS (XS) ANTIOXIDANT (AOX) USE - have been assembled from sections throughout this book.)

Nonetheless, there seems to be agreement that **the antioxidant N-acetylcysteine (NAC), a derivative of the naturally occurring amino acid cysteine, should be avoided by cancer patients because of studies showing interference with chemotherapeutic agents, such as cisplatin and doxorubicin.** (Olson et al, 1983) (Roller, Weller, 1998).

A 2005 report concluded that cancer patients should avoid antioxidant supplements while receiving chemotherapy or radiation treatment. (D'Andrea, 2005).

Also, **a Wall Street Journal article argued that antioxidants could block the beneficial effects of standard cancer therapy.** (Parker-Pope, 2005).

The debate continues and the opposite position was upheld in a 2008 article in which the *Journal of the National Cancer Institute* recently published <u>a review of randomized trial data, which suggested that</u> **cancer patients should avoid the routine use of antioxidant supplements because they may potentially decrease the efficacy of cancer therapy by protecting the tumor and reducing survival.** They looked at clinical trials investigating the impact of antioxidants on radiation therapy and found evidence suggesting that antioxidant supplementation reduced overall survival. (Lawenda et al, 2008).

Even modest quenching of oxygen radicals by dietary antioxidants could block completion of apoptosis. Administration of antioxidants subsequent to a mutagenic event may effectively intercept free radicals that are critical in promoting apoptosis. This imbalance may allow the rate of proliferation in tumors to exceed the capacity for apoptosis.

I believe that **peroxide is known to stimulate over 200 important metabolic transduction enzymes and removal or blockage of H_2O_2 formation (by antioxidants) could dangerously or fatally inhibit any or all of these enzymes.**

Any potential health supplements should not be allowed to be added to foods unless they have been shown to be beneficial, or at least proven not to be harmful." (Bjelakovic et al, 2007). People who take antioxidant vitamins such as A, C and E -- long touted as protecting against cancer, heart disease and other health problems - don't live any longer, new research shows. Worse yet, **there is actually evidence that they die younger than people who don't take vitamins.**

Danish researchers warned that consumers should be cautious about taking supplements containing nutrients. Supplements that millions of North Americans take to stave off disease and slow the aging process do not boost longevity and **appear to actually increase the risk of dying.** Bjelakovic's analysis, which pooled data from 68 studies involving more than 232,000 people, found no evidence that taking beta-carotene, Vitamin A or Vitamin E extends life span. (Bjelakovic et al, 2007). In fact, they found that antioxidant supplements increase mortality by 5%.

Cancer patients should avoid the routine use of antioxidant supplements during radiation and chemotherapy because the supplements may reduce the anticancer benefits of therapy, researchers concluded in a com-

mentary published online May 27, 2008 in the Journal of the National Cancer Institute.

Vitamin C supplements may significantly reduce the effectiveness of several anti-cancer drugs, according to a new study published 10/1/08.

"It is possible that vitamin C supplementation may alter the effectiveness of commonly used chemotherapeutic agents and adversely influence treatment outcome," the researchers write in the October 1, 2008 issue of *Cancer Research*.

In tests on isolated cancer cells in the laboratory, researchers found that **30 to 70 percent fewer of the cells were killed if pretreated with vitamin C.**

In studies of cancer cells in mice, studies found that tumors grew more rapidly if the animal was treated with chemotherapy and also given vitamin C supplements. (Agence France-Presse, First Posted 08:25:00 10/02/2008. Inquirer.net).

The new research shows that a number of chemotherapy drugs produce "oxygen free radicals." According to the study's theory, **vitamin C could "sop up the radicals," keeping cancer cells alive despite chemotherapy treatment.**

"The use of vitamin C supplements could have the potential to reduce the ability of patients to respond to therapy," said Dr Mark Heaney of Memorial Sloan-Kettering Cancer Center and **he advises his cancer patients to avoid supplemental vitamin C during chemotherapy.** "I recommend that my patients continue to eat a well-balanced diet that includes fruits and vegetables that contain vitamin C."

"Clearly, there remains an open question as to whether or not vitamin C supplementation is helpful or harmful in the treatment of patients with cancer. Until those questions are resolved with further clinical studies, **it would be inappropriate to recommend that patients take large quantities of vitamin C if they have cancer,"** Dr. Lichtenfeld told *Medscape Oncology*. (Heaney et al, 2008).

As reported on 2-04-09 in the journal Nature, Stanford researcher, Robert Cho, found that breast cancer stem cells make much higher levels of protective antioxidants than other cancer cells. **Use of a drug to block the antioxidant, glutathione, caused the cancer stem cells to become far more vulnerable to radiation**. Using cells from mice and human breast cancer, the antioxidant glutathione protected the cancer cells from being killed by radiation EMOD-induced apoptosis.

However, data from some studies indicate that **antioxidant supplementation at doses that are intermediate to dietary intakes (relatively low doses) and high supplemental doses may reduce the efficacy of x-irradiation against cancer cells.** (Sakamoto, Sakka, 1973) (Witenberg et al, 1999) or stimulate tumor cell growth (Prasad, Kumar, 1996).

The most concerning data are presented in a subsequent publication by Bairati et al. (Bairati et al, 2006) on the same cohort of patients. In this article, **they demonstrate that the patients who received antioxidants had statistically significant poorer overall survival. Some believe that this study is the most important randomized clinical trial, to date, on the use of a supplemental antioxidant and radiation therapy.**

Several other studies have provided evidence that antioxidants can decrease the effectiveness of radiation therapy. For example, Ferreira et al. randomly assigned 54 head and neck cancer patients who were undergoing radiation therapy to receive an oil-based oral rinse that contained either vitamin E or placebo before and after each daily dose of radiation. **Although the vitamin E supplementation was associated with a 36% reduction in symptomatic mucositis, the authors also reported a decrease in 2-year overall survival** (32% with supplemental vitamin E vs 63% with placebo; $P = .13$). This concerning decrease in overall survival, albeit **not statistically significant**, may have been confounded by the greater percentage of patients with stage 3 and 4 tumors found in the vitamin E group. (Ferreira et al, 2004).

Where do these findings leave us? With the results of Bairati et al, it appears that supplementation with beta-carotene is not justified for reduction in mucositis **given the concerns for a decrease in the efficacy of radiotherapy for head and neck cancers in addition to the concerns of increasing the risk of lung cancers in a group of patients who are already at an elevated risk.** Similarly, the results of Bairati et al with alpha-tocopherol in combination with the results observed by Ferreira et al suggest that additional randomized trials using antioxidants for normal tissue cytoprotection in patients with head and neck cancers are not warranted. Furthermore, the issue of patient self-supplementation with antioxidants during radiotherapy must also be addressed in more detail given the results of this study. **Without any definitive data on this issue, a reasonable approach would be to avoid unnecessary supplementation during and after radiotherapy.**

This **raises significant concerns about the possible inadvertent simultaneous protection of tumor tissues.**

In another study, **Lesperance et al.** investigated a historical cohort of 90 patients with nonmetastatic breast cancer who received conventional treatment (e.g., surgery, chemotherapy, radiation therapy, and hormonal therapy) either alone or in combination with high doses of beta-carotene, vitamin C, niacin, selenium, coenzyme Q10, and/or zinc. (Lesperance et al, 2002). **Breast cancer–specific survival (i.e., patients censored only at death from breast cancer) and disease-free survival were shorter in the nutrient-supplemented group than in the nonsupplemented group, but the differences were not statistically significant** (hazard ratio of breast cancer death = 1.75, 95% CI = 0.83 to 2.69, and hazard ratio of relapse = 1.55, 95% CI = 0.94 to 2.54, respectively). Despite the substantial limitations of these studies, **it is troubling that both reported results suggesting poorer survival with concurrent administration of antioxidants and cytotoxic therapy**, even though these results are at odds with other studies.

Studies using a mouse model with a mutated retinoblastoma (Rb) protein show that mice fed a diet low in vitamin E and other antioxidants had higher rates of apoptosis and reduced tumor volume. Other researchers have reported that **antioxidants such as vitamin E and N–acetylcysteine delay and inhibit apoptosis in a number of models, including pancreatic cells and PC-12 cells. There is some data in the literature suggesting that when we want to kill cells with chemotherapy or radiation, the mechanism we are using is the generation of excess levels of EMODs (ROS) that then activate cell death. If we gave antioxidants during these treatments, we would reduce the amount of cell death produced.**

Studies have investigated the effects of antioxidant supplementation on cancer therapy. Studies on cisplatin indicate that it kills breast cancer cells by apoptosis and necrosis, and that the addition of vitamin E blocks much of the apoptotic process. **High-dose vitamin E reduces the efficacy of cisplatin**, although the normal cells involved would be protected by vitamin E. Lymphoma cells treated with 5 Gy of radiation die or stop dividing, but **if N-acetylcysteine is added to the media, the lymphoma cells keep growing. Vitamin E succinate also protects cells against the effects of radiation in vitro.**

There has been no conclusive evidence to show which antioxidant doses or mixtures protect cells against DNA damage and lipid and protein oxidation but do not interfere with apoptosis signaling pathways. There may be a threshold beyond which DNA is protected against oxidants because the ROS oxidants produced are being quenched and there may be a higher dose needed to suppress signaling. **Oversupplementation may actually produce an environment that is beneficial to the tumor and allow it to survive.**

Conversely, **even modest quenching or reduction of EMODs by dietary antioxidants could block initiation or completion of apoptosis.**

Antioxidants, by preventing oxidant-mediated damage to diverse targets (DNA, RNA, proteins, and lipids), may logically play a protective role in healthy individuals; however, by inhibiting apoptosis, **these same antioxidants may exert a cancer-promoting effect in cancer patients and in individuals with precancerous DNA changes**.

Even though some speculate that early administration of antioxidants may help prevent the initiation and progression of cancer by quenching the action of potentially mutagenic reactive free radicals, **administration of antioxidants subsequent to a mutagenic event may effectively intercept free radicals (EMODs) that are critical in promoting apoptosis**. This imbalance may allow the rate of proliferation in tumors to exceed the capacity for apoptosis. It seems reasonable to suggest that **the potential risks and benefits of high-dose antioxidants in cancer patients should be approached with significant caution and indiscriminate use of antioxidant dietary supplements should be avoided.** (Zeisel, 2004).

Comprehensively, **the "antioxidant treatment" was found to have an effect both on reactive oxygen species levels** and glutathione peroxidase activity. The antioxidant treatment also reduced serum levels of IL-6 and TNF. Patients in both ECOG PS 0-1 and ECOG PS 2-3 responded to antioxidant treatment. (Mantovani et al, 2002). **Although this was a small study, it showed that antioxidants definitely reduce EMOD levels in cancer patients.**

Antioxidant vitamins can pose a significant potential danger to cancer patients both on and off of chemotherapy, radiation therapy and photodynamic therapy. While the intention of taking an antioxidant supplement would seem like a good idea, **voluminous research has shown that taking certain antioxidants with certain cancers actually block cancer cell kill and promote tumor spread.**

The Royal College of Radiologists advise patients to avoid antioxidant supplements, especially in high doses, during their conventional cancer therapy.

According to Breastcancer.org, **this can alter the cancer treatment process and seriously compromise prognosis and survival.** Taking any medication or antioxidant supplement can pose considerable <u>health</u> risks when undergoing cancer treatment. Thus, it may be prudent not take any unnecessary risks. (http://www.livestrong.com/article/318898-vitamins-cancer-chemotherapy/#ixzz1AZiaGLw0. accessed 1-9-11).

Antioxidant vitamins A, E, C, plus glutathione, and selenium are extremely dangerous to take with chemotherapy. According to Bastyr Center for Natural Health, these antioxidants reduce the desirable toxicity of chemotherapy, a necessary effect for killing cancer cells and shrinking tumors in the cancer patient. (D'Andrea, 2005). (http://bastyrcenter.org/content/view/902/. accessed 1-9-11).

These antioxidants actually protect the cancer cells by presenting a buffer between the healthy cells and the cancer-fighting oxygen free radicals (EMODS) in chemotherapy. **The vitamins work against both the patient's immune system and the chemotherapy actually providing an excellent environment for the cancer cells to flourish and grow.** (Parker-Pope, 2005).

Even cancer patients that are also deficient in nutrients are generally advised against taking antioxidant vitamins or mineral supplements on or off of chemotherapy treatments. **Multivitamin supplements for example, were shown to feed cancerous tumors.** Breastcancer.org suggests that the only vitamin that has not been linked to cancer spread is vitamin D. I believe that vitamin D is safe because it efficiently generates EMODs.

All other vitamins have shown considerable elevation of risk among patients with prostate and breast cancers with advanced metastases and premature death. Even multivitamins, which also contain antioxidants, are not recommended for cancer patients. (http://www.breastcancer.org/symptoms/types/recur_metast/ask_expert/conf_2007_10/question_24.jsp. accessed 1-9-11).

The following was taken from the website for the American Cancer Society: http://www.**cancer.org**/Treatment/TreatmentsandSideEffects/

TreatmentTypes/Chemotherapy/ChemotherapyPrinciplesAnIn-depthDiscussiono
ftheTechniquesanditsRoleinTreatment/chemotherapy-principles-selecting-chemo-
drugs-to-use?ssDomainNum=5c38e88&docSelected=chemotherapy-principles-add-
res&print=true. Last medical review and update 9/28/10. Accessed 1-9-11.

*Because most people think of vitamins as a safe way to improve health, it is not surprising that many people with cancer take high doses of one or more vitamins. But **few realize that some vitamins might make their chemotherapy less effective.***

- *If your doctor has not prescribed vitamins for a specific reason, it is best not to take any.*

- ***It is safest to avoid taking high doses of antioxidant vitamins during cancer treatment.** Ask your doctors if and when it might be safe to start such vitamins after treatment is finished.*

The American Cancer Society experts believe that antioxidant vitamins and supplements shouldn't be used during cancer treatment. A 2005 report in the medical journal *CA* cites several studies that show the use of vitamins by cancer patients doesn't help and may even cause harm.

Also, there is general agreement that **endogenous antioxidants such as glutathione and antioxidant enzyme-elevating agents may protect cancer cells against cytotoxic therapy**. (Pradad, 2004).

"Can vitamin and herbal supplements reduce the adverse effects of cancer treatment, decrease the risk of cancer recurrence or improve a patient's chances of survival? **We don't really know.** Research into these matters has been minimal," said senior author Cornelia (Neli) Ulrich, Ph.D., an associate member of the Hutchinson Center's Public Health Sciences Division. "While supplement use may be beneficial for some patients, such as those who cannot eat a balanced diet, **research suggests that certain supplements may actually interfere with treatment or even accelerate cancer growth**," she said in an article published Feb. 1, 2008 in the *Journal of Clinical Oncology*.

In reviewing **32 studies conducted between 1999 and 2006**, Ulrich and co-author Christine Velicer, Ph.D., formerly a postdoctoral fellow at the Hutchinson Center (now an epidemiologist at Merck Research Laboratory in North Wales, Pa.), found that many of **the nation's 10 million adult cancer survivors** use nutritional supplements. **I believe that this is a major problem, in that cancer patients may be at even greater danger by the use of antioxidant supplements, which favor cancer growth.**

Knowing about supplement use is crucial, she continues, because of potential adverse effects. **"Evidence clearly suggests the need for caution,"** Ulrich said. **"Some vitamins, such as folic acid, may be involved in cancer progression while others, such as St. John's wort, can interfere with chemotherapy.** However, we really need more research to understand whether use of these supplements can be beneficial or do more harm than good."

Concern has been expressed that **antioxidant supplement use might pose a risk for adverse effects** as well as provide possible benefits, especially in vulnerable populations **such as individuals who have been diagnosed with cancer** (Gottlieb, 1999).

Antioxidants could be beneficial in people with innate or acquired high baseline levels of reactive oxygen species but be harmful in people with lower innate levels. (Salganik, 2001).

Meta-analyses of randomized clinical trials have not shown that antioxidant supplements reduce cancer incidence. (Bjelakovic et al. 2004) (Bjelakovic et al, Lancet 2004) (Caraballoso et al, 2003) (Bjelakovic et al, 2006).

In the absence of good evidence of benefit, it is contrary to the principle of **primum non nocere** to advise patients to continue a potentially harmful intervention. In this report published in 2008, researchers cautioned that cancer patients should avoid use of antioxidant supplements during radiation and <u>chemotherapy</u>. According to the report's authors, **antioxidant supplements may reduce the anticancer effects of therapy** (Lawenda et al, 2008).

However, **concern has been expressed that the action of supplemental antioxidants might not be restricted to reducing the oxidative damage to normal tissues generated by radiation therapy and certain chemotherapeutic agents.** (D'Andrea, 2005) (Seifried et al, 2003).

Theoretically, **antioxidants can exert their effects on all tissues to some degree, thereby protecting tumor cells as well as healthy ones. Experimental and clinical studies** (Bairati et al, J Clin Oncol. 2005) (Ferreira et al, 2004) (Fantappie et al, 2004) (Sakamoto, Sakka, 1973) (Mothersill et al, 1986) (Wiernik et al, 1992) (Lesperance et al, 2002) (Lawenda et al, 2007) (Salganik, 2001) **lend support to this hypothesis, with some clinical data also suggesting that cancer patients who use antioxidant supplements during radiation or chemotherapy have worse survival than those who do not** (Bairati et al, J Clin Oncol. 2005) (Ferreira et al, 2004) (Lesperance et al, 2002) (Bairati et al, 2006).

Our studies provide evidence that **ascorbic acid by its antioxidative capacity reduces drastically the production of EMODs in mitochondria that are required for the execution of drug-induced apoptosis. The data consequently raises the question of whether a high intake of ascorbic acid during chemotherapy of tumors is beneficial.** (Llobet et al, 2008).

The **antioxidant**, rather than prooxidant, activities of quercetin on normal cells: - quercetin protects mouse thymocytes from glucose oxidase-mediated apoptosis. (Lee J, et al, 2003). **This indicates that the FRS drink advertised and promoted by Lance Armstrong is capable of blocking the oxidative killing of cancer cells. This also applies to the widely advertised OPC Factor product by Dr. Fredrich Vagnini, which contains a variety of "powerful" antioxidants.**

Some companies have claimed that acai berries can cure cancer. **The U.S. Food and Drug Administration (FDA) has found no evidence that acai can reduce or eliminate cancer cells.** In fact, the **Memorial Sloan-Kettering Cancer Center issued a statement that acai may lessen the positive effect of chemotherapy by interfering with the drugs used to eradicate the cancer.**

AARP's Drug Directory recommends using acai with caution if you are taking antineoplastic medications, antioxidants or anti-inflammatory drugs or herbs.

In the concluding sentence of this review, **the authors recommend that "Antioxidant and other nutrient food supplements are safe and can help to enhance cancer patient care"** (Simone et al, 2007).

Others caution antioxidant use in cancer patients. Such a recommendation merits close examination of the evidence because it is at odds with other authoritative reviews on this topic (D'Andrea, 2005) (Ladas et al, 2004) (Block et al, 2007) (Dennert, Horneber, 2006) (Sagar, 2005).

Kedar N. Prasad, PhD, at the Center for Vitamin and Cancer Research at the University of Colorado Health Sciences Center stated that **"It is likely that** recommendation of low doses of multiple vitamins containing low doses of micronutrients including antioxidants after therapy may increase the risk of recurrence of the primary tumor among those who are in remission.

On the other hand, **more than 60% of cancer patients use vitamins, and the majority combines them with standard therapy, mostly without the knowledge of their oncologists.** This practice may also be harmful because **a multiple-vitamin preparation may contain antioxidants such as gluta-thione-elevating agents, including alpha-lipoic acid and N-acetylcysteine (NAC), and antioxidant enzyme-elevating agents such as excess of sele-nium, which is a cofactor for glutathione peroxidase, or dietary antioxi-dants such as vitamin E or vitamin C, which, at low doses, may protect cancer cells against free radical damage produced by chemotherapeutic agents or x-irradiation.** Neither oncologists nor patients are aware of these potential dangers of taking antioxidants without any scientific rationale." (Pradad, 2004).

By increasing the number of reactive oxygen species (ROS) in cells, STA-4783 can tip tumors cells beyond the breaking point into a death path-way (apoptosis). While these cells die, normal cells have less ROS and can shield themselves against the drug's effects. Thus, the **induction of oxi-dative stress by elesclomol exploits this unique characteristic of cancer cells by increasing ROS levels beyond a threshold that triggers cell death.** (Kirshner et al, 2008).

Additional points *against* the use of antioxidants with chemo or radia-tion therapy

- Vitamin E reduces effectiveness of radiation therapy

When vitamin E is given to mice at dosages not likely to be achieved with normal supplementation in humans (e.g., dosage greater than 35,000 IU) it can **reduce the effectiveness of radiation therapy.** (Sakamoto, Sakka, 1973).

2) **NAC (N-acetylcysteine - a derivative of the naturally occurring amino acid cysteine) has not been shown to significantly effect treatment out-come and carries with it some risk of inhibiting chemotherapy agents** (e.g., cisplatin). (Olson et al, 1983) (Roller, Weller, 1998).

- Investigators compared plasma levels of antioxidants and oxidative stress bio-markers in **head and neck squamous cell carcinoma (HNSCC)** patients with healthy controls. **Seventy-eight HNSCC patients and 100 healthy controls** were included in this study. **High relative increase in plasma levels of d-ROMs and high relative decrease in FRAP during radiotherapy are also positively associated with survival. I believe that this important study shows that increased plasma EMODs and lowered plasma antioxidants are associated with increased survival in HNSCC.** (Sakhi et al, 2009).

In 2001, researchers from the National Cancer Institute (NCI) and the Southwest Oncology Group (SWOG) launched the massive **SELECT study (short for Selenium and Vitamin E Cancer Prevention Trial)** to find out whether taking <u>selenium</u> and <u>vitamin E</u> supplements could protect men from prostate cancer. **In October 2008, researchers halted the trial after early analysis showed the supplements weren't working, and in fact, in some cases, may have been doing more harm than good (i.e., increasing the risk of prostate cancer).**

**The less you know,
the less you question.**
R. M. Howes, M.D., Ph.D.
9/7/09

CHAPTER ONE:

Is there still a rising cancer problem?

In 1971, President Nixon launched the "War Against Cancer," which was designed to fight the escalating incidence of cancer that had reached epidemic proportions. For the past forty years, only incremental progress has been made in this overall crusade.

In developing countries, cancer is rising

About 10 percent of the 1.5 million people diagnosed with cancer in 2010 were younger than 45, more than 15,000 of them under 20.

Soon, cancer will overtake heart disease as the number one killer in America and it is on the rise in developing countries.

Contributing factors such as tobacco use, poor nutrition, physical inactivity, obesity, alcohol consumption, excessive sun exposure, prevention of certain chronic infections, and selected other environmental factors are getting increasing attention by the American Cancer Society.

While just 10 percent of all cancers in the economically developed world are a function of infection, that figure rises to one-quarter of all cancers in third world countries. Infectious agents, such as hepatitis B and C viruses, human papillomavirus (HPV), Epstein–Barr virus, certain other viruses, and *Helicobacter pylori* bacteria are known to increase cancer risk.

Many of these factors are potentially controllable; whereas, inherited genetic traits are not.

In third world countries, the biggest risk for men appears to be lung, stomach and liver cancers, and with women, it is breast, cervical and lung cancers. But, in economically developed nations, as of 2008, prostate, lung and colorectal cancers were the most prevalent among men, while breast, colorectal and lung cancers were the most common among women.

Even though we are frequently told that we are winning the war against cancer in the U.S., global disease figures in 2008 showed 12.7 million new cancer cases and 7.6 million cancer deaths and those numbers are predicted to nearly double by 2030, as the world's population both grows and ages. Dr. Otis W. Brawley, American Cancer Society chief medical officer, said, "About one-third of all cancer deaths that occurred worldwide in 2008 (equal to roughly 7,300 deaths per day) might have been avoided by focusing on preventable risk factors such as smoking, drinking, infection patterns and dietary habits."

The Global Cancer Facts & Figures report showed that "The majority of the world's new cancer cases and deaths (7.1 million and 4.8 million, respectively) are now occurring in economically developing countries and this reflects the growing adoption of unhealthy behaviors, such as smoking, sedentary lifestyles and poor diets, that typically accompany economic development." We can reduce cancer by decreasing tobacco-related cancers and by improving nutrition and increasing physical activity (exercise).

These are emerging priorities due to the relationship between smoking and obesity and their association with increased risk of getting cancer. Early detection can lead to more effective treatment with such things as cancer screening utilizing PAP smears, mammography and colonoscopy.

We are learning to pay attention to our health as never before. Environmental pollution is making it an increasingly dangerous world. We must protect our environment and in doing so, we protect our health. Strive to stay healthy. After all, health is wealth.

It has long been believed that antioxidant supplements like vitamins A, E and C might help slow or even prevent cancer and the formation of plaques within coronary arteries. Indeed, decades ago several epidemiological studies seemed to confirm that antioxidant vitamins could improve outcomes. As a result, millions of individuals (including many doctors, nurses and medical personnel) now routinely take vitamins A, E and C supplements.

Because of the impression that these antioxidants are good for their overall well being, they also recommend them to their patients and their families. Have they been misled?

Please note that not all vitamins are antioxidants and vitamin D3 is a very good example of an effective prooxidant.

One in eight women will get breast cancer

According to BBC News -Health - as of February 2011, a woman's risk of developing **breast cancer has risen to one in eight from one in nine**, stated Cancer

Research UK. The charity's figures show that breast cancer rates in the UK have increased by 3.5% in 10 years, from 42,400 new cases in 1999 to 47,700 in 2008. Women aged between 50 and 69 have seen the biggest rise in breast cancer rates of 6%.

Exercising and eating healthily can reduce the risk, cancer charities say. Cancer Research UK figures suggest that breast cancer is by far the most common cancer in women, accounting for almost a third of cases. Bowel cancer is the second most common, followed by lung.

Almost half of breast cancer cases in 2008 (48%) were in women aged between 50 and 69. A third were in women aged over 70, with 19% in women aged 25-49.

Previous research has shown that lifestyle factors and a family history of breast cancer increase a woman's risk of developing the disease. Sara Hiom, director of health information at Cancer Research UK, said that small changes in everyday habits can help to reduce cancer risk. "Cutting back on alcohol by keeping within government recommended limits of no more than 14 units a week (a small drink a day) helps.

"Taking more exercise and eating a diet high in fiber but low in saturated fat can help maintain a healthy weight - which in turn reduces breast cancer risk."

The figures from the World Cancer Research Fund suggest that making these simple changes in lifestyle could result in about 79,000 cases of all kinds of cancer being prevented in the UK each year. The WCRF says breast cancer cases specifically could be reduced by 42%. But, I have my doubts.

Obesity most likely increases the risk of cancer by raising levels of hormones such as the antioxidant, estrogen and insulin in the body. **High levels of these hormones, produced by the fat tissues, are common features of many cancers**. Please note that fat cells produce the antioxidant, estrogen, which feeds breast cancer. Excess body fat may also affect how the body processes fats and sugars and how the immune system functions.

Almost two out of every three women with breast cancer survive for more than 20 years and more than three-quarters of women with breast cancer survive for at least 10 years, says Cancer Research UK. Sara Hiom, from Cancer Research UK, urged women to get tested at the earliest possible stage.

Dr Rachel Greig, senior policy officer at Breakthrough Breast Cancer, said the figures were **a wake-up call** and should not be ignored. "More women are developing breast cancer and, although survival is improving thanks to breakthroughs in breast awareness, screening and treatment, we clearly have much further to go.

"A two-pronged attack is needed - commitment to research into the causes of breast cancer, supported by women arming themselves with knowledge of the risks that may contribute to the disease."

I believe that antioxidant stacking is proving to be a significant risk factor for cancer.

Breast cancer risk factors

You can do everything right and still get breast cancer.

1) Family history. A woman with a mother, sister or daughter with breast cancer has around double the risk of getting it herself than a woman with no family history.

2) Obesity. **Being overweight or obese is thought to increases the risk of postmenopausal breast cancer by up to 30%,** because excess body fat raises levels of hormones such as estrogen and insulin - common features of cancers.

3) Age. The older the woman, the higher her risk. Women aged 50-69 are most at risk, particularly those who have a late menopause.

4) Childbirth. The younger a woman has children, the lower her risk. Having children at all cuts the risk, as does breastfeeding.

5) Lifestyle. Regular physical exercise and a healthy diet helps reduce the risk by cutting dangerous fatty body tissues. Smoking is not advised.

6) HRT. Women using hormone replacement therapy have a 66% increased risk of breast cancer but the risk is temporary, returning to that of a never-user within five years of stopping.

7) Oral contraceptives. They increase risk by around a quarter but since users are generally younger women, their risk is relatively low.

8) Alcohol. Drinking as little as one alcoholic drink per day increases breast cancer risk by around 12%. Source: Cancer Research UK.

Over the past few decades it has become common practice by oncologists to advise patients who are undergoing chemotherapy not to take anti-oxidant supplements. The rational behind this advice is that chemotherapy destroys cancer cells by inducing free radicals and by promoting oxidation of the cancer cells. Antioxidants, on the contrary, do the exact opposite, i.e. they prevent free radicals (by binding to them or destroying their free radical character) and the oxidation of cells. Theoretically, therefore, it would seem to logically follow that antioxidants may interfere with chemotherapy and reduce its effectiveness.

Yet, this is a very confusing and controversial issue. Neither side of the argument has full support of the data. Ergo, one must go with the preponderance of the data and with common sense.

Ranks of cancer survivors growing fast

In 2011, the number of cancer survivors in the United States is increasing by hundreds of thousands a year, and **now includes roughly one in 20 adults**, health officials said Thursday. More people are surviving cancer, in part, because of earlier detection and better treatment, they said.

In 2007, there were about 11.7 million Americans with a history of cancer, the Centers for Disease Control and Prevention said. Forty years ago, the number of cancers survivors was about 3 million. That increased to 10 million in 2001 and to 11.4 million in 2006.

Healthy eating, less smoking and other preventive steps may also be playing a role in the increase, health officials said. "There are some cancers that we can't prevent and they are terrible tragedies," said CDC Director Dr. Tom Frieden. "But there are many that are preventable, or if caught early can result in much longer life."

Demographics are a factor in the survivor increase, too. **Cancer is most common in people 65 and older**, and the nation's elderly population is growing. The CDC said **7 million — 60 percent — of the cancer survivors were 65 or older.**

Women diagnosed with breast cancer made up the largest share of cancer survivors, at 22 percent, followed by men with prostate cancer, at 19 percent. The estimates from the CDC and the National Cancer Institute were based on information from nine U.S. cancer patient registries.

The survivor count includes anyone who had a cancer diagnosis, including people who had been successfully treated as well as those still getting treated or who may be dying from the disease. About 65 percent had survived for at least five years, and 40 percent for 10 years or more.

CHAPTER TWO:

Cancer Patients and Antioxidants

Do cancer patients take antioxidants?

On June 9, 2009, Denise Mann of CNN Health reported on antioxidants that may interfere with breast cancer treatment.

Despite evidence that antioxidants may be more harmful than helpful, many breast cancer patients take powerful antioxidant vitamins during radiation or chemotherapy. My previous research has unequivocally shown that antioxidants have considerable potential to do harm. As of Janurary 2011, eighty studies, out of 250, showed wide ranging adverse effects of the antioxidant vitamins A, C and E.

In 2009, Dr. Marisa Weiss, president and founder of the advocacy group Breastcancer.org and author of "Taking Care of Your Girls: A Breast Health Guide for Girls, Teens and In-Betweens, said, **"It is possible that if you are taking concentrated high-grade antioxidant vitamins in significant doses, it may interfere with your treatment."**

Dr. Weiss was referring to a study in the July 15, 2009 issue of the journal *Cancer*, in which 60.5 percent of women with breast cancer reported taking antioxidants, including vitamin E, vitamin C, beta carotene, and selenium, during their treatment. And 69.3 percent of those on antioxidants took high doses (anything more than the amount found in a Centrum multivitamin).

As stated before, research has shown that the rate of vitamin use is higher among cancer patients than in the general population. Researchers at the Fred Hutchinson Cancer Research Center in Seattle reviewed 32 studies conducted between 1999 and 2006 and found that **64 percent to 81 percent of cancer survivors in the studies were taking extra vitamins or minerals beyond multivitamins.** Whereas, in the general population, only 50 percent of American adults reported taking dietary supplements.

Again, the use of antioxidant vitamins in cancer patients exceeds their use in the general population.

The following study showed the prevalence of the problem. High does of antioxidants are taken by many breast cancer patients despite possible harmful consequences. Many women with breast cancer take antioxidant supplements while undergoing cancer treatment, even though **the consequences of doing so are unknown**. Published in the July 15, 2009 issue of *CANCER*, a peer-reviewed journal of the American Cancer Society, the study indicated that **additional research should be undertaken to determine the effects of antioxidant supplementation on the health and survival of breast cancer patients.**

Antioxidant supplements include vitamin C, vitamin E, beta-carotene, and selenium. They are found in individual supplements as well as in many multivitamins. **Many breast cancer patients believe that antioxidant supplements will protect them from the side effects of breast cancer treatment, help prevent breast cancer recurrence, and improve their overall health**. That has not been proven to be the case.

However, the actual effects of taking antioxidants during cancer treatment are poorly understood and the **findings to date are mixed. Some physicians strongly believe antioxidants may in fact interfere with radiation. Others know that some types of chemotherapy** attack tumor cells by generating EMODs (reactive oxygen species, ROS), very small molecules that play a role in cell kill.

Researchers led by Heather Greenlee, ND, PhD, Assistant Professor of Epidemiology and Medical Oncology (in Medicine) at Columbia University Mailman School of Public Health in New York, investigated the prevalence of antioxidant use in women with breast cancer who participated in the population-based Long Island Breast Cancer Study Project (LIBCSP). LIBCSP, which included more than 1,500 breast cancer patients. Dr. Greenlee's study was based on the **764 patients** who completed a follow-up interview and provided information on antioxidant supplement use.

Among the 764 patients studied, 663 women (86.8 percent) reported receiving chemotherapy, radiation, or hormone therapy for breast cancer. Of these 663 women, **six in ten (60.5 percent) reported using antioxidants during breast cancer treatment,** which included chemotherapy, radiation, and tamoxifen (anti-estrogen) therapy.

About seven in ten antioxidant users (69.3 percent) used high doses, defined as higher than the dose contained in a Centrum multivitamin. Women who took high doses of antioxidants during treatment were more likely to be using tamoxifen and to have a history of eating more fruits and vegetables, using herbal products, and engaging in mind-body practices.

"Given the common use of antioxidant supplements during breast cancer treatment, often at high doses and in conjunction with other complementary therapies, future research should address the effects of antioxidant supplementation on breast cancer outcomes," including whether antioxidants affect treatment toxicities, treatment efficacy, cancer recurrence, and survival. (Greenlee et al, 2009).

Dietary supplement use in adult cancer survivors

Investigators assessed dietary supplement use and its association with demographic and health-related characteristics among cancer survivors and investigated differences in supplement use patterns by cancer site with a cross-sectional survey.

The study included 1,233 adult (ages 30-69) **survivors** participating in the Penn State Cancer Survivor Study who underwent an interviewer-administered questionnaire.

Supplement use ranged from 50% among blood cancer survivors to 85% among melanoma skin cancer survivors, with an overall prevalence rate of 73%. Multivariate logistic regression revealed statistically significant associations between supplement use and older age (>or= age 50), higher levels of education and physical activity, female gender, lower body mass index, and white ethnicity.

Overall, a wide variety of supplements were reported, **although multivitamins, calcium and vitamin D combinations, and antioxidant vitamin combinations were the most prevalent. Seventy-eight percent of supplement users took more than one supplement.**

Patients should be cautioned against the use of individual supplements as well as combinations of different supplements containing nutrient quantities above recommended daily intake levels.

Furthermore, healthcare professionals should be receptive to questions and prepared to initiate conversations with patients about their use of dietary supplements (Miller et al, 2009).

Cheryl Rock, Ph.D., R.D., Professor, Department of Family and Preventive Medicine, University of California—San Diego, reported on antioxidant supplement use in cancer survivors and the general population. **Approximately one-half of the general population takes dietary supplements, and use is higher among individuals with health concerns, especially those diagnosed with cancer.**

Two recent studies, the Olestra Post-Marketing Surveillance Study (OPMSS) and the Women's Healthy Eating and Living (WHEL) Study, collected data on supplement use. Results from OPMSS indicate that predictors of antioxidant use are age, education, sex, and region of the United States. OPMSS participants reported taking multivitamins (41%), vitamin E (9.5%), vitamin C (17%), and ß-carotene (2%). Among users of supplements, the median dosage of vitamin C was 500 mg and that of vitamin E was 34 mg; Dr. Rock commented that each of these represents relatively modest intake from supplements.

The WHEL study examined data on women diagnosed with stage I, II, or IIA invasive breast cancer within the past 48 mo and after treatment. Results indicated that at baseline (1995–2002), there was a wide range of antioxidant dietary supplement use. **At baseline, 91% of women used dietary supplements**. Specific antioxidant dietary supplements used included multivitamins (59%), antioxidant mixtures (9.8%), selenium (10.1%), vitamin A and carotenoids (10.6%), vitamin C (41.6%), and vitamin E (45.8%).

Positive predictors of supplement use included older age (vitamins E and C), high levels of physical activity (vitamins E and C and multivitamins), and education and stage at diagnosis (multivitamins). Negative predictors of supplement use included race or ethnicity and BMI (vitamins E and C and multivitamins) and time since diagnosis (vitamins E and C). Motivations for supplement use included **beliefs** (impressions) that vitamin C and E increase general health, that vitamin E decreases menopausal symptoms, and that vitamin C improves immune functions.

Conclusions drawn from these studies suggest that **the prevalence of antioxidant dietary supplement use is higher among cancer survivors than among the general population, and that the supplements being used are increasingly complex mixtures of ingredients**. (Rock et al, 2004).

Widespread vitamin and mineral use among cancer survivors

Use of vitamin and mineral supplements among cancer survivors is widespread, despite inconclusive evidence that such use is beneficial, according to a comprehensive review of scientific literature conducted by researchers at Fred Hutchinson Cancer Research Center and published Feb. 1, 2008 in the Journal of Clinical Oncology.

"Can vitamin and herbal supplements reduce the adverse effects of cancer treatment, decrease the risk of cancer recurrence or improve a patient's chances of survival? **We don't really know.** Research into these matters has been minimal," said senior author Cornelia (Neli) Ulrich, Ph.D., an associate member of the Hutchinson Center's Public Health Sciences Division. "While supplement use may be beneficial for some patients, such as those who cannot eat a balanced diet, **research suggests that certain supplements may actually interfere with treatment or even accelerate cancer growth**," she said.

In reviewing **32 studies conducted between 1999 and 2006**, Ulrich and co-author Christine Velicer, Ph.D., formerly a postdoctoral fellow at the Hutchinson Center (now an epidemiologist at Merck Research Laboratory in North Wales, Pa.), found that many of **the nation's 10 million adult cancer survivors** use nutritional supplements. **I believe that this is a major problem, in that cancer patients may be at even greater danger by the use of antioxidant supplements, which favor cancer growth.**

They found 64 percent to 81 percent of cancer survivors overall reported using vitamins or minerals (excluding multivitamins), whereas in the general population only 50 percent of adults reported taking dietary supplements.

Survivors of breast cancer reported the highest use (75 percent to 87 percent), whereas prostate-cancer survivors reported the least (26 percent to 35 percent). Factors associated with the highest level of supplement use overall included a higher level of education and being female.

The researchers also found that many people initiate the use of vitamins and supplements after cancer diagnosis; between 14 percent and 32 percent start taking them **after learning they have cancer.**

"Cancer survivors report that they hope to strengthen their immune system with supplement use or gain a sense of control and empowerment," Ulrich said. However, **many cancer survivors who use supplements do not let their doctors know**; 31 percent to 68 percent of cancer patients and survivors who use supplements may not disclose this information or their doctors may fail to record it in their charts.

"This is disconcerting and suggests that many physicians may not recognize the importance of understanding whether their patients are taking supplements," Ulrich said.

Knowing about supplement use is crucial, she continues, because of potential adverse effects. **"Evidence clearly suggests the need for caution,"** Ulrich said.

"Some vitamins, such as folic acid, may be involved in cancer progression while others, such as St. John's wort, can interfere with chemotherapy. However, we really need more research to understand whether use of these supplements can be beneficial or do more harm than good."

Concern has been expressed that **antioxidant supplement use might pose a risk for adverse effects** as well as provide possible benefits, especially in vulnerable populations **such as individuals who have been diagnosed with cancer** (Gottlieb, 1999).

Use of antioxidant supplements during breast cancer treatment: a comprehensive review

An estimated 45-80% of breast cancer patients use antioxidant supplements after diagnosis, and use of antioxidant supplements during breast cancer treatment is common. Dietary supplements with antioxidant effects include vitamins, minerals, phytonutrients, and other natural products. We conducted a comprehensive review of literature on the associations between antioxidant supplement use during breast cancer treatment and patient outcomes.

METHODS: Inclusion criteria were: two or more subjects; clinical trial or observational study design; use of **antioxidant supplements (vitamin C, vitamin E, antioxidant combinations, multivitamins, glutamine, glutathione, melatonin, or soy isoflavones)** during chemotherapy, radiation therapy, and/or hormonal therapy for breast cancer as exposures; treatment toxicities, tumor response, recurrence, or survival as outcomes.

RESULTS: They identified 22 articles that met those criteria. Their **findings did not support any conclusions regarding the effects of individual antioxidant supplements during conventional breast cancer treatment on toxicities, tumor response, recurrence, or survival.** A few studies suggested that antioxidant supplements might decrease side effects associated with treatment, including vitamin E for hot flashes due to hormonal therapy and glutamine for oral mucositis during chemotherapy. Underpowered trials suggest that melatonin may enhance tumor response during treatment.

CONCLUSION: The evidence is currently insufficient to inform clinician and patient guidelines on the use of antioxidant supplements during breast cancer treatment. Thus, well designed clinical trials and observational studies are needed to determine the short- and long-term effects of such agents. (Greenlee, Hershman et al, 2009).

Other sides of the argument

On one side, Dr. D'Andrea takes a mechanistic view in saying "radiotherapy and many chemotherapy agents act by producing free radicals; some vitamins and supplements, including vitamins C and E, are antioxidants and bind to free radicals, preventing oxidative damage." She continues: **"There are considerable in vitro and animal data showing that vitamin C and other antioxidants can protect cells against radiation and chemotherapy.** It seems likely that they would therefore reduce treatment-related toxicities and there are promising, although not unequivocal, data that this indeed is the case. However, it also follows that **antioxidants might protect cancer cells, thereby reducing the oncologic effectiveness of cytotoxic therapy.** This is the reason why most oncologists discourage patients from using antioxidants during treatment." (D'Andrea, 2005).

Whereas, D'Incalci et al say that "Studies have explored the effect of predominantly antioxidant vitamins and folate on efficacy or toxicity mediated by cisplatin and anthracyclines. Cisplatin toxicity in rodents was ameliorated by vitamin E. The design of clinical studies of dietary agents in combination with cytotoxic agents has been very heterogeneous and results have been inconclusive." They conclude cautiously that "whilst preclinical experiments hint at a potential benefit of certain dietary agents, **the evidence emanating from clinical studies does not allow firm conclusions to be made.** Future studies should explore physiological doses of dietary agent and include pharmacokinetic and pharmacodynamic measurements." (D'Incalci et al, 2007.

To add even more confusion, Shacter et al examined the effects of oxidative stress on chemotherapy-induced cell killing. They found **that H_2O_2 (hydrogen peroxide) inhibits the ability of four different chemotherapy drugs (VP-16, doxorubicin, cisplatin, and AraC) to induce apoptosis in human Burkitt lymphoma cells.** H_2O_2 shifts the form of cell death from apoptosis to pyknosis/necrosis, which occurs after a significant delay compared with chemotherapy induced apoptosis. It can also lower the degree of cell killing by these drugs. These effects of H_2O_2 can be prevented by the antioxidant agents Desferal, Tempol, and dimethylsulfoxide. (Shacter et al, 2000).

Dr. Block and co-author Dr. Robert Newman, Professor of Cancer Medicine at M. D. Anderson Cancer Center said, "Their study, along with the evolving understanding of antioxidant-chemotherapy interactions, suggests that the **previously held beliefs about interference do not pertain to clinical treatment.**" (Block et al, 2007).

Antioxidants can promote cancer

Antioxidants, by preventing oxidant-mediated damage to diverse targets (DNA, RNA, proteins, and lipids), may play a protective role in healthy individuals with no existing cancer cells that must be eliminated; however, **by inhibiting apoptosis, these same antioxidants may exert a cancer-promoting effect in cancer patients and in individuals with precancerous DNA changes.**

Inhibition of apoptosis by antioxidants may explain why, in several studies in heavy smokers, **vitamin E and beta-carotene enhanced carcinogenesis in the lung** (DeLuca and Ross, 1996) **but decreased carcinogenesis in the prostate** (Heinonen et al, 1998) (where, presumably, smoking had not caused precancerous lesions that predated antioxidant treatment).

Thus, though early administration of antioxidants may prevent the initiation and progression of cancer by quenching the action of potentially mutagenic reactive free radicals, **administration of antioxidants subsequent to a mutagenic event may effectively intercept free radicals that are critical in promoting apoptosis.** This imbalance may allow the rate of proliferation in tumors to exceed the capacity for apoptosis. It seems reasonable to suggest that the potential risks and benefits of high-dose antioxidants need to be considered on a case-to-case basis, and indiscriminate use of antioxidant dietary supplements should be avoided.

Unfortunately, many studies attempting to evaluate so-called oxidative therapy have relied on studies done on terminal patients. Thus, results were naturally biased against oxidative therapy.

Please keep in mind, that as of 2011, no one has found a bonified (scientifically proven) so-called "miracle cure" for cancer.

Colon and liver cancer cells killed by EMODs and blocked by antioxidants (NAC)

Paradoxically, EMODs (reactive oxygen species, ROS) can promote normal cellular proliferation and carcinogenesis, and can also induce apoptosis of tumor cells. In this report, they studied the contribution of ROS to various cellular signals depending on the nature and the level of ROS produced. In nontransformed NIH 3T3 cells, ROS are at low levels and originate from NADPH oxidase. Hydrogen peroxide (H_2O_2), controlled by the glutathione system, is pivotal for the modulation of normal cell proliferation. **In CT26 (colon) and Hepa 1-6**

(liver) tumor cells, high levels of ROS, close to the threshold of cytotoxicity, are produced by mitochondria and H_2O_2 is controlled by catalase. **N-acetylcysteine, which decreases H_2O_2 levels, inhibits mitogen-activated protein kinase and normal cell proliferation but increases tumor cell proliferation as H_2O_2 concentration drops from the toxicity threshold.** In contrast, antioxidant molecules, such as **mimics of superoxide dismutase (SOD), increase H_2O_2 levels** through superoxide anion dismutation, as well as in vitro proliferation of normal cells, but **kill tumor cells.** CT26 tumors were implanted in mice and treated by oxaliplatin in association with one of the three SOD mimics manganese(III)tetrakis(4-benzoic acid) porphyrin, copper(II)(3,5-diisopropylsalicylate)2, or manganese dipyridoxyl diphosphate. After 1 month, the volumes of tumors were respectively 35%, 31%, and 63% smaller than with oxaliplatin alone (P < 0.001). Similar data were gained with Hepa 1-6 tumors. In conclusion, **antioxidant molecules may have opposite effects on tumor growth.** SOD mimics can act in synergy with cytotoxic drugs to treat colon and liver cancers (Laurent et al, 2005).

SOD mimetics kill cancer because they produce peroxide and antioxidants block cancer kill because they block EMODs, especially H_2O_2. This is a pattern I have seen repeated many times and convinces me that antioxidants are dangerous.

Memorial Sloan-Kettering Cancer Center said large doses of vitamin C might sabotage treatment

Because of their well-recognized antioxidant properties, vitamins A (beta-carotene), C, and E are often touted for their ability to protect the body against cancer. However, **new data have emerged suggesting that cancer patients who take high supplemental doses of vitamins A, C, and E might actually be doing more harm than good.**

The most recent research, presented at a meeting of the American Cancer Society by **oncologists from Memorial Sloan-Kettering Cancer Center in New York, suggests that cancer patients who take large doses of vitamin C— one gram (1,000 mg) or more daily—might sabotage their treatment** by helping cancer cells protect themselves from radiation and chemotherapy.

While these adverse effects have **not been proven conclusively**, researchers report that there are persuasive biological reasons to think large doses could be harmful. For example, scientists recently discovered that **cancer cells contain large amounts of vitamin C, which appears to protect them—just as it**

protects healthy cells—from oxygen damage to the genes. Several cancer therapies, particularly radiation, work by triggering oxygen damage (via EMODs) in cancer cells, helping to cripple and destroy them.

University of North Carolina's School of Public Health said vitamins A & E may undermine cancer treatment

Previous research in mice, conducted at the University of North Carolina's School of Public Health, has suggested that vitamins A and E may undermine the efficacy of cancer treatment as well. When the DNA of cells in both mice and humans has been damaged beyond repair, the cells undergo a natural process that forces them to destroy themselves. This process is called apoptosis. **The mouse study indicated that some antioxidant vitamins may suppress apoptosis, thereby reducing cancer cell death.**

No signs dietary supplements prevent bladder cancer

3-10-11 Popping vitamins, minerals or anti-inflammatory substances like garlic or fish oil doesn't appear to stave off bladder cancer, a large U.S. study shows.

The findings, published in the **Journal of Urology, are more evidence that the alleged anti-cancer effects of such supplements, found in some early studies, don't hold up.**

"If you're eating a good diet then taking extra supplements is not something that has proven health benefits," said Dr. Michael Pollak of McGill University in Montreal, a cancer prevention expert who wasn't involved in the new work.

"Going from sufficiency to excess is something that people had hoped would be an easy way to prevent cancer, but it just hasn't worked out," Pollak told Reuters Health.

The new results are based on data from more than **77,000 older men and women** in Washington State, who had filled out a detailed questionnaire about their health, diet and supplement intake at the outset of the study.

Over the following six years, **330 people developed bladder cancer. Whether or not they reported taking dietary supplements had no impact on their risk,** after accounting for age, smoking, fruit and vegetable intake and other factors.

"At this time we can't recommend taking any of these supplements to prevent bladder cancer," said Dr. James Hotaling, a urologist who worked on the study.

Hotaling and his colleagues looked at a wide range of substances, including multivitamins, several B vitamins, vitamin C, D, and E, calcium, magnesium, zinc, glucosamine, ginkgo biloba, fish oil and garlic.

"The number of patients who take these supplements is extremely high," said Hotaling, of the University of Washington School of Medicine in Seattle. "It has become a million-dollar industry, and there is not a lot of data to show that these supplements make a difference" in cancer, he said.

If eating extra vitamins actually protected against the disease, he added, it would not only save lives but also a lot of money. That's because patients with bladder cancer require repeated checkups to ensure the cancer doesn't return after they've had surgery.

According to the American Cancer Society (ACS), about one in 26 American men and one in 84 women get bladder cancer.

"No nutritional supplement has been proven to reduce risk of cancer and **the American Cancer Society does not recommend using supplements to prevent cancer,"** ACS's Eric Jacobs told Reuters Health in an e-mail.

It's not all bad news, however. **"Some of the things that are much harder to do than taking vitamins are actually much more effective, like stopping smoking or avoiding obesity,"** said Pollak. (SOURCE: http://bit.ly/i2WV6L Journal of Urology, online February 18, 2011).

Cancer cells need high amounts of vitamin C to thrive

Prior to the University of North Carolina study, **another mouse study suggested that tumor cells need high amounts of vitamin C to thrive**. Moreover, years ago, **two human studies found that smokers with high levels of beta-carotene in their blood had a higher risk of lung cancer (CARET study)**, compared with smokers with low levels of the antioxidant.

Cancer specialists still recommend eating a diet rich in fruits and vegetables, but many now caution their cancer patients to avoid taking high doses of vitamin supplements. Until we learn more, consider these precautions:

1. Do not take vitamin supplements unless your doctor has prescribed them.

2. Avoid taking high doses of antioxidant vitamins during radiation therapy or chemotherapy. After treatment is complete, ask your physician if it is safe to start taking vitamins.

3. Eat a balanced diet. Doing so should supply enough of the vitamins, minerals, and nutrients the body needs in the natural proportions

Cancer cells readily take up vitamin C in vitro (Baader et al, 1994) (Spielholz et al, 1997).

Thus, it appears that cancer cells like and need sugar and antioxidants, such as lactate, glutathione and vitamin C.

Studies have demonstrated high vitamin C concentrations in neo-plasms compared with the adjacent normal tissue (Langemann et al, 1989). The mechanism by which cancers accumulate vitamin C in vivo, however, is unknown. (National Cancer Foundation for Cancer Research.org website. Accessed 10-31-07)

Theoretical reason to avoid antioxidants in cancer patients

According to Institute of Medicine, a **dietary antioxidant is defined as "a substance in foods that significantly decreases the adverse effects of reactive species, such as reactive oxygen and nitrogen species, on normal physiological function in humans."** (Institute of Medicine, 2000).

This definition is part of the problem, in that it states that EMODs have adverse effects and completely ignores their many beneficial effects. Thus, if antioxidants are capable of "significantly decreasing" their adverse effects, it is logical that they will also "significantly decrease" the beneficial effects of EMODs, including the killing of cancer cells. In fact, that is at the heart of the arguments concerning the use of antioxidants in cancer patients.

Actually, the notion that "oxygen free radicals are bad and antioxidants are good" is an outdated concept based on the many documented in vivo beneficial roles for EMODs and their apparent low toxicity. (Howes, 2004) (Howes, 2009) (Howes, Philica. Feb 26, 2007) (Howes, Philica. April 5, 2007) (Howes, Philica. Feb 7, 2009)

The following organizations or groups either do not recommend anti-oxidant vitamins or have found inconclusive evidence of their benefit:

- **The American Cancer Society**
- **The American College of Cardiology**
- **The American Heart Association (AHA)**
- **The American Diabetes Association**
- **The National Cancer Institute (NCI)**
- **Institute of Medicine of the National Academies**
- **National Academy of Sciences**
- **The American Academy of Family Physicians**
- **The U.S. Food and Drug Administration (FDA)**
- **Food and Nutrition Board, Institute of Medicine**
- **The Food and Nutrition Board of the National Academy of Sciences**
- **American College of Cardiology Foundation Task Force on Clinical Expert Consensus Documents**
- **United States Preventive Services Task Force (USPSTF)**
- **The AHA Scientific Position of the American Heart Association**
- **The American College of Chest Physicians (ACCP)**
- **National Institutes of Health State-of-the-Science Conference**
- **Scientific Statement From the American Heart Association and the American Diabetes Association**
- **The American Cancer Society Guidelines on Nutrition and Physical Activity for Cancer Prevention**
- **The American Heart Association Atherosclerosis, Hypertension, and Obesity in Youth Committee, Council of Cardiovascular Disease in the Young, With the Council on Cardiovascular Nursing**
- **The Swedish Council of Technology Assessment**
- **The Medical Letter**
- **National Heart Foundation of Australia's Nutrition and Metabolism Advisory Committee**
- **The Oregon Health and Science University**
- **The Canadian Task Force on Preventive Health Care (CTFPHC)**
- **Food Standards Agency/ the British Nutrition Foundation (BNF)**
- **The Nutrition Committee of the American Heart Association Council on Nutrition, Physical Activity, and Metabolism**
- **Quackwatch**
- **The 2006 AHA Diet and Lifestyle Recommendations**
- **The American College of Cardiology/American Heart Association Task Force on Practice Guidelines**

- **The Physicians Health Study**
- **The 2008 VITAmins and Lifestyle (VITAL) study**
- **The Physicians' Health Study II Randomized Controlled Trial**

(Howes, Am J Cos Surg. 2009) (Howes, 2010) (Howes, 2010).

Antioxidants combat the effects of both endogenously and exogenously produced prooxidants. In the body, electronically modified oxygen derivatives (EMODs) [formerly called free radicals and reactive oxygen species (ROS)] appear as a natural consequence of energy production in the organism. EMODs (ROS) include superoxides, hydrogen peroxide, and the hydroxyl radical. These cellular oxidants arise from oxygen and appear constantly, in part, as a result of mitochondrial release of electrons from the electron transport chain and the reduction of oxygen molecules to superoxides. (Salganik, 2001).

In December of 1999, Salganik pointed out that, "**Almost all anticancer drugs kill cancer cells by way of apoptosis, and antioxidants like vitamin A and vitamin E dramatically reduce apoptosis in cancer cells." Patients should therefore avoid taking any more than a normal amount of these vitamins during chemotherapy treatment.** In short, do not add to normal intake but Dr. Salganik's advice went further indicating that "an antioxidant-depleted diet could improve cancer therapies."

Studies indicate that 40% of the U.S. population takes vitamin supplements, and scientific discussions have been directed toward antioxidants in particular. (Meyers et al, 1996).

Oxidative function and EMOD production are crucial for proper health. For example, oxidation processes are used by the body's immune systems to kill microorganisms, fungi, protozoans and viruses. (Howes, 2010) (Winkler et al, 1999).

Even though there may be growing scientific arguments that antioxidants, particularly the polyphenolic forms, may help lower the incidence of disease, such as certain cancers, cardiovascular and neurodegenerative diseases, DNA damage, or even have anti-aging properties, **questions remain as to whether some antioxidants or phytochemicals potentially could do more harm than good, as an increase in glycation-mediated protein damage (carbonyl stress) and some risk has been reported.** (Obrenovich et al, 2011).

For example, Centrum sells a phytosterol combo vitamin, which it claims is important for heart healthy purposes but there is no proof of this.

As of 2008, Dr Alison Ross, science information officer at Cancer Research UK, pointed out, **there is currently no evidence from clinical trials in humans that injecting or consuming vitamin C, or other antioxidants, is effective in treating cancer**. "**Some research even suggests that high doses of antioxidants can make cancer treatment less effective, reducing the benefits of radiotherapy and chemotherapy.**"

Beloved of health food shops and alternative therapists, antioxidant pills have been marketed as preventive therapies to ward off everything from cancer to the signs of aging. Until recently, the theory behind much of this seemed sound. Some studies had shown that people who eat a healthy balanced diet with plenty of fruit and vegetables were less likely to develop cancer and one benefit of these foods was thought to be the antioxidant chemicals they contain. So, why not get that benefit directly in a pill?

Yet, that assumption has not held up to rigorous scientific investigations.

Hundreds of large studies I collected have now compared the benefits of supplement pills against placebos and have conclusively shown that the benefits of a healthy diet are not shared by vitamin pills — and **in 80 cases they have been shown to be harmful**.

Dr Jennifer Lin and her colleagues at Brigham and Women's Hospital in Boston, Massachusetts, gave vitamins C, E, beta-carotene or placebos to 7,627 women who were at high risk of cardiovascular disease. After an average of 9.4 years' follow-up, 624 of the women had developed cancer, of which 176 died. But these cancer cases were distributed evenly between the different treatment groups, and **there was no statistical difference between the number of deaths among people taking single antioxidants or combinations and the group taking the placebos.** As of 2008, antioxidant **supplements did not reduce risk of developing cancer**. The researchers gave **vitamins C, E, beta-carotene** or placebo pills to patients and followed their progress for an average of **nearly 10 years**. The results showed that **the supplements, either on their own or in combination, did not protect the women against cancer**.

"Supplementation with vitamin C, vitamin E, or beta-carotene offers no overall benefits in the primary prevention of total cancer incidence or cancer mortality," the authors wrote in the **Journal of the National Cancer Institute**. "In our trial, **neither duration of treatment nor combination of the three antioxidant supplements had effects on overall fatal or nonfatal cancer events.**"

The results agree with those of **a separate randomized controlled clinical trial of vitamin C and E supplements, published in November. That study, which involved nearly 15,000 men in the US, found no cancer prevention effect from taking the supplements.**

The advice from Cancer Research UK is that supplements cannot take the place of eating a healthy diet. "The best way to get your full range of vitamins and minerals is to eat a healthy, balanced diet, with a variety of fruit and vegetables. Supplements do not substitute for a healthy diet, although some people may be advised to take them at certain times in their lives."

Vitamins A and E appear to keep cancer cells from dying through the natural protective process scientists call apoptosis. Giving patients those vitamins may prevent cancer cells from self-destructing and work against cancer therapy.

Fruit and vegetables do not reduce overall cancer risk

As of December of 2010, reducing smoking and alcohol consumption was a far better way to avoid cancer than eating large quantities of fruit and vegetables.

Eating lots of fruit and vegetables will do little to reduce your risk of developing cancer, according to a review of a decade of research involving more than a million people. It concluded that maintaining a healthy weight and cutting down on smoking and drinking are far better ways to ward off the disease, if one exercises.

Vegetables and fruit are important for a healthy diet but the review says **that eating increased amounts does not seem to offer much protection against cancer.**

Tim Key, an epidemiologist from Oxford University, said, "There's strong scientific evidence to show that, after smoking, being overweight and alcohol are two of the biggest cancer risks." (Key, 2011).

In an article published in the **British Journal of Cancer**, Key summarised the epidemiological evidence from more than a million people taking part in several dozen long-term research projects looking at the amount of fruit and vegetables people eat and their overall cancer risk. He also studied specific cancers of the gastrointestinal tract, lung and breast.

Key found little, if any, connection between eating lots of fruits and vegetables and the likelihood of developing cancer. "The conclusion implies that, at least in relatively well-nourished westernised populations, a general increase in total fruit and vegetable intake will not have a large impact on cancer rates. **A certain level of intake is necessary to prevent nutrient deficiencies, but intakes above that level do not make the relavant tissues 'super healthy.'**"

The studies included data from **the European Prospective Investigation into Cancer and Nutrition, the Pooling Project based at Harvard University**, and the National Institutes of Health and American Association of Retired Persons Diet and Health Study.

The idea that fruit and veg might help reduce cancer rates was first postulated in the 1970s, when the results of a small-scale study showed that, after controlling for smoking, people with reduced intakes of vitamin A were at increased risk of lung cancer. By the 1990s, scientists were concluding that "for most cancer sites, persons with low fruit and vegetable intake experience about twice the risk of cancer compared to those with a high intake, even after control for potentially confounding factors."

But these "case-control" studies – where people with a disease are matched with controls who do not have the disease – still suffered from confounding factors. "While a lot of those [earlier] case-control studies do try and adjust for how much people smoke and how much people drink, there's always a worry that you haven't completely adjusted for that because smoking and drinking have such a massive impact on the risk of those cancers," said Ed Yong, head of health evidence and information at Cancer Research UK.

Key said case-control studies can suffer from two main types of bias. "One is that people with cancer may be under treatment so it may affect how they remember what they used to eat in the years before they developed cancer. They may be feeling ill or under strong medical treatment."

A bigger problem is with the selection of the control group, which might not be entirely random. "People who come forward are those interested in health and related behaviours," said Key. "The controls may well appear to have a healthy diet because the potential controls with an unhealthy diet may have stayed in the pub eating chips and beans and not volunteered to be studied."

A better way to analyse the relationship between diet and cancer is to conduct "**prospective studies**", which ideally follow hundreds of thousands of people who don't have cancer. "They tell you what they eat and you follow them until, inevitably, some of them do develop cancer," said Key. "But you made the measurements when they're healthy, so the biases don't apply. **Those types of studies have been coming out in the last 10-15 years and have not supported the original findings** [from case-control groups]."

Key's review supports work published in April, 2010 in the Journal of the National Cancer Institute. Paolo Boffetta from the Tisch Cancer Institute at Mount Sinai School of Medicine in New York found that **eating a lot of fruit and vegetables has only "a very modest" protective effect against cancer.** That conclusion was **based on a decade of research on almost 500,000 people in 10 European countries.** (Key, 2011).

Despite the results of the studies, Yong said it was still a good idea for people get their minimum daily five portions of fruits and vegetables. "It's not a bad message because it could help people to lose weight, which is a massive cause of cancer, and it could displace other [unhealthier] things in their diet," he said. "There's no harm to eating lots of fruits and vegetables and there are benefits for other diseases as well, such as heart disease."

Doubt about antioxidants

Although antioxidants may be beneficial in deficiency diseases, the findings on antioxidants and diseases such as cancer, heart disease and strokes have been shocking. **The antioxidant marketing industry is in full stride and the best scientific evidence has passed unnoticed or has been denied or ignored.**

Antioxidants are not magic bullets

The latest scare has infuriated many in the vitamins industry and nutritionists such as Patrick Holford who believe there is a campaign by the medical establishment to discredit their products and their role in optimizing health. Mr. Holford said: **"Antioxidants are not meant to be magic bullets and should not be expected to undo a lifetime of unhealthy habits."**

Antioxidants were never intended for the prevention of chronic disease and mortality

Pamela Mason, of the industry-backed Health Supplements Information Service, said: **"Antioxidant vitamins, like any other vitamins, were never intended for the prevention of chronic disease and mortality."**

"Antioxidants are not the magic bullets that the supplement industry would like consumers to believe," said David Schardt, a nutrition expert with the consumer advocacy group, the Center for Science in the Public Interest. **"They're not even necessarily benign." OVERSTATED HEALTH CLAIMS: Makers can say a supplement addresses a nutrient deficiency, supports health, or reduces the risk of developing a problem, but then must say the product "is not intended to diagnose, treat, cure, or prevent any disease."**

They are intended for health maintenance on the basis of their various physiological roles in the body and in the case of antioxidant vitamins, this does, in appropriate amounts, include an unproven protective antioxidant effect in the body's tissues.

Can it be said that EVERYTHING causes death? You eat vitamins -- you will die, you do not eat them -- you will die, too! And about "prematurely" -- some people live longer than others no matter what they eat, or drink, or even smoke. So, what is one to do?

Dr. Krinsky, professor of biochemistry at Tufts University Boston, noted, "Many people are likely to continue to believe that these compounds (dietary antioxidants) have many health benefits, including the prevention of chronic disease, but "we were not able to find definitive proof of that hypothesis."

Maureen Storey, Ph.D., a nutritionist with the Georgetown Center for Food and Nutrition Policy, stated, **"You can get too much of a good thing." People who pop large amounts of vitamins or minerals--thinking that if a little is good, a lot is better--need to know that there are dangerous levels of these compounds.**

I have made the most important discovery that you have probably never heard of: antioxidant vitamins can lower EMODs to dangerously low levels and increase the risk of cancer, heart disease, strokes, sepsis, AIDS, malaria and overall mortality. I first introduced my theories in my prior books, U.T.O.P.I.A. and The Medical and Scientific Significance of Oxygen Metabolism.

In many cases, these antioxidant vitamins are no better than a dummy pill or placebo but they also have dangerous potential. I have now accumulated 80 studies showing that they had a higher rate of causing diseases than a placebo. That is shocking.

**The human body is simultaneously
a masterpiece of energy and
a mysterious miracle of matter.
It does and it thinks....
at least....I think it does.**
R. M. Howes, M.D., Ph.D.
9/7/09

CHAPTER THREE:

Heated debate of antioxidants
in cancer patients

We must keep an open mind as we evaluate the overall data.

We must find answers to the following questions:

- Does the co-administration of antioxidants, either singular or in combinations, decrease the effectiveness of chemotherapy and radiation therapy?

- Does the co-administration of antioxidants significantly increase the effectiveness of chemotherapy and radiation therapy and overcome the theoretical objections to their use?

- Does the co-administration of antioxidants mitigate some of the side effects of chemotherapy and radiation therapy and improve quality of life, while not reducing the intent of the cancer therapy?

- Does the co-administration of antioxidants favorably or unfavorably affect long-term survival rates, based on current scientific evidence?

Heated debate over antioxidant use in cancer patients

Heated debates have raged over the use of antioxidant supplements by cancer patients during chemo and radiation therapy. Scientists and oncologists are on both sides of this controversial area of oncology. However, **I believe that there is adequate research data, with its theoretical support, to arrive at a meaningful conclusion.** I have examined and reviewed this data in great detail and will show you the potential dangers of antioxidant use in cancer patients.

Past surveys indicate that antioxidant use is high in cancer patients and in medical personnel overall. It is time to bring these groups up to running speed with the current scientific evidence and to set the record straight.

Proponents of antioxidant use say, "Antioxidants are attractive to both clinicians and patients because these substances counteract free radicals and prevent them from causing tissue and organ damage." But, both the theoretical and the scientific based evidence for this position is lacking, although there have been some weak studies and biased reports still advocating antioxidant use by cancer patients.

Fans for antioxidant use argue that patients with cancer are taking antioxidant supplements in combination with conventional chemotherapy and radiotherapy to enhance their anticancer activity and reduce the side effects of conventional treatment. They claim that not all chemotherapy agents rely on oxidative stress for anticancer activity, so the risk for interaction with antioxidant supplements is also dependent on the type of conventional chemotherapy. They cite several studies showing **that plasma concentrations of antioxidants are depleted in individuals undergoing treatment for cancer;** some studies suggest that this reduction may be associated with therapy-related toxicities.

Yet, there have been few randomized controlled trials which investigated the efficacy of antioxidants as a treatment for cancer and most published trials have been epidemiologic case series or non-randomized trials. Clinical trials have yielded inconclusive and mixed results and all healthcare providers should be cautious before recommending antioxidant supplements during chemotherapy.

Whereas, opponents of their use argue that the protective mechanisms of antioxidants may not distinguish between normal and malignant cells, such that supplements may interfere with the anticancer activity of conventional therapies. Further, **results from large randomized controlled trials (ATBC study, the CARET study and the SELECT study), indicated that the use of beta-carotene and vitamin E (and perhaps selenium) supplements in conjunction with radiation therapy is contraindicated and should be avoided**. These three studies had a total of 82,980 human participants and were all shut down about 21 months early due to the fact that the supervisory physicians detected harmful effects of the antioxidants and felt it unethical to continue these studies. To me, this speaks volumes!

The ATBC study had 29,133 men participants. The CARET had 14,254 heavy smokers and 4,060 asbestos workers and the SELECT study had 35,533 men for a total of 82,980 participants in these studies. This is no longer debatable at this point. Yet, this data is still ignored and denied.

A major problem is that people have been erroneously led to believe that antioxidants are beneficial for their overall health and well being. They look at antioxidants as a form of harmless "natural" therapy rather than as being dangerous drugs or medicines. They therefore have an inaccurate and dangerous viewpoint.

We must learn to think of antioxidants as we do drugs. There is always a benefit/ risk ratio to consider.

A little antioxidant history

Once upon a time, just a few decades ago, the theoretical use of antioxidants seemed to be a good idea but hundreds of scientific studies have repeatedly failed to show any consistent, scientifically measurable benefit from taking antioxidant supplements.

Having failed to meet the "predictability requirements" of the scientific method, the free radical theory is no longer valid and I have endeavored to replace it with more advanced and improved theories.

The field of redox chemistry (oxidation/reduction chemistry) and antioxidant research is controversial and confusing to many scientists, medical personnel, nutritionists and clinicians because the study results have been confusing and conflicting, making reaching solid conclusions difficult as to antioxidant efficacy and safety. Antioxidants fall under the regulatory guidelines and category of "food" and can not be marketed or regulated like drugs for disease treatment, diagnosis, cure or prevention. Yet, **medicinal-sounding false claims abound extolling the wonders of antioxidants in disease prevention and cure, including the prevention and cure of cancer.**

Historically, electronically modified oxygen derivatives (EMODs, formerly called reactive oxygen species, ROS) were viewed in a negative light and they were seen as indiscriminately damaging agents, randomly ravaging cellular structure, components and function. Now, we know better and **these erroneous and outdated views of EMODs have been repudiated and partially corrected for those knowledgeable in the field.** Yet, strong market forces continue to flood antioxidant products upon the consumer market and to mislead the public and the medical community.

The primary query is, "Can antioxidants in any way protect cancer cells from being killed during cancer therapy and thus further endanger the survival of the patient?" The next big question is, "Can antioxidants safely reduce the adverse effects of chemotherapy, radiotherapy and photodynamic therapy (PDT) without reducing the cancer treatment efficacy?"

Can antioxidants negate current cancer therapies?

Prof Randolph M. Howes MD, PhD

A review of effective tumoricidal methods reveals a "commonality of cures," in that **many successful cytotoxic agents, procedures or methods have been shown to proceed via prooxidants (EMODs).**

These agents, in part, include the **anthracyclines (e.g., doxorubicin), platinum-containing complexes (e.g., cisplatin, carboplatin), alkylating agents (e.g., cyclophosphamide, ifosfamide), and cytotoxic antibiotics (e.g., bleomycin, mitomycin-C).** Please refer to the chemotherapy section.

My discussions will compare chemotherapy, radiation therapy, megadose intravenous vitamin C therapy, photodynamic therapy, sonodynamic therapy, Howes' singlet oxygen tumoricidal system, hyperbaric oxygen therapy and hydrogen peroxide therapy.

As a matter of fact, hypoxia and so-called antioxidants can effectively modify or block cancer cell kill by interfering with electronically modified oxygen derivative (EMOD)-induced apoptosis.

Contrary to the teachings of the free radical theory, certain prooxidants may offer unique tumoricidal properties and approach the Holy Grail for cancer treatments, allowing for selective killing of cancer cells while sparing normal cells.

Even though prooxidants, such as oxygen free radicals or reactive oxygen species, have been blamed for cancer causation, it has become increasingly apparent that the use of prooxidants for cancer therapy offers considerable clinical advantage and may present heretofore undiscovered safe and economical therapeutic promise.

I have investigated the over use of **supra-dietary doses of chemical antioxidants as a** possible cause for disease manifestation and coexistence. My case gets stronger and stronger all of the time. Vitamin A and carotenoids, vitamin C, vitamin E, selenium, and glutathione may alone or in combination, along with environmental antioxidants and preservatives, be "stacking" up against us.

The greatest controversy and arguments surround the **concomitant** administration of supra-dietary doses of antioxidant agents during chemotherapy, PDT and/or radiation therapy. Conventional oncologic therapies may be compromised by the cumulative antioxidant levels.

There are authors who claim that previous study results, which showed potential harm to cancer patients, have "over-hyped negative conclusions, presented sensational-but-flawed conclusions, and gave warnings that were overblown."

Nevertheless, "the data is the data" and it should not and can not be embellished, ignored nor denied.

The standard view is that chemotherapy, radiotherapy and photodynamic therapy kill cancer cells because they involve the production and action of EMODs. Ergo, **anything that interferes with EMOD production or activity (EMOD-induced apoptosis) must, to some degree, interfere with the efficacy of the cancer treatment.**

However, the complete and precise mechanisms critical for cellular suicide are still unknown. So, we must base our actions on that which we do know.

Apoptosis is a combination of several complex interconnected actions, especially redox involvement. Arguing which mechanism is more critical may not be important, and these clarified mechanisms should be connected and utilized in homeostatic maintenance for protection against pathogens and neoplasia. But, crystal clear answers to these arguments may be a long time forthcoming.

Actually, data from a limited number of randomized controlled trials have shown that high-dose antioxidant supplementation during radiotherapy decreases local tumor control and shortens the survival of cancer patients. Also, **because of the inconsistency in the overall data and in the interest of greatest safety for the patient, it would appear prudent that high doses of any antioxidant should be avoided during chemo, PDT or radiation therapy unless there is unequivocally clear evidence that the benefits outweigh the potential risk.**

Harman's free radical theory

**The free radi-crap theory is
the dropped end product of
Kerplunk Sphincteric Productions.**
R. M. Howes, M.D., Ph.D.
12/12/09

Harman's free radical theory hypothesized that diseases, such as cancer and aging, resulted from the random or "stochastic" accumulation of oxidative damage purportedly caused by EMODs, from environmental sources and from by-products of normal cellular metabolism. (Harman, 1956) (Harman, 1981) (Beckman, Ames, 1998) (Finkel, Holbrook, 2000) (Harman, 1961).

These alleged damaging derivatives of oxygen were defined as being inherently deleterious and harmful. However, this notion has been challenged by Howes. (Howes, 2006).

Apoptosis, in part, controls the neoplastic process as genetically damaged or mutated cells can be eliminated **by apoptosis. (White, McCubrey, 2001).**

Apoptosis, necrosis, and growth arrest have been shown to be regulated by EMOD levels. (Aw, 1999). (Kwon et al, 2003.

Apoptosis is largely based on oxygen free radicals released from the mitochondrial energy production pathway and EMODs serve as significant anti-tumorigenic signaling species. (Duranteau et al, 1998) (Valko et al, 2006).

Apoptosis involves caspases (cysteine proteases cleaving after particular aspartate residues), mitochondrial pathways and/or reactive oxygen species (EMODs), which are usually, but not always, key components. (Fiers, et al, 1999).

Many apoptogenic-inducing agents function as prooxidants in vitro. (Howes, Philica. Feb 26, 2007).

Most tumor cells are resistant to apoptosis. So, such resistance may be related to the particular properties of mitochondria in cancer cells that are distinct from those of mitochondria in non-malignant cells. Their resistance may also be due to their high antioxidant concentrations of vitamin C, lactate and glutathione.

EMOD generating agents have repeatedly been shown to kill cancer cells selectively, while sparing normal cells and this tumoricidal action can be blocked by antioxidants and accelerate cancer growth both in vitro and in vivo. (Begin, 1988) (Begin, 1987) (Das et al, 1987) (Lhuillery et al, 1997).

Since therapeutic agents (radiation, chemotherapy or PDT) work, at least in large part, by releasing free radicals (EMODs), it is logical that antioxidants likely interfere with their action.

EMOD levels and cellular redox tone may be uniquely exploitable targets in cancer chemoprevention via the stimulation or induction of cytoprotection in normal cells and/or the induction of apoptosis in transformed malignant cells.

What is apoptosis (cellular suicide)?

Two paths for apoptosis death

Apoptosis occurs primarily through two well-recognized pathways in cells, including the intrinsic, or mitochondrial-mediated, effector mechanism and the extrinsic, or death receptor–mediated, effector mechanism.

However, death not only can follow the well-characterized type I apoptotic pathway but also can proceed by nonapoptotic modes such as type II (macroautophagy-related) and type III (necrosis) or combinations thereof. In contrast to apoptosis, the induction of macroautophagy may contribute to either the survival or death of cells in response to a stressor.

Endogenous electronically modified oxygen derivatives (EMODs) participate in cell signaling and confer bacteriocidal activities to phagocytes. The burst of EMOD formation also allows organisms to kill invading cancer cells.

Prooxidants can be generated in the body as a result of purposeful (cancer killing), exogenous drug administration; i.e., chemotherapeutics. (Conklin, 2000).

This is the theoretical basis that the effects of chemotherapeutics, whose cytotoxicity depends either on EMOD generation or free radical intermediates, may be thwarted by antioxidants. (Conklin, 2004).

Another issue to consider is that nucleophilic antioxidants such as glutathione (GSH), n-acetylcysteine (NAC), and alpha-lipoic acid (ALA) can compete with chemotherapy drugs that act by nucleophilic substitution reactions, such as most alkylating compounds, thereby reducing their efficacy. (Conklin, 2004).

Individuals animals with low EMOD levels may become more prone to cancer by taking antioxidants, because of their already deficient EMOD production, which becomes further suppressed, thereby reducing the level of protective EMOD-induced apoptosis. (Salganik, 2001).

The generation of **excess levels of reactive oxygen species is important for activation of internal cell programs for cell suicide (apoptosis)** that are important protection mechanisms that kill cancer cells (Weijl, et al, 1997).

This mechanism (excess levels of reactive oxygen species) is critical for effective cancer chemotherapy and radiation treatment (Kuipers, Lafleur, 1998) (Blumenthal et al, 2000).

One of the important functions of apoptosis is the elimination of pre-neoplastic and neoplastic cells (Lowe et al, 1993) (Thompson, 1995) (Tomlison, Bodmer, 1995).

Many studies of cellular suicide have shown that **the** apoptotic **signaling cascade utilizes reactive oxygen species as essential intermediate messenger molecules** (Albright et al, 2003) (Vrablic et al, 2001) (Slater et al, 1995) (Johnson et al, 1996) (Sugiyama et al, 1996).

Arguments against prooxidant apoptosis

Antioxidant agents have a wide variety of biochemical actions and are capable of interfering selectively with EMOD initiation, propagation and termination and they are a part of the normal human diet. They have also been studied for their positive effects in the prevention or cure of some cancers, cardiovascular disease, age-related diseases, and other disorders. (Enger et al, 1995) (Jarvinen, 1995) (Taylor et al, 1995) (Frommel et al, 1995).

Antioxidants are believed to be balanced by EMODs generated from daily stresses, such as inflammation, cigarette smoke, exercise, detoxification, environmental chemicals, radiation, ultraviolet light, alcohol, and fatty diets. Some believe that antioxidants are balanced with EMOD levels to prevent disease and protect the cell. (Garewal, 1997).

Yet, **reduction in EMOD levels generated by chemotherapeutic agents has the same effect as a reduction in dose.** (Erhola et al, 1996).

Furthermore, the concentration of reactive oxygen species and its relationship to maximum drug effect determines the extent to which drug-nutrient interactions can interfere with this action. According to the Michaelis-Menten model:

Effect = (Maximal effect × [D]) / (KD + [D])

As drug dose (D) approaches maximum effect, changes in dose have a diminishing impact on effect. Based on this model, low-dose, fractionated regimens would be predicted to be more vulnerable to dosage variations resulting from drug-nutrient (chemotherapeutic drug produced EMOD-antioxidant) interactions.

Until such data is available, **considerations for utmost patient safety must prevail. The mechanisms of action of chemotherapeutic drugs and antioxidants are understood well enough to predict their apparent interactions and to suggest that considerable care should be exercised with respect to both clinical decisions and study interpretation.** (Chabner et al, 1990).

A number of authors express the belief that antioxidants do not interfere with chemotherapy or radiation and that at commonly used dosages they actually appear to enhance the success of these treatments. (Kagreud, Peterson, 1981) (Perez Ripoll et al, 1986) (Jaakkola et al, 1992) (Prasad et al, 1999) (Lamson, Brignall, 1999) (Moss, 2006).

This is counterintuitive to biochemical teachings.

Nonetheless, there seems to be agreement that **the antioxidant N-acetylcysteine (NAC), a derivative of the naturally occurring amino acid cysteine, should be avoided by cancer patients because of studies showing interference with chemotherapeutic agents, such as cisplatin and doxorubicin.** (Olson et al, 1983) (Roller, Weller, 1998).

A 2005 report concluded that cancer patients should avoid antioxidant supplements while receiving chemotherapy or radiation treatment. (D'Andrea, 2005).

Also, **a Wall Street Journal article argued that antioxidants could block the beneficial effects of standard cancer therapy.** (Parker-Pope, 2005).

Those who defend the use of antioxidants in cancer patients often point to older or prior studies which claim that antioxidants such as vitamin C, vitamin E, coenzyme Q10, glutathione, and selenium can reduce the toxicity of free radicals. (Weijl, et al, 1997) (Judy et al, 1984) (Sieja, Talerczyk, 2004) (Cascinu et al, 1995).

A 2007 article not only defends the use of antioxidants in cancer patients, it states that, "In 15 human studies, 3,738 **patients who took non-prescription**

antioxidants and other nutrients actually had increased survival." (Simone et al, 2007). This conclusion is in sharp contrast to the preponderance of the data (both in vitro and in vivo studies), which shows the strong possibility that antioxidants will negatively interfere with EMOD activated apoptosis.

The debate continues and the opposite position was upheld in a 2008 article in which the *Journal of the National Cancer Institute* recently published a review of randomized trial data, which suggested that **cancer patients should avoid the routine use of antioxidant supplements because they may potentially decrease the efficacy of cancer therapy by protecting the tumor and reducing survival.** They looked at clinical trials investigating the impact of antioxidants on radiation therapy and found evidence suggesting that antioxidant supplementation reduced overall survival. (Lawenda et al, 2008).

The use of nutritional supplements with antioxidant activity has the risk of interfering with the known actions of many chemotherapeutic agents that utilize EMODs as a mechanism for cytotoxicity. Even though they may improve their short-term tolerance to treatment and reduce toxicity symptoms, they may be increasing their vulnerability to a later recurrence or exacerbation as a result of having blocked the efficacy of their EMOD-producing drug.

However, **patients who have been asked to forego non-conventional supplements may surreptitiously use them anyway and risk undesirable interactions**. (Eisenberg et al, 1993).

Since many patients treat themselves with oral antioxidants during chemotherapy, clinicians need to formulate a credible position on this subject if they are to provide their patients with timely advice about the potential risks. (Labriola, 1999).

Oxygen dependence has also been established for a number of chemotherapeutic agents such as cyclophosphamide, carboplatin, doxorubicin, etc. and levels are different for each agent. Hypoxia can impart resistance to many chemotherapeutic agents (Teicher et al, 1990).

The chemotherapeutic agents doxorubicin, mitomycin C, etoposide and cisplatin are superoxide generating agents. (Yokomizo et al, 1995). Also, please see chapter thirteen.

In addition, tumor hypoxia can dramatically effect cytokines (interferon gamma and tumor necrosis factor-*a*) and alter Interleukins 2-induced activation of lymphokine-activated killer cells.

Studies on tumors of the uterine cervix have demonstrated that tumor hypoxia is independent of patient and tumor characteristics such as, patient age, menopausal status, and parity, International Federation of Gynecology and Obstetrics (FIGO) stage, clinical tumor size, histopathological and grade of malignancy. In fact, **tumor oxygenation was the strongest independent prognostic factor.** (Howes, 2004).

The role of heme and the mitochondrion in the chemical and molecular mechanisms of mammalian cell death induced by the artemisinin antimalarials

The artemisinin compounds are the frontline drugs for the treatment of drug-resistant malaria. They are selectively cytotoxic to mammalian cancer cell lines and have been implicated as neurotoxic and embryotoxic in animal studies. The endoperoxide functional group is both the pharmacophore and toxicophore, but the proposed chemical mechanisms and targets of cytotoxicity remain unclear. In this study we have used cell models and quantitative drug metabolite analysis to define the role of the mitochondrion and cellular heme in the chemical and molecular mechanisms of cell death induced by artemisinin compounds. **HeLa r(0) cells, which are devoid of a functioning electron transport chain,** were used to demonstrate that actively respiring mitochondria play an essential role in **endoperoxide-induced cytotoxicity (artesunate IC(50) values, 48 h: HeLa cells, 6 ± 3 µM; and HeLa r(0) cells, 34 ± 5 µM) via the generation of reactive oxygen species and the induction of mitochondrial dysfunction and apoptosis** but do not have any role in the reductive activation of the endoperoxide to cytotoxic carbon-centered radicals. However, using chemical modulators of heme synthesis (succinylacetone and protoporphyrin IX) and cellular iron content (holotransferrin), we have demonstrated definitively that free or protein-bound heme is responsible for intracellular activation of the endoperoxide group and that this is the chemical basis of cytotoxicity (IC(50) value and biomarker of bioactivation levels, respectively: 10**b**-(p-fluorophenoxy) dihydroartemisinin alone, 0.36 ± 0.20 µM and 11 ± 5%; and with succinylacetone, >100 µM and 2 ± 5%). (Mercer et al, 2011). **I believe that this shows that even the artesunate derivatives go through an endoperoxide form of an EMOD to activate apoptosis.**

Confusing data: antioxidants cure cancer and peroxide blocks apoptosis

To add to the confusion, among the many possible causes of cancer, reactive oxygen species (ROS) have been implicated in the onset and development of the disease. Some experimental studies support this premise, in part, by showing that antioxidants that prevent ROS damage can act as cancer preventive agents. **Once cancer has occurred, however, radiation therapy, photodynamic therapy and** many forms of chemotherapy rely on **EMOD (ROS) toxicity** to eliminate or destroy tumor cells.

Hydrogen peroxide and other EMODs have been shown to improve the response to radiation and to be proapoptotic through release of cytochrome *c* from mitochondria (Biaglow et al, 1989) (Biaglow et al, 1992) (Esposti et al, 1999) (Huang et al, 2000) (Kuninaka et al, 2000).

Cellular reducing metabolites, or antioxidants, such as glutathione, ascorbate, and NADPH alter cellular responses to the alleged damaging effects of EMODs (Deneke, 2000) (Sastre et al, 2000).

Reactive oxygen species (electronically modified oxygen derivatives, EMODs) are produced by normal cellular processes and the action of many chemotherapy drugs depend on increased production of EMODs to kill cancer cells. Any agent or process which neutralizes or quenches EMOD production can theoretically modify their influence or have a negative impact on their effectiveness. **Adding to the confusion, some investigators argue that oxidants, such as hydrogen peroxide, can block apoptosis and phagocytic uptake of killed cancer cells.** (Shacter et al, 2000) (Senturker et al, 2002).

**For the energy of the sun to get to me,
at the very least,
its flavorful photons must be gathered by the earth,
converted by excited chlorophyll,
confined within leafy floral carbohydrates,
which become directly ingested and
reprocessed by ravenous fauna,
ultimately being locked in lipids and packaged in proteins.
Whereupon, I can pick it, pluck it or kill it.
Then, devour it
and absorb its life sustaining radiance.
Bon Apetite'
But sometimes it's hard to get the taste
out of your mouth.**
R. M. Howes, M.D., Ph.D.
9/27/09

In the 1950s Dr. Reginald Holman treated the implanted tumors of experimental rats, by adding a dilute solution of hydrogen peroxide to their drinking water. Hydrogen peroxide, an oxidant, delivers a primary redox (reduction/oxidation) signal in the body. The treatment cured more than half the rats (50-60%) within a period of two weeks to two months, with complete disappearance of the tumors. Holman also reported four human case studies, concerning people with advanced inoperable cancer. Two patients showed marked clinical improvement and tumor shrinkage. He published his findings in *Nature*. (Holman RA. 1957) (Holman RA. A method of destroying a malignant rat tumour in vivo. Nature . 1957. 4568, 1033)

CHAPTER FOUR:

Peroxide, the magnificent

Hydrogen peroxide has tumoricidal activity

Antitumor effects of H_2O_2 in vivo

Glucose oxidase, covalently coupled to polystyrene microspheres (GOL), produced H_2O_2 at an average rate of 3.6 nmol/min per 10(9) beads under standard assay conditions. Injection of $1.3 \times 10(10)$ to $1.1 \times 10(11)$ GOL i.p. prolonged the survival of mice by 27 percent after injection of 10(6) **P388 lymphoma cells** in the same site, consistent with destruction of 97.6 percent of the tumor cells. Placing mice for several hours in 100 percent O_2, the probable rate-limiting substrate for GOL, afforded a 42 percent prolongation of survival from P388 lymphoma, consistent with destruction of 99.6 percent of the tumor cells. When the P388 inoculum was 10(5), 10(4), or 10(3) cells, GOL led to long-term survival (presumed cure) of 23 percent, 77 percent, and 92 percent of the mice, respectively, consistent with reduction of the injected tumor dose to less than 10 cells. Subcutaneous growth of 10(5) P388 cells (approximately 300 lethal dose to 50 percent of mice) was suppressed in 83 percent of mice by admixture of GOL with the tumor cell inoculum. GOL alone had no effect against a more peroxide-resistant tumor, P815 mastocytoma. However, P815 cell glutathione reductase could be inhibited in vivo by well-tolerated doses of the antitumor agent, 1,3-bis(2-chloroethyl)- 1-nitrosourea (BCNU). BCNU alone cured few mice with P815. Together, BCNU and GOL apparently cured 86 percent of mice injected with 10(6) P815 cells i.p. The protective effect of GOL was abolished by boiling it to inactivate the enzyme, by co-injection of catalase coupled to latex beads, or by delaying the injection of tumor cells for 3 h, by which time the beads had formed aggregates. Soluble glucose oxidase, in doses threefold higher than that bound to GOL, had no detectable antitumor effect. A single injection of preformed H_2O_2 readily killed P388 cells in the peritoneal cavity, but only at doses nearly lethal to the mice. In contrast, GOL had very little toxicity, as judged by the normal appearance of the mice for over 400 d, gross and microscopic findings at autopsy, and various blood tests. GOL injected i.p. remained in the peritoneal cavity, where it was gradually organized into granulomata by macrophages, without generalized inflammation. Thus, **a H_2O_2 generating system confined to the tumor bed exerted clear-cut antitumor effects with little toxicity to the host.** (Nathan, Cohn, 1981).

Earlier, in 1979, Nathan et al, wrote of extracellular lysis of cancer cells by macrophages and granulocytes. (Nathan et al, 1979).

Nathan and Cohn's work suggested that "hydrogen peroxide could exert a direct anti-tumor effect in vivo and thereby prolong the survival of the patient." They suggested that "hydrogen peroxide can synergize in vivo with certain anti-tumor drugs already in use." (Nathan, Cohn, 1981).

In 1989, Samoszuk et al. took cell cultures and treated them to low concentrations of hydrogen peroxide, which caused a substantial killing of the infected cells after 15 minutes of incubation. They concluded that, "The significance of our observation is that it provides a rationale for investigating new therapeutic modalities designed specifically to deliver cytotoxic quantities of hydrogen peroxide to Hodgkin's disease." (Samoszuk et al, 1989).

In 1998, Nicholson et al. found that hydrogen peroxide would kill giant cell tumors in vitro, adding to the spectrum of its tumoricidal activity. (Nicholson et al, 1998).

And in 2001, hydrogen peroxide was injected into tumor cells to cause tumor cell death, without generating dangerous by-products. (Symonds et al, 2001).

In studies initiated in 2003, Howes injected hydrogen peroxide and hypochlorous acid (to produce excited singlet oxygen, delta species) into human squamous cell carcinoma in athymic mice and had a 22% cure rate in the first pilot study. (Howes, 2005).

H_2O_2 concentration determines its effect on cell proliferation

The induction of apoptosis in Jurkat T-lymphocytes with 50 microM hydrogen peroxide was associated with caspase activation. Caspase activity was first detected 3 h after treatment, and the morphological features of apoptosis were apparent by 6 h. At higher concentrations of hydrogen peroxide there was no detectable caspase activity, and the cells died by necrosis. Cells treated with hydrogen peroxide were impaired in their ability to undergo Fas-mediated apoptosis. This appeared to be the result of direct inhibition of the cysteine-dependent caspases. The cells were able to recover and undergo apoptosis at later times. Therefore, **hydrogen peroxide has two distinct effects. It initially inhibits the caspases and delays apoptosis. Then, depending on the degree of the initial oxidative stress, the caspases are activated and the cells die by apoptosis, or they remain inactive and necrosis occurs.** (Hampton, Orrenius, 1997).

I believe that this is consistent with the work of Davies, who showed that cellular responses were concentration dependent. Low levels allowed for cellular proliferation, intermediate concentrations caused cellular arrest and high levels caused apoptosis or necrosis. (Davies, 1999).

Intravenous hydrogen peroxide

The Baylor University Medical Center in Texas (the Baylor group) led pioneering work utilizing hydrogen peroxide to treat cancer and other common diseases. Their initial work in the early 1960s found that regional intra-arterial infusion of hydrogen peroxide increased cancer cell sensitivity to radiation therapy. They conducted animal and human trials and found peroxide to be a source of oxygen. I consider their work on EMODS as ground breaking.

Many clinical and experimental applications of hydrogen peroxide have been demonstrated. In over 300 patients regional intra-arterial hydrogen peroxide has potentiated the effect of radiation therapy in situations of malignancy involving the head, neck, pelvis and retro-peritoneum. (Mallams et al, 1965).

Increased localization of radioactive isotopes in malignant tumors had been achieved by regional and intra-arterial infusion of hydrogen peroxide. (Finney et al, 1961)   (Finney et al, 1965).

Even though the Baylor group's work on hydrogen peroxide was ground breaking, it has remained in obscurity. Still, it teaches the therapeutic potential of hydrogen peroxide in the treatment of cancer, wound healing, atherosclerosis, shock management and infectious diseases. Peroxide has been used widely in Europe and has had a promising record of safety and effectiveness.

Hydrogen peroxide: general info

Hydrogen peroxide appears to have medical attributes but has received little support in Western "modern" medicine. The reason may be simple. **Hydrogen peroxide cannot be patented. Hydrogen peroxide (H_2O_2) is a moderately strong oxidant that induces apoptosis of tumor cells in vitro.** (Fang et al, 2002).

Some investigators believe that AIDS and cancer can be helped with hydrogen peroxide because of its induction of interferon-gamma production and it interactions which can produce a wide variety of oxygen derivatives. (Manakata et al, 1985).

Davies has shown that cellular division or cell death is EMOD concentration dependent, when utilizing the EMOD, H_2O_2. Cellular responses go from proliferation, to arrest, to apoptosis. (Davies, 1999).

Hydrogen peroxide has been accused of acting as a "genotoxicant or epigenetic" agent but although H_2O_2 can cause DNA damage, it is, at best, a very weak mutagen in mammalian cells. (Takeuchi et al, 1997).

Use of hydrogen peroxide in treating cancer

The following were part of a review of "Can Oxygen Cure Cancer?" http://www.amazon.com/dp/1594771774/ref=pe_606_12214760_pe_ar_t1 Accessed 8-07-09.

In 2001, a group of **researchers from the Department of Life Sciences at Nottingham Trent University injected hydrogen peroxide solutions in solid tumors in mice and found the solutions had the potential to cause tumor cell death without generating dangerous by-products.** They were impressed concluding that hydrogen peroxide was a potential cytotoxic agent. Hydrogen peroxide used as an anti-cancer drug is cheap and cost effective.

In 2003, Jackson State University in Mississippi explored the combined effect of oxidative stress with hydrogen peroxide, Nigella sativa, a medicinal herb from the Middle East, on breast cancer. **The combination of hydrogen peroxide, ethanol, and Nigella sativa could inactivate MCF-7 cancer cells.** (Farah and Begum, 2003).

Carolinas Medical Center in Charlotte, NC, investigated the efficiency of using hydrogen peroxide as an adjuvant therapy after extended local curettage (scraping away lesions) for benign cell tumors of the bone. Cell cultures taken from the tumor tissue of six patients was cultured and treated with hydrogen peroxide for 2 minutes. **Hydrogen peroxide was very effective in killing giant tumors of bone.** (Nicholson et al, 1998).

Researchers in 1989, found that peroxidase in Hodgkin's disease sensitizes the tumor cells to killing by low levels of hydrogen peroxide. The idea was to deliver cytotoxic quantities of hydrogen peroxide to Hodgkin's disease.

Dr. Carl F Nathan and Dr. Zanvil A Cohn wrote, "**Hydrogen peroxide contributes to the lysis [destruction] of tumor cells by macrophages [immune cells] and granulocytes [white blood cells] in vitro.**" They found that 8

milligrams of hydrogen peroxide was able to kill more than 90 percent of P338 lymphoma cells. (Nathan, Cohn, 1981).

http://www.med.cornell.edu/research/cnathan/

Tottori University School of Medicine **in Japan in 1966, fifteen patients suffering from maxillary cancer (cancer of the nasal cavity) were given intra-arterial infusions of hydrogen peroxide daily for ten days** followed by daily injections of mitomycin C, an antibiotic showing anti-tumor activity. Of the fifteen cases treated with hydrogen peroxide and Mutamycin, **eight showed almost a complete disappearance of the tumor, while six experienced a partial reduction.** One had little change. The changes involve either an actual shrinking of the tumor or a softening of a hard tumor.

The Tottori group stated, "Enhancement of the anti-cancer agent was observes. We have also proven clinically that the method [does not] cause danger in each individual patient." (Sasaki et al, 1967).

During a Baylor University cancer study of inoperable abdominal tumors, **intra-arterial hydrogen peroxide and irradiation was administered.** The researchers wanted to see if hydrogen peroxide could shrink the tumors and make them amenable to surgery. Two of the three experience shrinkage of the tumor and underwent successful operations to remove the tumors. One of the patients experience no shrinkage and was sent home. He began to improve over the next several months and the tumor began shrinking considerably. The doctors removed the shrunken tumor.

Dr J.W Finney, in 1962 stated, **"The use of Hydrogen Peroxide as a source of oxygen in a Regional Intra-arterial Infusion System revealed that cancer cells become more sensitive to irradiation in the presence of increased oxygen tension produced by hydrogen peroxide."** The researchers noted increased regional oxygenation, which led them to believe that there is an increased therapeutic ratio in malignant tumors receiving radiation when oxygen levels of the affected area are increased with hydrogen peroxide.

Oxidative therapies increase the activity of immunocompetent cells, stimulate the release of cytokines, upregulate the body's antioxidant system and induce mild activation of the immune system. Activating the patient's neuro-endocrine system causes the patient to experience less pain and greater sense of well-being.

Vitamin C IV megadoses and hydrogen peroxide

Vitamin C (ascorbate, ascorbic acid) has had a controversial history in the prevention of cancer. One clinical case report showed that vitamin C together with other oxidants, when added adjunctively to first-line chemotherapy, prevented recurrence in two ovarian cancer patients. (Drisko et al, 2003).

This high dose, intravenous vitamin C therapy was believed to operate through the generation of hydrogen peroxide. Ascorbate-mediated cell death was due to protein-dependent extracellular H_2O_2 generation (i.e., EMOD prooxidant generation). Ascorbate, an electron-donor in such reactions, ironically initiates prooxidant chemistry and H_2O_2 formation. It was concluded that ascorbate at pharmacologic concentrations in blood is a pro-drug for H_2O_2 delivery to tissues. (Buettner, Jurkiewicz, 1996) (Halliwell, 1990).

Vitamin C acts as a cosubstrate for hydroxylase and oxygenase enzymes for the biosynthesis of procollagen, carnitine, and neurotransmitters. (Levine, 1986).

These enzymes produce EMODs and ascorbate acts as a cosubstrate for them and thus, acts as a prooxidant. (Chen et al, 2005).

At pharmacologic concentrations, ascorbate acts as a prooxidant, hydrogen peroxide generating agent, which exhibits selective cytotoxicity towards a wide variety of cancer cells in vitro and in vivo. (Chen et al, 2007) (Chen et al, 2008).

Even though there is much to be discovered in the ascorbate and hydrogen peroxide system, this appears to be an area of great potential. (Levine et al, 2008).

Yet, in contrast, several vitamin C and iron cosupplementation studies, both in animals and humans, indicate that **vitamin C inhibits rather than promotes iron-dependent oxidative damage.** (Carr, Frei, 1999).

Linking EMOD levels, apoptosis and cancer proliferation

Paradoxically, EMODs (reactive oxygen species, ROS) can promote normal cellular proliferation and carcinogenesis, and can also induce apoptosis of tumor cells. In this report, they study the contribution of ROS to various cellular signals depending on the nature and the level of ROS produced. In non-transformed NIH 3T3 cells, ROS are at low levels and originate from NADPH oxidase. Hydrogen peroxide (H_2O_2), controlled by the glutathione system, is pivotal for the modulation of normal cell proliferation. In CT26 (colon) and Hepa 1-6 (liver) tumor cells, high levels of ROS, close to the threshold of cytotoxicity, are produced by mitochondria and H_2O_2 is controlled by catalase. **N-acetylcysteine, which decreases H_2O_2 levels, inhibits mitogen-activated protein kinase and normal cell proliferation but increases tumor cell proliferation as H_2O_2 concentration drops from the toxicity threshold.** In contrast, antioxidant molecules, such as **mimics of superoxide dismutase (SOD), increase H_2O_2 levels** through superoxide anion dismutation, as well as in vitro proliferation of normal cells, but **kill tumor cells.** CT26 tumors were implanted in mice and treated by oxaliplatin in association with one of the three SOD mimics manganese(III) tetrakis(4-benzoic acid) porphyrin, copper(II)(3,5-diisopropylsalicylate)2, or manganese dipyridoxyl diphosphate. After 1 month, the volumes of tumors were respectively 35%, 31%, and 63% smaller than with oxaliplatin alone (P < 0.001). Similar data were gained with Hepa 1-6 tumors. In conclusion, **antioxidant molecules may have opposite effects on tumor growth.** SOD mimics can act in synergy with cytotoxic drugs to treat colon and liver cancers. (Laurent et al, 2005). **SOD mimetics kill cancer because they produce peroxide and antioxidants block cancer kill because they block EMODs, especially H_2O_2. This is a pattern I have seen repeated many times and convinces me that antioxidants are dangerous.**

Howes' rational for EMOD benefits and antioxidant harm

One of the important functions of apoptosis is the elimination of pre-neoplastic and neoplastic cells. (Thompson, C. B., 1995).

Some cancer cells are more sensitive to generated reactive oxygen species, and this may be a useful difference that can be exploited when seeking to kill cancer cells but spare normal cells.

Apoptosis itself is largely based on EMODs (free radicals) released from mitochondria. ROS generation in mitochondria no longer appears to be **a precise mechanism used in signaling pathways such as apoptosis**, as demonstrated in **cardiomyocytes.** (Duranteau et al, 1998).

In most forms of cell suicide, **the signaling cascade utilizes reactive oxygen species as essential intermediate messenger molecules** (Albright, C. D., 2003) (Vrablic, A. S., 2001) (Slater, A. F., 1995) (Johnson, T. M., 1996) (Sugiyama, H., 1996).

Even modest quenching of oxygen radicals by dietary antioxidants could block completion of apoptosis. Administration of antioxidants

subsequent to a mutagenic event may effectively intercept free radicals that are critical in promoting apoptosis.

Oxidants can also activate lymphocytes, which then use EMODs (ROS) as weapons against infection (Reth, M., 2002).

Apoptosis, necrosis, and growth arrest can all be regulated by ROS (EMODs). (Aw, 1999).

A growing body of evidence shows that ROS (EMODs) within cells act as secondary messengers in intracellular signalling cascades which induce and maintain the oncogenic phenotype of cancer cells, however, ROS (EMODs) can also induce cellular senescence and apoptosis and can therefore function as anti-tumorigenic species. (Valko et al, 2006).

Administration of antioxidants subsequent to a mutagenic event may effectively intercept free radicals that are critical in promoting apoptosis. **This imbalance may allow the rate of proliferation in tumors to exceed the capacity for apoptosis. It seems reasonable to suggest that the potential risks and benefits of high-dose antioxidants need to be considered on a case-to-case basis, and indiscriminate use of antioxidant dietary supplements should be avoided.**

Antioxidants can promote cancer

Antioxidants, by preventing oxidant-mediated damage to diverse targets (DNA, RNA, proteins, and lipids), may play a protective role in healthy individuals with no existing cancer cells that must be eliminated; however, **by inhibiting apoptosis, these same antioxidants may exert a cancer-promoting effect in cancer patients and in individuals with precancerous DNA changes.**

Inhibition of apoptosis by antioxidants may explain why, in several studies in heavy smokers, **vitamin E and beta-carotene enhanced carcinogenesis in the lung.** (DeLuca et al, 1996) (where, presumably, precancerous lesions caused by smoking predated antioxidant treatment) **but decreased carcinogenesis in the prostate.** (Heinonen et al, 1998) (where, presumably, smoking had not caused precancerous lesions that predated antioxidant treatment).

Antioxidant blocking of EMODs can block apoptosis

Thus, **some cancer cells may be more sensitive to generated reactive oxygen species (EMODs), and this may be a useful difference that can**

be exploited when seeking to kill cancer cells but spare normal cells.
Even a moderate increase in the accumulation of oxygen radicals in malignant cells
of animals fed an antioxidant-poor diet could increase reactive oxygen species to
the critical level required for progression of apoptosis. Conversely, **even modest
quenching of oxygen radicals by dietary antioxidants could block completion of apoptosis.**

**Tumor cell anti-oxidant defenses. Inhibition of the glutathione redox
cycle enhances macrophage-mediated cytolysis**. (Nathan et al, vol 153, 1981)

The basis of resistance to oxidative injury was studied in **six murine tumor cell
lines (TLX9, P388, YAC, P815, J774 and NK lyphoma cell lines)** that differed 54-fold in their resistance to enzymatically generated H_2O_2. The logarithm of
the flux of H_2O_2 necessary to cause 50 percent lysis of the tumor cells correlated
with their content of glutathione (r = 0.91). The protective role of glutathione was
analyzed by blocking GR and GPO, the catalysts of the glutathione redox cycle.
This was facilitated by the demonstration that the anti-neoplastic agent 1,3-bis-
(2- chloroethyl)-l-nitrosourea (BCNU) was a potent inhibitor of GR in intact tumor cells. BCNU inactivated tumor cell GR with a 50 percent inhibitory dose of
11 muM and a t(l/2) of inhibition of 30 s. Complete inhibition of GR was attained
with no effect on GPO or catalase. Tumor cells whose GR was inactivated by
BCNU could be lysed by fluxes of H_2O_2 to which they were otherwise completely
resistant. They could be killed by phorbol myristate acetate (PMA)-stimulated, ba-
cilli Calmette-Guerin-activated macrophages in numbers which were otherwise
insufficient, and by nonactivated macrophages, which otherwise were ineffective.
BCNU-treated target cells were also much more sensitive to antibody-dependent,
macrophage-mediated cytolysis. However, such tumor cells were no more sensitive
than controls to lysis by alloreactive T cells or by antibody plus complement. Next,
we deprived tumor cells of selenium by passage in selenium-deficient mice. GPO
was inhibited 85 percent in such cells, with no effect on GR or catalase. Tumor
cells with reduced GPO activity were markedly sensitized to lysis by small fluxes of
H_2O_2 or by PMA-stimulated macrophages or granulocytes. In contrast, inhibition of
catalase with aminotriazole had no effect on the sensitivity of three tumors to peroxide-mediated lysis, and had modest effects with two others. Thus, the oxidation-
reduction cycle of glutathione serves as one of **the major defense mechanisms
of tumor cells** against three related forms of oxidant injury: lysis by fluxes of
H_2O_2 by PMA-triggered macrophages, and by macrophages in the presence of antitumor antibody. (Nathan et al, vol 153, 1981).   **This clearly illustrates the role
of antioxidants, such as glutathione or selenium, as a cancer cell defense
or protective system.**

Nathan et al. state that, "If the biochemical basis of cytotoxicity is known in a given experimental setting, it becomes feasible to hypothesize the pathways the target cell might employ to reduce or escape injury. If such pathways are identified, means can be sought to block them. EMODs, including H_2O_2, appear to be preeminently involved in the cytotoxicity of activated macrophages in the presence of PMA or anti-tumor antibody. Tumor cells are likely to possess several mechanisms, enzymatic and nonenzymatic, for disposal of H_2O_2." **Just as with bacterial pathogens, cancer cells endeavor to protect themselves from death activation by EMODs and this is accomplished via antioxidants or antioxidant enzymes.**

The GPO-deficient tumor cells were much more sensitive to lysis by enzymatically generated H_2O_2 and by PMA-triggered granulocytes and macrophages. **Other substances which might serve as protective antioxidants in tumor cells include other peroxidases, superoxide dismutase, vitamins C and E, free and protein cysteine, and unsaturated fatty acids.**

Antioxidant systems, such as glutathione redox agents, act to protect cancer cells against EMOD activated apoptosis and cancer cell death. This is illustrated by the following paper on " Potentiation and protection of doxorubicin cytotoxicity by cellular glutathione modulation."

One of the proposed mechanisms of doxorubicin cytotoxicity is generation of activated oxygen species, all of which are either free radical or potentially free radical species. Glutathione is an intracellular sulfhydryl-containing tripeptide that is known to detoxify free radicals and the damage they produce. The cytotoxicity of doxorubicin was evaluated following treatment with agents that will either elevate intracellular glutathione (2-oxothiazolidine-4-carboxylate) or deplete intracellular glutathione levels correlate with doxorubicin cytotoxicity, i.e., **elevated glutathione provides protection and decreased glutathione levels increase cytotoxicity**. (Russo, Mitchell, 1985).

Since glutathione disulfide and glutathione are a pivotal redox pair, the modulation of intracellular glutathione levels is shown to change the cytotoxicity of drugs dependent on the redox cycle, such as **adriamycin and bleomycin, as well as the oxygen dependent drug neocarzinostatin.**

In general, **GSH depletion has been demonstrated to further enhance the cytotoxicity of several chemotherapy drugs and nitroimidazole hypoxic cell radiosensitizers. Conversely, GSH elevation affords varying degrees of protection**. (Mitchell et al, 1989).

SECTION TWO:

EMODs - a primary means of killing cancer

CHAPTER FIVE:

EMODs and controlling apoptosis

Tumor cells have a complex array of genetic changes and develop an alteration in the metabolism of oxygen, having a higher steady state of EMOD production. The altered oxygen metabolism of cancer cells is not subject to the high genetic variability of tumors and serves as a point of selectivity in cancer therapy and protection of normal cells.

Role of vitamin and mineral supplementation and aspirin use in cancer survivors

Multivitamins and multiminerals are widely used in the United States, but their efficacy and, perhaps more importantly, **the potential for harm in individuals who have cancer** have received relatively little study. Beyond their general effects on health, the use of vitamins and minerals by patients with cancer has unique implications because of their potential direct effects on existing cancers, effects on factors that may influence carcinogenesis, such as immunity, and interactions with treatment. Some evidence suggests that vitamin D at higher than standard doses may improve cancer-specific and overall survival for several cancer sites. **Besides vitamin D, there is little evidence that nutritional supplements lower the risk of recurrence or improve survival from cancer**, although some benefits may be possible in specific subgroups. **Some data suggest that higher than standard doses of some vitamins or minerals could even enhance carcinogenesis or worsen survival in patients with cancer.**

For example, evidence suggests that although folate supplementation administered in preneoplastic stages may lower the risk of colorectal cancer, **excessive folic acid in patients with established cancer may be harmful.**

For prostate cancer, some preliminary evidence indicates that excess consumption of one or a combination of components in a multivitamin/ multimineral may accelerate cancer progression and increase fatality.

Use of aspirin is proven to lower risk of colorectal cancer, and recent evidence suggests that aspirin use in patients with colorectal cancer improves cancer-specific and overall survival, especially in patients with tumors that express cyclooxygenase-2 (COX-2). The potential beneficial or adverse effects of dietary supplements and aspirin in survivors of cancer warrant further study. (Giovannucce, Chan, 2010).

Why EMODs can kill cancer cells and not harm normal cells

Cancer cells have high prooxidant levels and this presents a point of selective kill of the cancer cells by EMOD induction of apoptosis. In other words, if we add EMODs to cancer cells, we can get them to kill themselves, without having the same effect on normal cells. This whole concept is key to a future successful cancer eradication and prevention program. I will have to include some biochemistry at this point but will try to keep it to a minimum or I will follow the complicated sections with common sense explanations.

NAC modulates doxorubicin-induced oxidative stress and antioxidant vitamin concentrations in liver or rats.

Doxorubicin (DOX) is a chemotherapeutic agent, and is widely used in cancer treatment. The most common side effect of DOX was indicated on cardiovascular system by experimental studies. There are some studies suggesting oxidative stress-induced toxic changes on liver related to DOX administration. The aim of the present study was to evaluate whether antioxidant N-acetylcysteine (NAC) relieves oxidative stress in DOX- induced liver injury in rat. **Twenty-four male rats** were equally divided into three groups. First group was used as a control. Second group received single dose of DOX. NAC for 10 days was given to constituting the third group after giving one dose of DOX. After 10 days of the experiment, liver tissues were taken from all animals. Lipid peroxidation (LP) levels were higher in the DOX group than in control whereas **LP levels were lower in the DOX+NAC group than in control**. Vitamin C and vitamin E levels were lower in the DOX group than in control whereas **vitamin C and vitamin E levels were higher in the DOX+NAC group than in the DOX group**. Reduced glutathione levels were higher in the DOX+NAC group than in control and DOX group. Glutathione peroxidase, vitamin A and b-carotene values were not changed in the three groups by DOX and NAC administrations. In histopathological evaluation of DOX group, there were mononuclear cell infiltrations, vacuolar degeneration, hepatocytes with basophilic nucleus and sinusoidal dilatations. The findings were totally recovered by NAC administration. In conclusion, **N-acetylcysteine induced modulator effects on the doxorubicin-induced hepatoxicity by inhibiting free radical production and supporting the antioxidant vitamin levels** (Kockar et al, 2010).

I believe that the presence of **NAC** 'saves' other antioxidants, such as vitamin C and E, from being used up or decreased by interactions with EMODs. This is a clear example of how "stacking" works. The stronger antioxidants attack EMODs first, then the lesser active antioxidants attack the EMODs. They have a cumulative effect and one can overload with them.

Flavone inhibition of tumor growth via apoptosis in vitro and in vivo

Colorectal carcinoma is a human malignant tumor, which is very resistant to currently available methods of treatment. Therefore, developing an effective agent with anti-colorectal carcinoma activity is important. In the present study, 8 structurally related flavones including flavone, 3-OH flavone, 5-OH flavone, 7-OH flavone, quercetin, kaempferol, quercetin, and morin were used to study their effects on **colorectal carcinoma cells (HT29, COLO205, COLO320-HSR)**. Results of MTT assay indicated that flavone shows the most potent cytoxic effect among them on these three cell types. The cytotoxicity induced by flavone is mediated by inducing the occurrence of apoptosis characterized by the appearance of DNA ladders, apoptotic bodies and hypodiploid cells. Activation of caspase 3 protein procession and enzyme activity with inducing cleavage of caspase 3 substrates PARP was identified in flavone-treated cells, and an inhibitory peptide Ac-DEVD-FMK for caspase 3, but not Ac-YVAD-FMK for caspase 1, attenuates the cytotoxic effect of flavone in COLO205 and HT29 cells. Elevation of p21 but no p53 protein was observed in flavone-treated cells. Increasing intracellular peroxide level was detected in flavone-treated cells by DCHF-DA assay, and **antioxidants such as tiron, catalase, SOD, PDTC, but not DPI, suppress flavone-induced cytotoxic effect**. In vivo anti-tumor study indicates that flavone exhibits ability to inhibit tumor formation elicited by s.c. injection of COLO205 cells in nude mice, and apoptotic cells and an increase in p21, but not p53, protein were observed in tumor tissues derived from flavone-treated group. Additionally, flavone induced apoptosis in primary colon carcinoma cells COLO205-X with appearance of DNA ladders, caspase 3 protein procession, PARP protein cleavage, and an increase in p21 (not p53) protein. These data provide evidence to suggest that flavone is an effective agent to induce apoptosis in colorectal carcinoma cells in vitro and in vivo; activation of caspase 3, **EMOD (ROS) production**, and increasing p21 protein are involved. (Chen et al, 2004). **This is another example of EMOD induction of apoptosis via a so-called antioxidant. This finding has seriously complicated the interpretation of the data and has led to misreading of the effects of an-**

tioxidants. If antioxidants work, they kill cancer via EMODs. Otherwise, they antioxidatively protect cancer cells.

N-acetylcysteine amide decreases oxidative stress but not cell death induced by doxorubicin in H9c2 cardiomyocytes.

While doxorubicin (DOX) is widely used in cancer chemotherapy, long-term severe cardiotoxicity limits its use. This is the first report of the chemoprotective efficacy of a relatively **new thiol antioxidant, N-acetylcysteine amide (NACA),** on DOX-induced cell death in **cardiomyocytes.** We hypothesized that NACA would protect H9c2 cardiomyocytes from DOX-induced toxicity by reducing oxidative stress. Accordingly, we determined the ability of NACA to mitigate the cytotoxicity of DOX in H9c2 cells and correlated these effects with the production of indicators of oxidative stress.

RESULTS: DOX at 5 microM induced cardiotoxicity while 1) increasing the generation of reactive oxygen species (ROS), 2) decreasing levels and activities of antioxidants and antioxidant enzymes (catalase, glutathione peroxidase, glutathione reductase) and 3) increasing lipid peroxidation. **NACA at 750 microM substantially reduced the levels of ROS and lipid peroxidation, as well as increased both GSH level and GSH/GSSG ratio. However, treating H9c2 cells with NACA did little to protect H9c2 cells from DOX-induced cell death.**

CONCLUSION: Although **NACA effectively reduced oxidative stress in DOX-treated H9c2 cells, it had minimal effects on DOX-induced cell death.** NACA prevented oxidative stress by elevation of GSH and CYS, reduction of ROS and lipid peroxidation, and restoration of antioxidant enzyme activities. Further studies to identify oxidative stress-independent pathways that lead to DOX-induced cell death in H9c2 are warranted (Shi et al, 2009).

I believe that this data shows that those recommending **NAC** to prevent or protect against the adverse oxidative side effects of **DOX** are wrong. It blocks EMODs but does not prevent killing of cardiomyocytes. Therefore, one does not need to protect against EMODs in this case. Also, this may indicate that the **NACA** could protect the cancer cells against **EMOD** induced apoptosis and not protect against the adverse effects of **DOX**.

See also: Keeping cancer from coming back. Should cancer survivors take vitamin supplements? Aspirin may be a better bet. Harv Health Lett. 2010 Oct;35(12):3.

Human colon cancer cells killed by EMODs

Cancer cells, relative to normal cells, have altered mitochondrial electron transport chains (ETC) that are more likely to form EMODs, reactive oxygen species (ROS; i.e., O_2^- and H_2O_2) resulting in a condition of chronic metabolic oxidative stress, that maybe compensated for by increasing glucose and hydroperoxide metabolism.

ETC inhibitors produce more prooxidants and more human colon cancer cell kill. **Treatment of HT29 and HCT116 cancer cells with Antimycin A (Ant A) or rotenone (Rot) increased carboxy-dichlorodihydrofluorescein diacetate (H2DCFDA) and dihydroethidine (DHE) oxidation, caused the accumulation of glutathione disulfide and enhanced 2DG-induced cell killing**. This study showed that the killing of human colon cancer cells was enhanced by sugar deprivation and increasing EMOD levels. (Fath et al, 2009).

Sugar (glucose) deprivation increases EMODs and cancer cell kill: blocked by NAC

Cancer cells (vs. normal cells) demonstrate evidence of oxidative stress, increased glycolysis, and increased pentose cycle activity. In cancer cells, glucose deprivation as well as treatment with 2-deoxyglucose (2 DG) has been shown to induce oxidative stress and cytotoxicity. Additionally, **transformed cells have been shown to be more susceptible to glucose deprivation (and 2DG-)-induced cytotoxicity and oxidative stress than untransformed cells.** Results support the hypothesis that cancer cells have a defect in mitochondrial respiration leading to increased steady state levels of O_2^- and H_2O_2, and glucose metabolism is increased to compensate for this defect.

This can be used to enhance and induce radio/chemosensitization. (Simons et al, 2009).

I believe that this relates to diabetes, in that, low sugar levels (sugar deprivation) produces adequate EMOD levels; whereas, high glucose levels (hyperglycemia) produce an EMOD insufficiency and allows for disease manifestation, such as atherosclerosis and cancer.

Paclitaxel (PTX) increases EMOD breast cancer cell kill: blocked by NAC

Inhibitors of glucose (i.e., 2-deoxy-d-glucose, 2DG) and hydroperoxide (i.e., l-buthionine-S,R-sulfoximine, BSO) metabolism were utilized in combination **with a chemotherapeutic agent, paclitaxel (PTX), thought to induce oxidative stress,** to treat breast cancer cells.

Antioxidants, including N-acetylcysteine and polyethylene glycol-conjugated catalase and superoxide dismutase, inhibited the toxicity of 2DG + PTX and suppressed parameters indicative of oxidative stress in cancer cells. In short, the antioxidant, NAC, shields the killing of the breast cancer cells by EMODs. (Hadzic et al, 2010). **This study strongly supports the view that apoptosis of human cancer cells is responsive to EMOD production, especially hydrogen peroxide and that antioxidants, such as NAC, can block their apoptotic effect.**

Human epithelial, colon and breast cancer cells protected by antioxidant enzyme, SOD

Investigators determined whether oxidative stress mediated by O_2^- and H_2O_2 contributed to the differential susceptibility of **human epithelial cancer cells** to glucose deprivation, the oxidation of DHE (dihydroethidine; for O_2^- and CDCFH(2) [5- (and 6-)carboxy-2',7'-dichlorodihydrofluorescein diacetate; for hydroperoxides] was measured in **human colon and breast cancer cells** (HT29, HCT116, SW480 and MB231) and compared with that in normal human cells [FHC cells, 33Co cells and HMECs (human mammary epithelial cells)]. SW480 is the human colon adenocarcinoma cell line.

Overexpression of manganese SOD (superoxide dismutase) and mitochondrially targeted catalase significantly protected HCT116 (colon cancer) and MB231 (breast cancer cells) cells from glucose-deprivation-induced cytotoxicity and oxidative stress and also protected HT29 cells from 2DG-induced cytotoxicity. These results show that **cancer cells (relative to normal cells) demonstrate increased steady-state levels of**

EMODs (ROS, reactive oxygen species; i.e. O_2^- and H_2O_2) that contribute to differential susceptibility to glucose-deprivation-induced cytotoxicity and oxidative stress. (Aykin-Burns et al, 2009).

This study clearly shows that by eliminating superoxide and hydrogen peroxide, with the antioxidant enzymes SOD and catalase, EMOD induced apoptosis of human colon and breast cancer cells is blocked by these antioxidant enzymes.

Sugar deprivation plus cisplatin increases EMOD production and head and neck cancer cell kill: blocked by NAC

Exposure of **human head and neck cancer cells (FaDu)** to the combination of 2DG and cisplatin resulted in a significant decrease in cell survival when compared with 2DG or cisplatin alone. **Simultaneous treatment with the thiol antioxidant N-acetylcysteine (NAC) inhibited parameters indicative of oxidative stress, as well as protected FaDu cells from the cytotoxic effects of cisplatin alone and the combination of 2DG and cisplatin.**

Exposure of human head and neck cancer cells to 2-deoxy-d-glucose (2DG) combined with cisplatin enhances cytotoxicity via metabolic oxidative stress. (Simons et al, 2007).

Here again, the antioxidant, NAC, protected human head and neck cancer cells from being killed via EMOD induced apoptosis.

Cisplatin combined with zidovudine enhances cytotoxicity and oxidative stress in human head and neck cancer cells: blocked by NAC.

Oxidative stress and mitochondrial dysfunction in cancer cells represent features that may be exploited therapeutically. We determined whether agents that induce mitochondrial dysfunction, such as zidovudine (AZT) and cisplatin (CIS), could enhance killing of **human head and neck cancer cells via oxidative stress**. AZT and/or CIS-induced cytotoxicity was determined using clonogenic survival, mitochondrial membrane potential was analyzed to investigate mitochondrial function, and glutathione was measured to determine thiol metabolism perturbations. AZT+CIS significantly increased toxicity and reduced mitochondrial membrane potential in **FaDu, Cal-27, and SQ20B head and neck cancer cells** while increasing the percentage of glutathione disulfide (%GSSG). Treatment with the thiol antioxidant **N-acetylcysteine (NAC) reversed the loss of mitochondrial membrane potential and the increase in %GSSG and partially protected FaDu and Cal-27 cells from AZT+CIS.** Finally, an inhibitor of glutathione synthesis, I-buthionine-[S,R]-sulfoximine, sensitized the cells to AZT+CIS-induced cytotoxicity, which was partially reversed by NAC. These results suggest that exposure of cancer cells to agents that induce mitochondrial dysfunction, such as AZT, causes significant sensitization to CIS-induced toxicity via disruptions in thiol metabolism and oxidative stress. These findings provide a biochemical rationale for evaluating agents that induce mitochondrial dysfunction in combination with chemotherapy and inhibitors of glutathione metabolism in **head and neck cancer.** (Mattson et al, 2009).

Human pancreatic cancer cells killed by EMODs and dicumarol: blocked by MnSOD

Dicumarol is a naturally occurring anticoagulant derived from coumarin that induces cytotoxicity and oxidative stress in human pancreatic cancer cells. (Cullen et al, 2003).

Dicumarol decreased clonogenic survival equally in both MDA-MB-468 NQO1(-) and MDA-MB-468 NQO1+ breast cancer cells. Dicumarol, with the addition of mitochondrial electron transport chain blockers, decreased clonogenic cell survival in human pancreatic cancer cells and increased superoxide levels.

Overexpression of manganese superoxide dismutase (MnSOD) and mitochondrial-targeted catalase with adenoviral vectors reversed the dicumarol-induced cytotoxicity and reversed fluorescence of the oxidation-sensitive probe. Investigators concluded mitochondrial production of EMODs mediates the increased susceptibility of cancer cells to dicumarol-induced cytotoxicity. (Du et al, 2006). **Again, EMODs induce cancer cell apoptosis, which can be blocked by antioxidants or antioxidant enzymes. The effect is the same whether EMODs are negated by antioxidant vitamins or antioxidant enzymes.**

Human osteosarcoma cancer cells killed by EMODs: blocked by MnSOD and catalase

The hypothesis that glucose deprivation-induced cytotoxicity in transformed human cells is mediated by mitochondrial $O_2^{\cdot-}$ and H_2O_2 was first tested by exposing glucose-deprived SV40-transformed human fibroblasts (GM00637G) to electron transport chain blockers (ETCBs) known to increase mitochondrial $O_2^{\cdot-}$ and H_2O_2 production (antimycin A (AntA), myxothiazol (Myx), or rotenone (Rot)).

Glucose deprivation in the presence of AntA also significantly enhanced cytotoxicity and parameters indicative of oxidative stress in several different **human cancer cell lines** (PC-3, DU145, MDA-MB231, and HT-29). In addition, **human osteosarcoma cells lacking functional mitochondrial electron transport chains (rho0) were resistant to glucose deprivation-induced cytotoxicity and oxidative stress in the presence of AntA.**

In the absence of ETCBs, overexpression of manganese containing superoxide dismutase and/or mitochondrial targeted catalase using adenoviral vectors significantly protected PC-3 cells from toxicity. This suggests that mitochondrial $O_2^{\cdot-}$ and H_2O_2 significantly contribute to glucose deprivation-induced cytotoxicity and metabolic oxidative stress in human cancer cells. (Ahmad et al, 2005).

Again, we see that EMODs are responsible for induction of cancer cell apoptosis and that this effect can be blocked by antioxidants.

Cancer cells are low in antioxidant enzymes and high in antioxidants

Total superoxide dismutase (SOD) and manganese superoxide dismutase (Mn SOD) specific activities were measured in tissue homogenates and in isolated mitochondria from normal rat liver and three Morris hepatomas of different growth rates. **Total SOD and Mn SOD specific activities were decreased in all tumor homogenates when compared to normal liver; the lowest activity was associated with the fastest growing tumor.** (Bize et al, 1980).

I have found that cancer cells also protectively concentrate antioxidants such as lactate, vitamin C and glutathione. I believe that this is a protective response by the cancer cells to block their demise via EMOD induced apoptosis. Interestingly, certain bacteria have evolved the synthesis of catalase to prevent their death via hydrogen peroxide.

EMODs may activate tumor suppressor genes

Reactive oxygen species are widely generated in biological systems. Consequently humans have evolved antioxidant defense systems that donate electrons for EMOD production. **Intracellular production of active oxygen**

species such as $-OH$, O_2^- and H_2O_2 is associated with the arrest of cell proliferation. Similarly, generation of oxidative stress in response to various external stimuli has been implicated in the activation of transcription factors and to the triggering of apoptosis. Investigators reviewed how free radicals induce DNA sequence changes in the form of mutations, deletions, gene amplification and rearrangements. **These alterations may result in the initiation of apoptosis signalling leading to cell death, or to the activation of several proto-oncogenes and/or the inactivation of some tumor suppressor genes.** The regulation of gene expression by means of oxidants, antioxidants and the redox state remains as a promising therapeutic approach. **Several anticarcinogenic agents have been shown to inhibit reactive oxygen species production and oxidative DNA damage, inhibiting tumor promotion. (RMH Note: this is merely showing that a low level of EMODs "allows" for the development of neoplasia and not that EMODs are causing cancer).**

EMOD scavenging enzymes reduce apoptosis

In addition, **recombinant vectors expressing radical-scavenging enzymes reduce apoptosis.** In conclusion, oxidative stress has been implicated in both apoptosis and the pathogenesis of cancer providing contrived support for two notions: free radical reactions may be increased in malignant cells and oxidant scavenging systems may be useful in cancer therapy. (Mates et al, 2000).

The EMOD spectrum from full health to serious diseases

In a similar manner, I believe that ROSI syndrome represents a spectrum of insufficiencies, from the mild to the severe. Mild EMOD insufficiency results in increased infections and skin cancer manifestation, whereas severe cases result in fatal cancer proliferation, increased metastasis and overwhelming infections and sepsis.

Non-melanoma Skin Cancer Linked to Risk of Other Cancers

A study published in the *Journal of the National Cancer Institute* 9/3/08 found that **people with a history of** basal or squamous cell skin cancer **(also known as non-melanoma skin cancer) were at an increased risk of developing other cancers later on.** The research suggests genetic factors may put some people at a higher cancer risk than others. **I believe that it is due to an overall EMOD insufficiency which will allow for the development of other cancers or for the manifestation of the coexistent diseases I have discussed.**

"There appears to be a heightened overall cancer risk associated with non-melanoma, and the evidence seems to indicate that genetic factors are involved," said lead researcher Anthony J. Alberg, PhD, from the Medical University of South Carolina.

Alberg, along with colleagues from the National Cancer Institute, Johns Hopkins University, and Medical University of South Carolina, used data from the CLUE (Give Us a Clue to Cancer and Heart Disease) II cohort study to compare risk in **769 non-melanoma cancer survivors and 18,405 individuals who never had the disease."** The researchers tracked the two groups **over a period of 16 years** – from May 1989 to December 2005 -- and found that those **patients with a history of skin cancer had about twice the risk of developing another type of cancer**, even after adjusting for other risk factors, including age, sex, body mass index, education, skin type, sunburn history, and smoking history. "We found that even after adjusting for all factors, there was a doubling of risk for subsequent cancers among non-melanoma patients," said Alberg.

The most frequently diagnosed cancers were also the most common in the United States: lung, colorectal, breast, and prostate cancer. Unsurprisingly, the increased risk was highest for melanoma, a cancer that is also linked to sun exposure, but the increased risk for other cancers remained statistically significant even when the researchers removed melanoma from the group.

Patients who were diagnosed with non-melanoma skin cancer at an earlier age -- in the 25-44 year age group – were more likely to be diagnosed with a subsequent cancer later on – a pattern that researchers think points to a genetic susceptibility in some people to develop cancer. **I attribute it to an EMOD insufficiency.**

Skin Cancer May Increase Risk of Other Cancers

A new study on January 7, 2009, from the US suggests that **people who have had nonmelanoma skin cancer (NMSC) may be at increased risk of developing** other cancers, including those that affect other parts of the body. **People with a history of non-melanoma skin cancer were found to face a two-fold increase in the risk of subsequent cancers**. Previous research has suggested that non-melanoma skin cancer survivors are at increased risk of developing melanoma in the future, but the researchers found that the disease also increases the risk of other forms of cancer.

The study is the work of Dr Jiping Chen of the National Cancer Institute in Bethesda, Maryland, and Dr Anthony Alberg of the Medical University of South

Carolina, and colleagues, and is published on August 26 in the online issue of the *Journal of the National Cancer Institute.*

Previous research has already shown a link between a history of NMSC and increased risk of developing melanoma, a rarer but more malignant form of skin cancer that causes most deaths from skin cancer, but it is not clear whether NSMC is also a risk factor for cancers that affect other parts of the body.

Chen and Alberg and colleagues analyzed data from a prospective cohort study known as **CLUE II,** which is based in Washington County, also in Maryland. They found **769** people in the cohort had been diagnosed with NMSC during a 16 year follow up period since the study started in 1989, and 18,405 people had no history of the disease over the same period. They then compared the risk of developing other types of cancer in the two groups.

The results showed that:

- **The overall rate of cancer diagnosis was 293.5 cases per 10,000 person-years in the NMSC group and 77.9 per 10,000 in the non-NMSC group**.
- After adjusting for other known cancer risk factors such as age, sex, body mass index (BMI), smoking status, and educational level, **people with a history of NMSC were twice as likely to develop other cancers as people with no such history.**
- The increased risk was unaffected by the removal of melanoma from the list of other cancers.
- **The figures were the same for both types of NMSC, basal cell and squamous cell carcinoma.**
- The strongest link between a history of NMSC and the risk of developing other cancers was in participants aged 25 to 44.

The authors concluded that:

"This community-based, prospective cohort study provides evidence for an association between an NMSC diagnosis and an increased risk of sub-sequent cancer, even after adjusting for individual-level risk factors."

Speculating on the finding that the younger participants with a history of NMSC were the ones most likely to develop other cancers, the authors **suggested it could be because of an inherited predisposition to cancer.**

Discussing the limitations of the study, the editors suggested that people with a history of NMSC might be more likely to receive a diagnosis for another cancer because they are more closely monitored. Also, the people studied in this cohort were all from one county in Maryland and may not be representative of the population as a whole. And finally, the adjustments that were made to eliminate factors such as skin type and sunburn history had to include assumptions because a lot of the data was missing for those factors.

(Chen J et al, 2008).

General discussion of cancer and oxygen

Cancerous cells are always being created in the body. It's an ongoing process that has gone on for eons. Specific parts of your immune system are designed to seek out and destroy cancer cells.

Poor oxygenation comes from a buildup of carcinogens and other toxins within and around cells, which blocks and then damages the cellular oxygen respiration mechanism. Clumping up of red blood cells slows down the bloodstream, and restricts flow into capillaries. This also causes poor oxygenation. Even lack of the proper building blocks for cell walls, essential fatty acids, restricts oxygen exchange.

(This is why the flax oil in cottage cheese treatment popular in Europe - 2 tablespoons of organic, refrigerated flax oil or freshly ground flax seed mixed in some cottage cheese - has become a well known cancer treatment. It provides essential fatty acids needed by cell walls so that oxygen can enter the cells.)

Decades ago, two researchers at the National Cancer Institute, Dean Burn and Mark Woods, (Dean translated some of Warburg's speeches) conducted a series of experiments where they measured the fermentation rate of cancers that grew at different speeds. What they found **supported Dr. Warburg's theory. The cancers with the highest growth rates had the highest fermentation rates. The slower a cancer grew, the less it used fermentation to produce energy**.

Dr. Otto Warburg, director of the Max Planck Institute for Cell Physiology in Berlin, stated in 1966 that the primary precondition for development of cancer is a lack of oxygen at the cellular level. (Warburg, 1996).

Naturally Warburg's contention was challenged and tested by other scientists.

Some researchers claimed his theory was not valid after they had measured a particularly slow growing cancer, and found no fermentation at all. And if cancer could grow with no fermentation, then fermentation, or lack of oxygen respiration, was not the cause of cancer. Dean Burn and Mark Woods checked those results.

Using more sophisticated equipment, they determined that the equipment these researchers used to measure fermentation levels was not accurate enough to detect fermentation at low levels. Their testing, using newer and more accurate equipment, showed that **even in those very slow growing cancer cells, fermentation was still taking place, at very low levels.**

Pietro Gullino, also at the National Cancer Institute, devised a test which showed **that this slow growing cancer always produced fermentation lactic acid.** Silvio Fiala, a biochemist from the University of Southern California, also confirmed that this slow growing cancer produced lactic acid, and that its oxygen respiration was reduced.

Further research into Warburg's theory showed that when oxygen levels were turned down, cells began to produce energy anaerobically. *They ultimately became cancerous when levels went low enough. It took a reduction of 35% in oxygen levels for this to happen.* **NOTE: RMH. This is the point I believe that low oxygen levels lead to low or insufficient EMOD levels, which allows neoplasia to manifest itself.**

J. B. Kizer, a biochemist and physicist at Gungnir Research in Portsmith, Ohio explains, "Since Warburg's discovery, this difference in respiration has remained the most fundamental (and some say, only) physiological difference consistently found between normal and cancer cells. Using cell culture studies, I decided to examine the differential responses of normal and cancer cells to changes in the oxygen environment.

"The results that I found were rather remarkable. I found that... **"High O_2 tensions were lethal to cancer tissue, 95 percent being very toxic**, whereas in general, **normal tissues were not harmed by high oxygen tensions**. Indeed, some normal tissues were found to require high O_2 tensions. It does seem to demonstrate the possibility that if the O_2 tensions in cancer tissues can be elevated, then the cancer tissue may be able to be killed selectively, as it seems that the cancer cells are incapable of handling the O_2 in a high O_2 environment." **RMH Note: the high oxygen levels results in higher EMOD levels, which induce apoptosis in the cancer cells and are handled readily by normal cells.**

RMH NOTE: This, I believe, is a classic example of EMOD induced apoptosis.

Low oxygen levels in cells may be a fundamental cause of cancer. **RMH Note: I do not look at it as a cause of cancer but rather as a condition which "allows" for the development of cancer.** There are several reasons cells become poorly oxygenated. An overload of toxins clogging up the cells, poor quality cell walls that don't allow nutrients into the cells, the lack of nutrients needed for respiration, poor circulation and perhaps even low levels of oxygen in the air we breathe. **RMH NOTE: Any factor which produces an EMOD insufficiency will allow for cancer formation.**

Cancer cells produce *excess lactic acid* as they ferment energy. Lactic acid (an antioxidant) is toxic, and tends to prevent the transport of oxygen into neighboring normal cells. Over time as these cells replicate, the cancer may spread if not destroyed by the immune system. **I believe that the antioxidant, lactic acid, provides for an EMOD insufficiency, which is needed to sustain the cancer cells and avoid EMOD induced apoptosis.**

Dr. Joachim Varro discovered in 1974 a peroxide intolerance in tumor cells and proposed that ozone and hydrogen peroxide may induce metabolic inhibition in certain types of cancerous growths. (Varro, 1974). And, **he was right.**

With low O_2, cells mutate and with high O_2, cells stop (reportedly)

We also need to discuss the antioxidant, lactic acid.

RMH Note: Lactic acid is an antioxidant and it is in this capacity that it is advantageous for cancer cells to produce it, such that EMODs can be kept at sub-apoptotic levels. Salts of lactic acid are used in foods as a humecticant and an antioxidant which can increase the effect of other antioxidants.

Chemotherapy and radiation are used because cancer cells have higher standing levels of EMODs than normal cells and therefore die first.

However, chemo and radiation **damage respiratory enzymes** in healthy cells, and overload them with toxins, so they may be more likely to develop into cancer. The underlying cancer causing conditions are worsened, not improved. The immune system and its prooxidant content are reduced and the cancer usually returns quickly a second time unless you make changes to support the prooxidant status of your body.

The implication of this research is that an effective way to support the body's fight against cancer would be to **get as much oxygen as you can** into healthy cells, and improving their ability to utilize oxygen and generate EMODs. Raising the oxygen levels of normal cells would help prevent them from becoming cancerous. This is discussed in my book, Antioxidant Overkill.

And increasing oxygen levels in cancer cells to high levels could help kill those cancer cells.

A nurse who works in medical research said, *"It's so simple. I don't know why I never thought of it before. When we're working with cell cultures in the lab, if we want the cells to mutate, we turn down the oxygen. To stop them, we turn the oxygen back up."* Note: I do not have a source for this quote.

Ma Lan, MD and Joel Wallach DVD, point out that one type of white blood cells kills cancer cells by injecting oxygen creating hydrogen peroxide into the cells.

It is not easy to get **additional oxygen** into cells. Most approaches don't work well. **Breathing oxygen is still limited by the amount of hemoglobin available, and pH levels.** Dr. Whittaker points out, quite rightly, that liquid oxygen supplements that release oxygen into the blood, *can't* get oxygen into the cells.

He explains that a delivery mechanism is needed to transport oxygen into cells. And though the typical oxygen supplement gets oxygen into the blood, that doesn't mean it gets into the cells. However, there is a lot more to this oxygenation story.

Tumor necrosis factor (TNF) and oxygen free radicals

During various biological processes as inflammation or septic shock, free radical damages are produced by a direct production of oxygen radicals by phagocytes, but also by a TNF-mediated generation in target cells. **Antioxidants have been demonstrated as protective against TNF cytotoxicity.** We try to measure directly the free radical produced by **murine recombinant TNF on L929 cells**, by detecting the direct light produced by decomposition of superoxide using an adapted chemiluminometer. We measure also the chemiluminescence after addition of luminol. These techniques demonstrate the effective production of oxygen radicals. Unfortunately they have a rather poor specificity and sensitivity. So we use the protective effect of antioxidants on cytotoxicity to investigate the origin of the productive mechanism. We evaluate cytotoxicity of 1 U/ml TNF on L929 murine fibroblasts after 24 hours incubation with actinomycin D by the MTT and Cr51 release. Using the MTT test we observe that **addition of thiourea or catalase has the better protecting effect when Cu-Zn SOD had few effect**. Reversely, using the Cr51 release we observe a good protective effect of Cu-Zn SOD simultaneously with a good protective effect of catalase. So the difference in the effect of various antioxidant agent do not permit to identify the species generated, but depend more on the ability of the antioxidant to reach the cell compartment tested by the method (membrane, or mitochondria). **The oxidative effect of TNF is beneficial in physiological condition to destroy cancerous or virus infested cells infested by virus inside the body.** But this effect can be deleterious in situation of deficiency in some antioxidant. TNF-induced free radicals can increase the replication of virus as HIV-1 and destroy immunocompetent cells as T cells. This last action explains the defect in cellular immunity observed in oxidative stress and the immunostimulatory effect of many antioxidants. (Ferlat et al, 1993).

Oxygen radicals have been found to trigger cell death by apoptosis in several phenotypes of tumor-killing lymphocytes. (Hansson et al, 1996) (Hansson et al, 1999) (Betten et al, 2001), **in addition to inducing the disappearance of critical signal transduction structures on remaining viable cells** (Betten et al, 2001) (Aoe et al, 1995) (Otsuji et al, 1996).

Arguments against EMOD induced apoptosis

Oxygen radicals have been proposed to significantly contribute to cytotoxic lymphocyte dysfunction in several forms of human cancer, including solid cancers such as melanoma, colorectal cancer, renal cell cancer, and prostate cancer. (Kono et al, 1996) (Rabinowich et al, 1996) (Healy et al, 1998), **as well as in hematological malignancies such as acute and chronic myelogenous leukemias.** Therefore, understanding the molecular events underlying radical-induced lymphocyte inactivation could be useful in identifying therapeutic strategies to alleviate cancer-related immunosuppression. **I believe that these results have been misinterpreted in view of the crucial role of EMODs in apoptosis induction.**

It is concluded that **caspase activation is a late event during oxygen radical-induced lymphocyte apoptosis and that the role of caspases is rather in the execution phase than in the induction phase of apoptosis.** In contrast, PARP/AIF axis may be critically involved in initiating phagocyte-mediated, oxygen radical-induced lymphocyte apoptosis. (Fredrik et al, 2006).

127

Prof Randolph M. Howes MD, PhD

Hydrogen Peroxide Enhances Tumor Necrosis Factor-Alpha Toxicity in Inducing Human Vascular Endothelial Cell Apoptosis: Reversal with Propofol

TNF is a cytokine.

Investigators designed the present study to test the hypothesis that oxygen free radicals can enhance tumor necrosis factor (TNF)-alpha cellular toxicity, which might be reversed by **propofol, an anesthetic with antioxidant properties**, in human vascular endothelial cell line ECV304. Cultured ECV304 were either not treated, treated with 10 μM of hydrogen peroxide (H_2O_2), treated with TNF-alpha (40 ng/mL) alone, TNF-alpha in the presence of 10 μM of H_2O_2 (H+T), or propofol plus H_2O_2 for 24 h. Cell viability was measured by lactate dehydrogenate (LDH) assay. Cell apoptosis was assessed by flow cytometry and terminal deoxynucleotidyl transferase (TdT)-mediated deoxyuridine triphosphate (dUTP) nick end-labeling. The **antiapoptotic Bcl-2 and pro-apoptotic Bax protein** expressions were measured by immunocytochemical analysis. **Increases in apoptosis, Bax, lipid peroxidation product malondialdehyde, LDH, and decreases in Bcl-2, superoxide dismutase, and glutathione peroxidase were observed in TNF-**alpha **–treated cells. H_2O_2 10 μM did not cause significant lipid peroxidation** as compared with control but further enhanced TNF-alpha –induced lipid peroxidation, upregulated Bax, and down-regulated Bcl-2 expression and enhanced TNF-alpha–induced cell apoptosis. **Propofol 50 μM attenuated TNF-**alpha **and H_2O_2-induced cell apoptosis,** accompanied by decreases in malondialdehyde and LDH production and restoration of Bcl-2 expression. Propofol exerts protective effects against H_2O_2-enhanced TNF-alpha cell toxicity by reducing oxidative injury.

The vascular endothelium plays an important role in maintaining cardiovascular homeostasis, including important functions such as the regulation of vascular tone and tissue perfusion, vascular permeability, myocardial function, blood fluidity, anticoagulant activity, and inflammatory responses. Various forms of endothelial cell injury occur in patients with shock, sepsis, and, in particular, during myocardial ischemia reperfusion injury, such as in patients undergoing cardiac surgery using cardiopulmonary bypass (Verrier et al, 1996).

One study suggests that circulatory pro-apoptotic inflammatory cytokines (such as tumor necrosis factor [TNF]-alpha) and EMODs (reactive oxygen species, ROS), which are increased during myocardial ischemia reperfusion injury and atherosclerosis, promote cardiomyocyte apoptosis subsequent to the induction of endothelial cells apoptosis.(Scarabelli et al, 2001).

Thus, inhibition of TNF-alpha– and ROS-induced endothelial cells apoptosis may represent an effective therapy for myocardial ischemia reperfusion injury.

Propofol, an IV anesthetic with potential antioxidant property, has a chemical structure similar to that of phenol-based free-radical scavengers, such as vitamin E, and reduces free radicals. (Murphy et al, 1992).

Propofol has been shown to attenuate hydrogen peroxide (H_2O_2)-induced mechanical and metabolic derangements in the isolated rat heart. Our study showed that propofol can dose-dependently reduce TNF-alpha –induced human umbilical vein endothelial cells (HUVECs) apoptosis *in vitro*, and the effect was more profound at concentrations $\geq$50 µM. **TNF-alpha and EMODs (ROS) may work synergistically in inducing endothelial cell apoptosis.** It is unknown, however, whether ROS enhancements of TNF-alpha cellular toxicity was mediated through enhanced lipid peroxidation or primarily through the modulation of pro- and antiapoptotic proteins. **Apoptosis caused by TNF-alpha and H_2O_2 were reduced significantly by the addition of propofol.**

As an aside, propofol has been implicated in the death of Michael Jackson.

EMODs (ROS), which could be generated by TNF-alpha in many tissue and cell types, plays an important role in inducing cell apoptosis. Studies have shown that both the application of exogenous antioxidants such as vitamin E and the over-expression of endogenous antioxidant proteins such as Bcl-2, SOD, catalase, GSH, or GSH-Px can attenuate apoptosis induced by lipopolysaccharide and cytokines such as TNF in different cell types.

H_2O_2 10 µM induced only a small amount of cell apoptosis. **The H_2O_2 concentration (10 µM) used in this study is in the smallest range that induces minimal endothelial cell apoptosis but not necrosis.** (Burlacu et al, 2001).

Interestingly, H_2O_2, when used at such a small concentration (i.e., 10 µM), profoundly augmented TNF-alpha –induced vascular endothelial cell apoptosis. The possible mechanism for this phenomenon is likely that application of H_2O_2 could result in increased intracellular Bax and decreased Bcl-2 levels, which may make the cells more vulnerable to TNF- alpha.

A novel finding of the current study is that **H_2O_2, at a trace concentration (10 µM), did not cause significantly enhanced lipid peroxidation in ECV304 cells** and markedly exacerbated TNF-alpha–induced increases in ECV304 cell lipid peroxidation and pro-apoptotic Bax protein, leading to enhanced cell apoptosis. **Propofol attenuated H_2O_2-mediated exacerbation of TNF- alpha effects.**

In summary, results from the current study indicate that **H_2O_2 could enhance TNF-** alpha **–induced vascular endothelial cell apoptosis. Propofol can attenuate TNF-alpha and H_2O_2 cellular toxicity. I believe that this indicates the dangers of propofol in patients with precancerous or cancerous growths. It would block the killing of cancer cells.**

TNF Blockers May Increase Cancer Risk in Kids

On August 5, 2009, it was reported that kids and teens treated with drugs called tumor necrosis factor (TNF) blockers may be at an increased risk for lymphoma and other cancers, according to the US Food and Drug Administration (FDA), which is updating black box warnings for the drugs.

The FDA's decision is based on a yearlong review of the childhood cancer risk associated with **TNF blocker drugs, which are used to treat rheumatoid arthritis, Crohn's disease, and other inflammatory diseases.**

These drugs -- which include adalimumab (Humira), etanercept (Enbrel), certolizumab pegol (Cimzia), golimumab (Simponi), and infliximab (Remicade) -- work by blocking tumor necrosis factor, a protein that's overproduced in some immune system diseases. The FDA started investigating the drugs in 2008 after evidence suggested that **interfering with TNF may also increase the risk of some life-threatening infections and certain cancers. I believe that this is due to the blocking of TNF, which generates EMODs, and the creation of an EMOD insufficiency state, and the patient is unable to fight infections and allows cancer development.**

This analysis found **children and teens taking these drugs had an increased risk of cancer, with cases occurring on average after 30 months of treatment. About half were lymphomas, and some were fatal.** The FDA said it was working with TNF drug manufacturers, including Johnson & Johnson, Abbott, and Wyeth, to better understand the childhood cancer risk associated with these drugs.

Cancers in children often are hard to recognize. Parents should be sure that their children have regular medical check-ups and watch for any unusual signs or symptoms that do not go away. These may include:

- an unusual lump or swelling
- unexplained paleness and loss of energy easy bruising
- an ongoing pain in one area of the body
- limping
- unexplained fever or illness that doesn't go away
- frequent headaches, often with vomiting
- sudden eye or vision changes
- sudden unexplained weight loss

These symptoms are more likely to be caused by something other than cancer, but they should be checked out by your child's doctor.

Prooxidant thymoquinone induces apoptosis in colorectal cancer cells

Thymoquinone triggers inactivation of the stress response pathway sensor *CHEK1* and contributes to apoptosis in colorectal cancer cells

There are few reports describing the role of p53-dependent gene repression in apoptotic cell death. To identify such apoptosis-associated p53 target genes, we used **the pro-oxidant plant-derived drug thymoquinone** and compared p53+/+ and p53–/– colon cancer cells HCT116. The p53 wild-type (wt) status correlated with more pronounced DNA damage and higher apoptosis after thymoquinone treatment. A significant up-regulation of the survival gene *CHEK1* was observed in p53–/– cells in response to thymoquinone due to the lack of transcriptional repression of p53. In p53–/– cells, transfection with p53-wt vector and CHEK1 small interfering RNA treatment decreased CHEK1 mRNA and protein levels and restored apoptosis to the levels of the p53+/+ cells. p53–/– cells transplanted to nude mice treated with thymoquinone up-regulated CHEK1 expression and did not undergo apoptosis unlike p53+/+ cells. Immunofluorescence analysis revealed that the apoptosis resistance in p53–/– cells after thymoquinone treatment might be conveyed by shuttling of CHEK1 into the nucleus. We confirmed the *in vivo* existence of this CHEK1/p53 link in **human colorectal cancer**, showing that tumors lacking p53 had higher levels of CHEK1, which was accompanied by poorer apoptosis. CHEK1 overexpression was correlated with advanced tumor stages, proximal tumor localization, and worse prognosis. We suggest that the inhibition of the stress response sensor CHEK1 might contribute to the antineoplastic activity of specific DNA-damaging drugs. (**Gali-Muhtasib** et al, 2008).

Methylglyoxal-induced apoptosis in human prostate carcinoma

Investigators examined the cellular effects of methylglyoxal (MG), a toxic physiological metabolite, on human prostatic cancer PC-3 cells. **Methods:** The effects of MG on cell growth and viability were evaluated first, and then its effects on the cell cycle and the glycolytic process were analyzed by Western blots and specific assays. Possible MG-induced apoptosis was also assessed by DNA analysis using agarose gel electrophoresis. **Results:** MG ^{3}3 mM caused severe growth inhibition, resulting in nearly 100% cell death by 24h. The time course study revealed that expression of cyclin D_1, cdk2, and cdk4 was significantly (>50%) downregulated in 3 h of MG (3 mM) exposure, followed by the dephosphorylation of retinoblastoma protein by 6 h. Both the glyceraldehyde 3phosphate dehydrogenase activity and the cellular lactate level were also reduced by ~50 and 80%, respectively, following 6-hour MG exposure. **Induction of apoptosis by MG was indicated by partial degradation of poly(ADP-ribose) polymerase and further confirmed by discrete DNA fragmentation detected on an agarose gel. Conclusion:** MG is capable of inducing apoptosis in prostatic cancer PC-3 cells, due primarily to a blocking of the cell cycle progression (G_1 arrest) and glycolytic pathway. Therefore, **MG could be a potent apoptosis inducer**, which may have a potential for prostate cancer treatment. (Milanesa et al, 2000).

Influence of methylglyoxal on antioxidant enzymes and oxidative damage

The effect of different doses of methylglyoxal (50–400 mg/kg body wt.) were examined using enzymes involved in the antioxidant function, glutathione (GSH) content and lipid peroxidation in the liver and spleen of Swiss albino mice (7–8 week old) after 6, 12 and 24 h. Significant changes were observed predominantly in the liver. The specific activities of superoxide dismutase (SOD), glutathione-S-transferase (GST), catalase, glyoxalase I (gly I) and glyoxalase II (gly II) were found to decrease in the liver. The mode and magnitude of change in the specific activities was seen to depend on the dose of methylglyoxal and the time after its administration. Methylglyoxal also decreased the GSH content and enhanced the lipid peroxidation in the liver. These findings are suggestive of the adverse effect of methylglyoxal on the antioxidant defense system. It is likely that **methylglyoxal undergoes a redox cycle and generates the free radicals** which in turn lower the antioxidant status in animals. The increased levels of lipid peroxidation provide support for the involvement of free radical processes in the detrimental effects of methylglyoxal. The response of DT-diaphorase (DTD) seems to be adaptive. (Dharamainder et al, 1997).

EMOD-induced apoptosis in human leukemia cells (Camptothecin, CPT)

Investigators used a human leukemia cell line that, after homologous recombination knockout of the gp91-phox subunit of the phagocyte respiratory-burst oxidase cytochrome b-558, **mimics chronic granulomatous disease** (X-CGD) to study the role of oxygen radicals in apoptosis. **Camptothecin (CPT),** a topoisomerase I inhibitor, induced significantly more apoptosis in PLB-985 cells than in X-CGD cells. Sensitivity to CPT was enhanced after neutrophilic differentiation, but was lost after monocytic differentiation. No difference between the two cell lines was observed after **treatment with other apoptosis inducers, including etoposide, ultraviolet radiation, ionizing radiation, hydrogen peroxide, or 7-hydroxystaurosporine.** After granulocytic differentiation of both cell lines, CPT still induced apoptosis, suggesting independence from replication in fully differentiated and growth-arrested cells. **Pyrrolidine dithiocarbamate (an antioxidant inhibitor of NF-kappaB) and catalase partially inhibited CPT-induced DNA fragmentation in granulocytic-differentiated PLB-985 cells,** but had no effect in X-CGD cells. Flow cytometry analysis revealed that reactive oxygen intermediates were generated in CPT-treated PLB-985 cells. These data indicate that **oxygen radicals generated by NADPH oxidase may contribute directly or indirectly to CPT-induced apoptosis in human leukemia and in neutrophilic-differentiated cells.** (Hiraoka et al, 1998). **I believe that these same EMOD producers could be used clinically to prevent or treat various malignancies. This study supports the role for EMOD induced apoptosis.**

Lack of Oxygen - the potential ability of cancer survival and spread

On Sept. 18, 2009, HealthDayNews published a report on a lack of oxygen as a supporting factor for cancer survival and metastasis. A sad fact of cancer is that some tumor cells spread, signaling a worse prognosis for the patient, while others don't. An enduring question in cancer research has been, "Why?"

"If you look at the public health problem of cancer, it's mostly due to cancer that has spread," says Dr. Max Sung, medical director of the Ruttenberg Cancer Treatment Center at the Mount Sinai Medical Center in New York City. "If there's a mechanism by which these cancer cells that have spread can be destroyed, that would be wonderful. The next best thing is to see if we could prevent the primary tumor from spreading in the first place."

An article appearing in the Sept. 18, 2009 issue of *Nature* looked into just this issue: why tumor cells spread and how that deadly process can be prevented. **Scientists already knew tumor cells that don't have enough oxygen, a condition known as hypoxia, have a greater tendency to spread than those with a regular supply of oxygen.** Now scientists have shown that **tumor cells that are deprived of oxygen also seem to have the ability to zoom in on certain organs, which explains why certain types of cancer tend to spread to certain parts of the body**.

Breast cancer, for instance, has a preference for bone marrow, lungs and the liver.

"This adds a novel dimension to our insight. It has shown that, not only do tumor cells acquire the ability to spread, but they also acquire the ability to home in on certain organs," says Rene Bernards, author of an accompanying article in the journal and a professor of molecular carcinogenesis at The Netherlands Cancer Institute in Amsterdam.

When faced with hypoxia, tumor cells respond by increasing production of a protein called hypoxia-inducible factor (HIF), which in turn binds to and activates different genes. The von Hippel-Lindau (VHL) tumor suppressor gene produces proteins that prevent cells from becoming malignant. It is also part of the oxygen-sensing machinery of the cell that controls the levels of the HIF.

"The question is 'What is the relationship of this gene to the tumor cells spreading?'" Sung says. In this study, the researchers introduced VHL into kidney cancer cells (which normally lack a copy of this gene) and then looked for changes in the activity of thousands of other genes under conditions of adequate oxygen. To their surprise, they found that VHL reduced the production of a receptor protein called CXCR4, which is known to be over-expressed in those breast cancer cells that spread to the bone. The CXCR4 acts as a sort of homing system. **"Now it turns out that if tumor cells become starved of oxygen, that they begin to express CXCR4, which allows tumor cells to migrate specifically to other organs,"** Bernards explains.

The findings do open up the possibility of gene therapy to correct the situation sometime in the future. At the same time, the results cast doubt on the concept of angiogenesis, which posits that cutting off blood supply to a tumor will shrink or kill it. **Oxygen is carried via the bloodstream.** "Although the concept that oxygen deprivation promotes tumor metastasis is not altogether novel, this is still an interesting and important study," says Charles Graham, assistant professor of anatomy and cell biology at Queen's University in Ontario. "The idea of using angiogenesis inhibitors to deprive tumors of their blood [and hence oxygen] supply as a therapeutic approach has been around for quite a while. However, this and **other studies... indicate that reducing the blood supply to a tumor may have unintended consequences, as it may promote the spread of malignant cells."**

There are other unresolved issues. "A key question that follows is whether these changes have already taken place in the primary tumor, allowing it to spread to a specific secondary site, or whether primary tumor cells that are carried to secondary organs undergo these changes after they have been exposed to the new environment," Bernards writes in his commentary.

The current results seem to suggest the changes leading to this deadly cascade happen early on. This supports research that Bernards and his colleagues previously conducted that was also published in *Nature*. "We showed that breast cancer comes in two flavors even if they are small primary tumors, either of good prognosis or bad prognosis. Even if the primary tumor is still small, it has either already decided very early in its life

that it will become malignant and aggressive and metastatic or has started out on a relatively benign path," he says.

"In a way, that is good news for cancer patients because you can determine up front whether a cancer is likely to metastasize to other parts of the body or not, and we can adjust the chemotherapy requirements to this insight."

(Bernards, Sung, 2003).

Onion oil EMOD-induced apoptosis blocked by NAC and glutathione

Protective effects of Allium vegetables against cancers have been shown extensively in experimental animals and epidemiologic studies. We investigated cell proliferation and the induction of apoptosis by onion oil extracted from Allium cepa, a widely consumed Allium vegetable, in human lung cancer A549 cells. GC/MS analysis suggested that propyl sulfides but not allyl sulfides are major sulfur-containing constituents of onion oil. Onion oil at 12.5 mg/L significantly induced apoptosis (13% increase of apoptotic cells) as indicated by sub-G1 DNA content. It also caused cell cycle arrest at the G2/M phase; 25 mg/L onion oil increased the percentage of G2/M cells almost 6-fold compared with the dimethyl sulfoxide control. The action of onion oil may occur via a reactive oxygen species–dependent pathway because **cell cycle arrest and apoptosis were blocked by the antioxidants N-acetylcysteine and exogenous glutathione.** Marked collapse of the mitochondrial membrane potential suggested that **dysfunction of the mitochondria may be involved in the oxidative burst and apoptosis induced by onion oil.** Expression of phospho-cdc2 and phospho-cyclin B1 were downregulated by onion oil, perhaps accounting for the G2/M arrest. Overall, these results suggest that onion oil may exert chemopreventive action by inducing cell cycle arrest and apoptosis in tumor cells. (Wu et al, 2006).

Phytosterols (plant antioxidant sterols) do not have anti-carcinogenic activity

Much interest has focused on the cholesterol-lowering effects of phytosterols (plant sterols) but limited data suggests they may also possess anti-carcinogenic activity. Conjugated linoleic acids (CLA), sourced from meat and dairy products of ruminant animals, has also received considerable attention as a potential anti-cancer agent. Therefore, the aims of this project were to (i) examine the effects of phytosterols and CLA on the viability and growth of human intestinal Caco-2 cells and (ii) determine their potential genoprotective (comet assay), COX-2 modulatory (ELISA) and apoptotic (Hoechst staining) activities. Caco-2 cells were supplemented with the phytosterols campesterol, b-sitosterol, or b-sitostanol, or a CLA mixture, or individual CLA isomers (c10t12-CLA, t9t11-CLA) for 48 h. The three phytosterols, at the highest levels tested, were found to reduce both the viability and growth of Caco-2 cells while CLA exhibited isomer-specific effects. None of the phytosterols protected against DNA damage. At a concentration of 25 µM, both c10t12-CLA and t9t11-CLA enhanced ($P < 0.05$) oxidant-induced, but not mutagen-induced, DNA damage. Neither the phytosterols nor CLA induced apoptosis or modulated COX-2 production. In conclusion, **campesterol, b-sitosterol, b-sitostanol, c10t12-CLA, and t9t11-CLA were not toxic to Caco-2 cells, at the lower levels tested, and did not exhibit potential anti-carcinogenic activity.** (Daly et al, 2009).

Green tea has no effect on risk of breast cancer

Although many *in vitro* and animal studies have demonstrated a protective effect of green tea against breast cancer, findings from epidemiological studies have been inconsistent, and whether high green tea intake reduces the risk of breast cancer remains unclear.

Methods: In this Japan Public Health Center-based Prospective Study, **581 cases of breast cancer were newly diagnosed in 53,793 women during 13.6**

years' follow-up from the baseline survey in 1990 to 1994. After the five-year follow-up survey in 1995 to 1998, 350 cases were newly diagnosed in 43,639 women during 9.5 years' follow-up. The baseline questionnaire assessed the frequency of total green tea drinking while the five-year follow-up questionnaire assessed that of two types of green tea, *Sencha* and *Bancha/Genmaicha*, separately.

Results: Compared with women who drank less than one cup of green tea per week, the adjusted hazard ratio (HR) for women who drank five or more cups per day was 1.12 (95% confidence interval (CI) 0.81 to 1.56; *P* for trend = 0.60) in the baseline data. Similarly, compared with women who drank less than one cup of *Sencha* or *Bancha/Genmaicha* per week, adjusted HRs for women who drank 10 or more cups per day were 1.02 (95% CI 0.55 to 1.89; *P* for trend = 0.48) for *Sencha* and 0.86 (0.34 to 2.17; *P* for trend = 0.66) for *Bancha/Genmaicha*. No inverse association was found regardless of hormone receptor-defined subtype or menopausal status.

Conclusions: In this **population-based prospective cohort study in Japan we found no association between green tea drinking and risk of breast cancer.** (Iwasaki et al, 2010).

Insufficient and conflicting evidence for green tea consumption and cancer prevention

Tea is one of the most commonly consumed beverages worldwide. Teas from the plant Camellia sinensis can be grouped into green, black and oolong tea. Cross-culturally tea drinking habits vary. **Camellia sinensis contains the active ingredient polyphenol, which has a subgroup known as catechins. Catechins are powerful antioxidants.** It has been suggested that green tea polyphenol may inhibit cell proliferation and observational studies have suggested that green tea may have cancer-preventative effects.

OBJECTIVES: To critically assess any associations between green tea consumption and the risk of cancer incidence and mortality.

SEARCH STRATEGY: We searched eligible studies up to January 2009 in the Cochrane Central Register of Controlled Trials (CENTRAL), MEDLINE, EMBASE, Amed, CancerLit, Psych INFO and Phytobase and reference lists of previous reviews and included studies.

SELECTION CRITERIA: We included all prospective, controlled interventional studies and observational studies, which either assessed the associations between green tea consumption and risk of cancer incidence or that reported on cancer mortality.

DATA COLLECTION AND ANALYSIS: At least two review authors independently applied the study criteria, extracted data and assessed methodological quality of studies. Due to the nature of included studies, which were mainly epidemiological, results were summarized descriptively according to cancer diagnosis.

MAIN RESULTS: Fifty-one studies with more than 1.6 million participants were included. Twenty-seven of them were case-control studies, 23 cohort studies and one randomized controlled trial (RCT). *Twenty-seven studies tried to establish an association between green tea consumption and cancer of the digestive tract, mainly of the upper gastrointestinal tract, five with breast cancer, five with prostate cancer, three with lung cancer, two with ovarian cancer, two with urinary bladder cancer one with oral cancer, three further studies included patients with various cancer diagnoses.* The methodological quality was measured with the Newcastle-Ottawa scale (NOS). The 9 nested case-control studies within prospective cohorts were of high methodological quality, 13 of medium, and 1 of low. One retrospective case-control study was of high methodological quality and 21 of medium and 5 of low. **Results from studies assessing associations between green tea and risk of digestive tract cancer incidence were highly contradictory. There was limited evidence that green tea could reduce the incidence of liver cancer. The evidence for esophageal, gastric, colon, rectum, and pancreatic cancer was conflicting.** In prostate cancer, observational studies with higher methodological quality and the only included RCT suggested a decreased risk in men consuming higher quantities green tea or green tea extracts. **However, there was limited to moderate evidence that the consumption of green tea reduced the risk of lung cancer, especially in men, and *urinary bladder cancer or that it could even increase the risk of the latter.* There was moderate to strong evidence that green tea consumption does not decrease the risk of dying from gastric cancer. There was limited moderate to strong evidence for lung, pancreatic and colorectal cancer.**

AUTHORS' CONCLUSIONS: There is insufficient and conflicting evidence to give any firm recommendations regarding green tea consumption for cancer prevention. The results of this review, including its trends of associations, need to be interpreted with caution and their generalisability is questionable, as the majority of included studies were carried out in Asia (n = 47) where the tea drinking culture is pronounced. **Desirable green tea intake is 3 to 5 cups per day (up to 1200 ml/day), providing a minimum of 250 mg/**

day catechins. If not exceeding the daily recommended allowance, those who enjoy a cup of green tea should continue its consumption. Drinking green tea appears to be safe at moderate, regular and habitual use. (Boehm et al, 2009).

H_2O_2 is poorly reactive and present throughout the human body

Hydrogen peroxide (H_2O_2) is widely regarded as an alleged cytotoxic agent whose levels must be minimized by the action of antioxidant defense enzymes. In fact, **H_2O_2 is poorly reactive in the absence of transition metal ions. Exposure of certain human tissues to H_2O_2 may be greater than is commonly supposed: substantial amounts of H_2O_2 can be present in beverages commonly drunk (especially instant coffee), in freshly voided human urine, and in exhaled air.** Levels of H_2O_2 in the human body may be controlled not only by catabolism but also by excretion, and H_2O_2 could play a role in the regulation of renal function and as an antibacterial agent in the urine. Urinary H_2O_2 levels are influenced by diet, but under certain conditions might be a valuable biomarker of 'oxidative stress'. (Halliwell et al, 2000).

This proapoptotic activity is at least partly mediated by H_2O_2, because catalase blocks apoptosis completely in some cells and partially in others. **The addition of EGCG to cultured cells causes the overexpression of many genes, and some of these genes are not activated in the presence of catalase.** I believe that this emphasizes the caution that should be exercised in the use of antioxidants.

I believe that **peroxide is known to stimulate over 200 important metabolic transduction enzymes and removal or blockage of H_2O_2 formation could dangerously or fatally inhibit any or all of these enzymes.**

In summary, **there is only a moderate increase in antioxidant capacity after tea consumption** because the bioavailability of tea polyphenols is low. **I believe that the prooxidative activities may be important in the anticancer activity of tea and EGCG in vivo.** Green tea and green tea polyphenols inhibit tumorigenesis at different organ sites, including the skin, lung, oral cavity, esophagus, stomach, liver, pancreas, and prostate.

Like most investigators, they have overly complicated the issue and have been blind to the fact that all that is necessary for tumoricidal activity is to increase EMOD levels, especially of H_2O_2 and singlet oxygen. This is

what I did with my singlet oxygen delivery system. **All of the above work is supportive of my Unified theory.**

Superoxide dismutase (SOD) produces hydrogen peroxide

The principal source of hydrogen peroxide in mitochondria is thought to be from the dismutation of superoxide via the enzyme manganese superoxide dismutase (MnSOD). However, the nature of the effect of SOD on the cellular production of H_2O_2 is not widely appreciated. **The current paradigm is that the presence of SOD results in a lower level of H_2O_2 because it would prevent the non-enzymatic reactions of superoxide that form H_2O_2.** The goal of this work was to: a) demonstrate that SOD can increase the flux of H_2O_2 and b) use kinetic modelling to determine what kinetic and thermo-dynamic conditions result in SOD increasing the flux of H_2O_2. We examined two biological sources of superoxide production (xanthine oxidase and coenzyme Q semiquinone, CoQ(*-) that have different thermodynamic and kinetic properties. We found that **SOD could change the rate of formation of H_2O_2 in cases where equilibrium-specific reactions form superoxide with an equilibrium constant (K) less than 1.** An example is the formation of superoxide in the electron transport chain (ETC) of the mitochondria by the reaction of ubisemi-quinone radical with dioxygen. We measured the rate of release of H_2O_2 into culture medium from cells with differing levels of MnSOD. We found that **the higher the level of SOD, the greater the rate of accumulation of H_2O_2.** Results with kinetic modelling were consistent with this observation; the steady-state level of H_2O_2 increases if K<1, for example CoQ(*-)+O(2)-->CoQ+O(2)(*-). However, when K>1, e.g. xanthine oxidase forming O(2)(*-), SOD does not affect the steady state-level of H_2O_2. Thus, **the current paradigm that SOD will lower the flux of H_2O_2 does not hold for the ETC.** These observations indicate that MnSOD contributes to the flux of H_2O_2 in cells and thereby is involved in establishing the cellular redox environment and thus the biological state of the cell. (Buettner et al, 2006). **This confirms my belief that SOD is a prooxidant and not an antioxidant.**

SOD over expression increases peroxide levels and suppresses prostate cancer cells

This study investigated the role of the antioxidant enzyme manganese superox-ide dismutase (MnSOD) in **androgen-independent human prostate cancer (PC-3) cells'** growth rate in vitro and in vivo. **MnSOD levels were found to be lower in parental PC-3** cells compared to nonmalignant, immortalized human prostate epithelial cells (P69SV40T). To unravel the role of MnSOD in the prostate cancer phenotype, PC-3 cells were stably transfected with MnSOD cDNA plasmid. The MnSOD protein and activity levels in clones overexpressing MnSOD were increased seven- to eightfold. These cell lines showed elongated cell doubling time, reduced anchorage-independent growth in soft agar compared to parental PC-3 (Wt) cells, and reduced growth rate of PC-3 tumor xenografts in athymic nude mice. Flow cytometric studies showed an increase in membrane potential in the MnSOD-overexpressing clone (Mn32) compared to Wt and Neo cells. Also, **production of extracellular H_2O_2 was increased in the MnSOD-overexpressing clones**. As determined by DNA cell cycle analysis, the proportion of cells in G(1) phase was enhanced by MnSOD overexpression. Therefore, MnSOD not only regulates cell survival but also affects PC-3 cell proliferation by retarding G(1) to S transition. Our results are consistent with **MnSOD being a tumor suppressor gene in human prostate cancer**. (Venkataraman et al, 2005). **I believe that this again confirms my theory that EMODs control and curtail cancer growth. The increased SOD resulted in increased peroxide levels, which in turn suppressed tumor growth, via EMOD-induced apoptosis.**

EMOD rise increases tumoricidal response

It has been hypothesized that **exposure of cells to hyperthermia results in an increased flux of reactive oxygen species (ROS), primarily superoxide anion radicals**, and that increasing antioxidant enzyme levels will result in protection of cells from the toxicity of these ROS. In this study, the prostate cancer cell line, PC-3, and its manganese superoxide dismutase (MnSOD)-overexpressing clones were subjected to hyperthermia (43 degrees C, 1 h). Increased expression of MnSOD increased the mitochondrial membrane potential (MMP). **Hyperthermic exposure of PC-3 cells resulted in increased ROS production**, as determined by aconitase inactivation, lipid peroxidation, and H2O2 formation with a reduction in cell survival. In contrast, PC-3 cells overexpressing MnSOD had less ROS production, less lipid peroxidation, and greater cell survival compared to PC-3 Wt cells. **Since MnSOD removes superoxide, these results suggest that superoxide free radical or its reaction products are responsible for part of the cytotoxicity associated with hyperthermia and that MnSOD can reduce cellular injury and thereby enhance heat tolerance** (Venkataraman et al, 2004). **In light of their data showing that SOD increases peroxide formation in the ETC, this study shows that increased EMODs increase tumoricidal activity and cancer kill and that reduced EMODs reduces an apoptotic response.**

Myeloperoxidase causes H$_2$O$_2$-induced apoptosis of HL-60 human leukemia cells

Investigators examined the mechanism of H$_2$O$_2$-induced cytotoxicity and its relationship to oxidation in human leukemia cells. The **HL-60 promyelocytic leukemia cell line** was sensitive to H$_2$O$_2$, and at concentrations up to about 20-25 micrometer, the killing was mediated by apoptosis. There was limited evidence of lipid peroxidation, suggesting that the effects of H$_2$O$_2$ do not involve hydroxyl radical. When HL-60 cells were exposed to H$_2$O$_2$ in the presence of the spin trap alpha-(4-pyridyl-1-oxide)-N-tert-butylnitrone (POBN), we detected a 12-line electron paramagnetic resonance spectrum assigned to the POBN/POBN(.) N-centered spin adduct previously described in peroxidase-containing cell-free systems. Generation of this radical by HL-60 cells had the same H$_2$O$_2$ concentration dependence as initiation of apoptosis. In contrast, studies with the **K562 human erythroleukemia cell line**, which is often used for comparison with the HL-60, and with high passaged HL-60 cells (spent HL-60) studied under the same conditions failed to generate POBN(.). Cellular levels of antioxidant enzymes superoxide dismutase, glutathione peroxidase, and catalase did not explain the differences between these cell lines. **Interestingly, the K562 and spent HL-60 cells, which did not generate the radical, also failed to undergo H$_2$O$_2$-induced apoptosis.** Based on this we reasoned that the difference in H$_2$O$_2$-induced apoptosis might be due to the enzyme myeloperoxidase. Only the apoptosis-manifesting HL-60 cells contained appreciable immunoreactive protein or enzymatic activity of this cellular enzyme. **When HL-60 cells were incubated with methimazole or 4-aminobenzoic acid hydrazide, which are inhibitors of myeloperoxidase, they no longer underwent H$_2$O$_2$-induced apoptosis. Hypochlorous acid stimulated apoptosis in both HL-60 and spent HL-60 cells, indicating that another oxidant generated by myeloperoxidase induces apoptosis and that it may be the direct mediator of H$_2$O$_2$-induced apoptosis.** Taken together these observations indicate that H$_2$O$_2$-induced apoptosis in the HL-60 human leukemia cell is mediated by myeloperoxidase and is linked to a non-Fenton oxidative event marked by POBN(.). (Wagner et al, 2000). **This emphasizes the role of EMOD-induced apoptosis in cancer cell kill. I have seen this over and over.**

Changing an antioxidant to a prooxidant

Increasing SOD in general causes a non-cytotoxic, growth inhibitory effect. They have shown that **increasing SOD while at the same time inhibiting peroxide removal changes the non-cytotoxic effect to a cytotoxic effect. I believe that this is simply due to a concentration effect.** Removal of peroxide can be inhibited by drugs like BCNU, which among other effects also inhibits the activity of the protein glutathione reductase (GR). Inhibition of GR prevents the conversion of GSSG back to GSH and thus interferes with the removal of peroxides by the GPx pathway. Thus, they have used adenoviral MnSOD (Ad*MnSOD*) plus BCNU to successfully treat animal xenograft models of human head and neck cancer. (Weydert et al, 2003).

As mentioned above, even though they were able to demonstrate a significant growth inhibitory effect of Ad*MnSOD* by itself, **they did not think that this treatment would be an effective clinical antitumor therapy.** This is because when they stop injecting the adenovirus, the cancer cells may start proliferating again. The resumption of proliferation is likely because the adenovirus does not integrate into the genome, but replicates episomally. Thus, with time in a dividing cell population, the transgene is diluted. **In humans, they cannot give more than a few injections of the adenovirus, because an immune response is mounted against the virus.** This presumed lack of a persistent growth regulatory effect prompted us to try a different approach to circumvent this shortcoming: combination of adenovirus with cytotoxic anticancer agents. In this approach, the short life of the adenovirus is not a shortcoming, but a benefit. The adenovirus is given, causes cell killing in conjunction with the cytotoxic agent, and then disappears. Thus, any negative effect of the adenovirus will not linger.

The enzymatic effect of MnSOD protein is to dismute superoxide radical into hydrogen peroxide. **If we inhibit hydrogen peroxide removal, then we should kill the cancer because of direct toxicity or hydrogen peroxide-mediated damage.** They have tested their anticancer concept *in vitro* in stable plasmid transfected rat glioma cells and found very positive results. (Zhong et al, 1995).

The higher the MnSOD levels, the higher the killing they observed in cells treated with 1,3-bis(2-chloroethyl)-1-nitrosourea (BCNU). BCNU is a clinically used anticancer drug that causes alkylation and also **inhibits glutathione reductase** (GR). **If GR is inhibited, cells cannot remove hydrogen peroxide.** (Zhong et al, 1995). This work led them to believe that Ad*MnSOD* plus BCNU could be used in the treatment of oral cancer and they have shown that this is a successful combination in this cancer. (Weydert et al, 2003).

This therapy relies on the endogenous levels of superoxide radical to act as a substrate for SOD. They have observed even greater antitumor efficacy in human breast cancer xenograft models by increasing the levels of superoxide radical so there is more substrate for the SOD. **Superoxide radical were increased by giving adriamycin or ionizing radiation.** Thus, a very effective treatment of breast cancer was obtained by giving Ad*MnSOD*, waiting two days to induce the

MnSOD, and then giving BCNU followed by ionizing radiation. **I believe that all of this served to increase H_2O_2 level, which was the tumoricidal agent.**

One of the problems with understanding this therapy is that BCNU has other effects besides inhibition of GR. In order to study whether the effects of BCNU are due to GR inhibition, they have also inhibited GR with more specific reagents. They have shown that inhibition of GR with siRNA also leads to increased killing when given with Ad*MnSOD*. This observation suggests that at least part of the antitumor effect observed with BCNU is due to inhibition of GR and thus inhibition of peroxide removal. **Again, I believe that this illustrates the tumoricidal activity of H_2O_2.**

There are a myriad of ways one could use the antioxidant pathways to treat cancer. One could try the two other forms of SOD and indeed CuZnSOD has been shown to have a similar anticancer effect as MnSOD. **A second important strategy would be to inhibit as many of the peroxide removing pathways as possible.** For example, since MnSOD is a mitochondrial protein, **inhibition of peroxide removing enzymes** in the mitochondria would be predicted to be particularly effective. **There are at least four of these proteins: GPx1, GPx4 (long form), Prx3, and Prx5.** Similarly, overexpression of CuZnSOD should be effective with inhibition of cytosolic peroxide removing proteins like GPx1, GPx4 (short form), and Prx2.

Apparently, it has never occurred to Oberley or Buettner that all that has to be done to kill cancer is to effectively increase EMOD levels, especially those of H_2O_2 and singlet oxygen.

Techniques to deliver SOD should also be considered. Different gene therapies need to be investigated besides adenovirus. Moreover, SOD can be delivered as a drug via the various SOD mimetic compounds and this technique may allow a higher percentage of cancer cells to be treated. Similarly, inhibition of peroxide removing proteins can be accomplished either with drugs or with molecular biological techniques such as siRNA or antisense oligos.

Another possibility is to decrease the SODs, rather than increase. It has already been shown that all three SODs are necessary for cell health and thus decreasing SOD should also kill cancer cells. SOD could be decreased by techniques like siRNA or antisense oligos. Of course, this could only work if cancer cells were killed more than normal cells. This is a possibility since in general **normal cells have more SOD, particularly MnSOD, than cancer cells**. Indeed, this difference in antioxidant levels between normal and cancer cells is what makes these possibilities so attractive. I believe that **the lower SOD cancer cell level is another example of the cancer cell trying to protect itself from EMOD activated apoptotis, similar to the fact that cancer cells have higher levels of antioxidants such as glutathione, vitamin C and lactic acid.**

Antitumor therapy via enzymatic generation of hydrogen peroxide

Hydrogen peroxide (H_2O_2) is a strong oxidant that induces apoptosis of tumor cells in vitro. Here, we investigated the antitumor activity of an H_2O_2-generating enzyme, D-amino acid oxidase (DAO), and its conjugate with polyethylene glycol (PEG; PEG-DAO). Compared with DAO, PEG-DAO showed improved pharmacokinetic parameters in mice after i.v. injection. PEG-DAO administered i.v. accumulated selectively in tumor tissue with insignificant accumulation in normal organs and tissues. To generate cytotoxic H_2O_2 at the tumor site, PEG-DAO was first administrated i.v. to tumor-bearing mice. After an adequate lag time, the substrate of DAO, D-proline, was injected i.p. This treatment resulted in significant suppression of tumor growth compared with tumor growth in control animals (not given treatment; $P < 0.001$). Similar treatment with native DAO showed no effect under the same conditions. Oxidative metabolites were significantly increased in solid tumors by administration of PEG-DAO followed by D-proline ($P < 0.002$, compared with the group receiving no treatment), as evidenced by thiobarbituric acid-reactive substance assay. This treatment did not affect results from the metabolites in the liver and kidney. These findings suggest that tumor-targeted delivery of DAO is accomplished by using pegylated enzyme and thereby taking advantage of the enhanced permeability and retention effect in solid tumor. **PEG-DAO thus delivered together with D-proline produces remarkable antitumor activity via extensive generation of H_2O_2.** (Fang et al, 2002).

Catalase blocks H_2O_2 tumoricidal activity

N-ß-Alanyl-5-S-glutathionyl-3,4-dihydroxyphenylalanine **(5-S-GAD) exhibits selective cytotoxicity toward certain human tumor cell lines. 5-S-GAD has been shown to release hydrogen peroxide autonomously.** Hydrogen peroxide is converted to water and oxygen by catalase. The purpose of this study is to determine whether or not 5-S-GAD exhibits **selective cytotoxicity toward tumor cells** with low catalase levels, but not toward ones with high catalase levels. They transfected **MDA-MB-435S cells** (originally a model for **metastatic human breast cancer but now genetically tests more closely to human melanoma cell lines**), which are sensitive to 5-S-GAD, with catalase cDNA to establish high catalase producer cells, and then examined their 5-S-GAD sensitivity.

Similarly, they repressed catalase expression in T47D cells, which are insensitive to 5-S-GAD, by catalase RNA interference to create low catalase producer cells, and then examined their 5-S-GAD sensitivity. They show that **the overexpression of catalase made MDA-MB-435S cells insensitive to 5-S-GAD**, whereas **the suppression of catalase made T47D cells sensitive to 5-S-GAD. The cellular catalase level was found to be crucial for cell sensitivity to 5-S-GAD** (Nishikawa et al, 2004).

Catalase over-expression blocks apoptosis and increases tumor growth

Glucocorticoids are used for the treatment of lymphoid neoplasms, taking advantage of the well-known ability of these compounds to cause apoptosis in lymphoid tissues. Previously, we have shown that **dexamethasone, a synthetic glucocorticoid, causes a down-regulation of several antioxidant defense enzymes and proteins, including catalase and thioredoxin, concomitant with the induction of apoptosis in WEHI7.2 mouse thymoma cells.** To test whether this down-regulation plays a critical role in the mechanism of steroid-induced apoptosis, WEHI7.2 cells were transfected with rat catalase. Two clones, expressing 1.4-fold and 2.0-fold higher catalase specific activity, respectively, when compared with vector-only transfectants were selected for further study. An increase to 1.4-fold parental cell catalase activity delayed cell loss after dexamethasone treatment, whereas a 2.0-fold parental catalase activity prevented dexamethasone-induced cell loss for 48 h after treatment. Dexamethasone treatment of the WEHI7.2 cells stimulated a release of cytochrome *c* into the cytosol. **Catalase-overexpressing cells showed a delay or lack of cytochrome c release from the mitochondria, which correlated temporally with the delay or prevention of cell loss in the culture after dexamethasone treatment.** A decreased amount of cell death from WEHI7.2 cells overexpressing catalase was also seen in tumor xenografts in severe combined immunodeficient mice when compared with tumors from vector-only transfected cells. Similarly, thioredoxin-overexpressing WEHI7.2 cells, shown previously to be apoptosis resistant, showed decreased cell death in tumor xenografts. This resulted in larger tumors from cells overexpressing these proteins. Cell death in control transfectant tumor xenografts was primarily attributable to apoptosis. In contrast, the cell death we observed in tumors from thioredoxin- or catalase-overexpressing cells had a higher frequency of a nonapoptotic, nonnecrotic type of cell death termed

para-apoptosis. These data suggest that: (*a*) **oxidative stress plays a critical role in steroid-induced apoptosis prior to the commitment of the cells to undergo apoptosis; and (*b*) resistance to oxidative stress can**

contribute to tumor growth. (Tome et al, 2001). I believe that again this emphasizes the true nature of EMOD induced apoptosis in tumor cells.

NAC is shown to abolish the anticancer effect of vitamin D3

The synergistic interaction was accompanied by **increased oxidative stress,** as manifested by glutathione depletion and was **abolished by exposure to the thiol antioxidant N-acetylcysteine.** The hormone, on its own, brought about an increase in the cellular redox state as reflected in the ratio between oxidized and reduced glutathione and glyceraldehyde-3-phosphate dehydrogenase, and **a reduction in the expression of the antioxidant enzyme Cu/Zn superoxide dismutase.** These results support the notion that the interplay between active vitamin D derivatives and other anticancer agents such as immune cytokines and anticancer drugs plays a role in the in vivo anticancer activity of vitamin D and that **reactive oxygen species are involved in the anticancer activity of vitamin D on its own and in its cross-talk with other anticancer modalities** (The role of reactive oxygen species in the anticancer activity of vitamin D. A. Ravid and R. Koren. Recent Results Cancer Res. 2003;164:357-67). **Again, NAC is shown to abolish the anticancer effect of EMODs and represents a danger if used in patients with neoplasia. Note that NAC reduces SOD levels, which would decrease peroxide production.**

With retinoblastoma, we have tissue which uses more oxygen that any other in the body on a per gram basis. Yet, it has an extremely rare occurrence rate of cancer, which is contrary to the teachings of the Free Radi-crap theory.

I believe that this is analogous to the fact that tumors are rare in the brain, heart, thyroid and the retina, even though they have the highest oxygen consumption levels, with high EMOD generation (and low antioxidant levels) in the body. Ergo, tumorigenesis is not related to EMOD levels.

Antioxidants blocked cancer cell apoptosis

Studies have investigated the effects of antioxidant supplementation on cancer therapy. Studies on cisplatin indicate that it kills breast cancer cells by apoptosis and necrosis, and that the addition of vitamin E blocks much of the apoptotic process. High-dose vitamin E reduces the efficacy of cisplatin, although the normal cells involved would be protected by vitamin E. Lymphoma cells treated with 5 Gy of radiation die or stop dividing, but if *N*-acetylcysteine is added to the media, the lymphoma cells keep growing.

Vitamin E succinate also protects cells against the effects of radiation in vitro. I believe that this answers the questionable use of antioxidants during chemotherapy and irradiation. There is no conclusive evidence to show which antioxidant doses or mixtures protect cells against DNA damage and lipid and protein oxidation but do not interfere with apoptosis signaling pathways. **Over supplementation may actually produce an environment that is beneficial to the tumor and allow it to survive.**

Despite the findings, however, patients still are consuming vast numbers of these antioxidant vitamins, and there may be no way to persuade them to stop.

Elesclomol (formerly STA-4783) oxidative EMOD apoptosis: blocked by NAC

Elesclomol (formerly STA-4783) is a novel small molecule undergoing clinical evaluation in a pivotal phase III melanoma trial (SYMMETRY). **In a phase II randomized, double-blinded, controlled, multi-center trial in 81 patients with stage IV metastatic melanoma, treatment with elesclomol plus paclitaxel showed a statistically significant doubling of progression-free survival time compared with treatment with paclitaxel alone.**

Although elesclomol displays significant therapeutic activity in the clinic, the mechanism underlying its anticancer activity has not been defined previously. Here, we show that **elesclomol induces apoptosis in cancer cells through the induction of oxidative stress.** Treatment of cancer cells in vitro with elesclomol resulted in the rapid generation of reactive oxygen species (ROS) and the induction of a transcriptional gene profile characteristic of an oxidative stress response. Inhibition of oxidative stress by the antioxidant N-acetylcysteine blocked the induction of gene transcription by elesclomol. In addition, **N-acetylcysteine blocked drug-induced apoptosis**, indicating that ROS generation is the primary mechanism responsible for the proapoptotic activity of elesclomol. Excessive ROS production (above normal cell levels) and elevated levels of oxidative stress are critical biochemical alterations that are found in cancer cells. Thus, the **induction of oxidative stress by elesclomol exploits this unique characteristic of cancer cells by increasing ROS levels beyond a threshold that triggers cell death.** (Kirshner et al, 2008).

Synta anticancer mechanism: STA-4783 causes EMOD apoptosis: blocked by NAC

The following was excerpted from an article by Mike Nagle dated Oct. 1, 2007.

Although it is over forty years since scientists realised cancer cells don't have the anti-oxidant protective capabilities of normal cells, it seems that only one pharma company has developed a drug to exploit this fact. Synta Pharmaceuticals, based in Massachusetts, US, is preparing to test its lead drug, STA-4783, on skin cancer patients in the final stage of clinical development.

"We are all taught free radicals are really bad, but scientists have found that cancer cells have increased levels of ROS and their ability to keep that in check is severely compromised," explained Dr Tony Williams, vice president of clinical research at the company.

By increasing the number of reactive oxygen species (ROS) in cells, STA-4783 can tip tumors cells beyond the breaking point into a death pathway (apoptosis). While these cells die, normal cells have less ROS and can shield themselves against the drug's effects.

In fact, when the drug has been tested in normal cell lines, there is no measurable increase in ROS levels, according to Williams.

Although the interest in this mechanism has rocketed in recent years (in 2006, there were over 3500 papers in journals about it, almost doubling the total number ever), Synta claims to be the only pharmaceutical industry pursuing it.

Williams explained that although some anticancer drugs increase ROS levels indirectly to a lesser extent, none do it as or directly, like Synta's molecule. The drug is not potent enough to work as a monotherapy unless the dose is dangerously high, said Williams; instead the drug is seen as a method of increasing a cell's sensitivity to chemotherapy. In this setting, it has shown promising results in clinical studies so far. Dr Williams was speaking to DrugResearcher.com before presenting the Phase II trial results to delegates at the European Congress of Clinical Oncology (ECCO) in Barcelona, Spain.

"The median progression free survival was 1.8 months in the group who got chemotherapy alone, but 3.7 months in the group who got the combination," he said. **"This doubling in progression free survival is impressive for this cancer,** and the result was achieved without substantial additional toxicity."

He added: "Progression-free survival was linked to improvements in overall survival. Patients on the experimental combination survived on average for 12 months after being diagnosed, while those getting only paclitaxel survived on average 7.8 months. **This is the first time an improvement in survival has been seen in a randomised, double-blind, multi-centre controlled trial for metastatic melanoma."**

While investigating the drug's mechanism, the team at Synta discovered that **once melanoma cells are exposed to the drug, levels of Heat Shock Protein 70 (Hsp70) shoot up over 300-fold in just one to three hours.** However, this is a "futile response," said Williams and over the next two to three hours, a switch inside the cell's mitochondria is triggered and the cells begin to die.

Although Hsp70 is not the target of the drug, as some have mistakenly thought, the increase in Hsp70 is, however, useful as a biomarker to prove the therapy is working. **For example, if the drug is given alongside antioxidants (such as NAC, N-AcetylCysteine), no extra Hsp70 is produced and the cells survive as normal.**

Williams said the company is unwilling to disclose the target as yet but hopes to soon once the programme is fully protected in terms of intellectual property (IP).

NAC is normally administered to people who have taken a paracetamol (acetaminophen) overdose, and Williams assured DrugResearcher.com that normal dietary levels of antioxidants shouldn't prevent STA-4783 from working, although he did say that **patients in the upcoming Phase III trial were told not to take any vitamin E supplements (an antioxidant).**

Melanoma is easily treated with surgery in its early stages and five-year survival rates are 99 per cent for localised disease, according to the American Cancer Society. However, once the cancer progresses to later stage, metastatic disease, survival rates plummet to just 15 per cent. STA-4783 is being tested in patients with advanced disease (stage IV metastatic melanoma), who desperately need more treatment options.

Most of the world's biggest pharma companies are developing drugs for melanoma. Pfizer's CP-675206 (tremelimumab/ticilimumab) and Bristol-Myers Squibb's (BMS) ipilimumab are both in Phase III clinical trials, the latter being developed in conjunction with Medarex. The drugs are antibodies against cytotoxic T-lymphocyte antigen-4 (CTLA-4), which is thought to suppress the immune system's T cell response to cancer.

AstraZeneca is testing a MEK inhibitor in Phase II trials. MEK is so called after the MAPK/ERK kinase pathway it belongs to. This cascade of extracellular signal-regulated kinases (ERK) or mitogen-activated protein kinases (MEPK) are thought to be involved in a number of processes that promote cancer, including cell growth and survival.

Novartis is utilising a different target in the same pathway, namely b-RAF kinase to design melanoma drugs. RAF265 is currently in Phase I clinical trials. Roche and Plexxikon's PLX4032/R7204 is at the same stage of development and targets the same protein.

Genzyme is looking at a transforming growth factor (TGF)-beta inhibitor, GC-1008, as a means of treating melanoma in Phase I/II clinical trials. Astellas Pharma's YM155, a survivin expression inhibitor is in Phase II trials.

With these and other melanoma drugs filling oncology pipelines globally, the outlook for patients with advanced melanoma might not be so bleak in the future.

This is not as good as the Howes singlet oxygen generating system.

CHAPTER SIX:

EMODs and spontaneous cancer regression

EMODs cause spontaneous regression of cancer (melanoma)

Investigators described before that **oxidative burst of granulocytes is cytotoxic for melanoma B16F10 and for Walker 256 carcinoma (W256)**. Therefore, we assumed that granulocytes could also be important mechanism of the host defense against tumor. In current study we report **massive granulocyte infiltration at the site of W256 transplanted in the hind limb of Sprague–Dawley associated with spontaneous tumor regression observed for 22/25 rats (87%). Peripheral blood granulocytes of these animals were highly cytotoxic for W256 cells cultured in vitro**. After the tumor disappearance the inflammatory oxidative burst of the granulocytes ended. Distraction of granulocytes from the tumor by s.c. Sephadex injection decreased the incidence of the W256 regression to only 7/25 animals (30%). These results suggest that **innate immunity based on immune competent granulocytes may be the cause of well known phenomenon of spontaneous regression of W256 carcinoma.** (Jaganjac et al, 2008).

Hyperthermia inhibits tumor growth with EMODs

Also, we must remember that hyperthermia has tumoricidal properties, which is, in part, due to increased EMODs.

Tumor cells are selectively inhibited by hyperthermia (41–42.5°C) in the same conditions where normal cells are not damaged. At higher temperature, also normal cells are injured. In spite of the large number of reports on the cytotoxic effect of hyperthermia the mechanisms of heat cytotoxicity are yet unclear. It appears plausible that concomitant phenomena, triggered by heat, and related each other, may be involved. The major points on this subject are the following: **Heat appears to increase the flux of oxygen free radicals mediating, at least in part, the cytotoxicity.** (Pietrangeli, Mondovi, 2008).

Hyperthermia speculation

A similar correlation has been reported between the speed of aging and body temperature. It is most apparent in cold-blooded organisms, which change their metabolic rate in accordance with their body temperature. **When**

earthworms adapt to a temperature rise from 15 to 30°C, its tissues undergo a 28% increase in the level of superoxide dismutase and its oxygen consumption rises by 135%. Since this level of increased oxygen consumption cannot be accounted for by the rise in superoxide dismutase activity, it has been proposed to be the reason for the considerably higher lifespan of the earthworm at 15°C. **I believe that this is the reason that we have developed a febrile response to infections and pathogen protection. This may also be the beneficial basis of hyperthermia therapy.**

Non-protein anti-oxidants may increase lifespan in short-living strains of mice by 30 to 33%. Experiments on transgenic animals are very promising but inconsistent. In a very early study of superoxide dismutase, the DNA of copper-bearing superoxide dismutase was implanted in drosophila by genetic engineering methods. This genetic modification resulted in its **increased activity and modest, but significant, lifespan increase**. Drosophila with complementary copies of genes of superoxide dismutase and catalase lived longer than control animals by 20 to 37%. Additionally, transgenic drosophila demonstrated signs of improved age-related characteristics; decreased accumulation of carbonyl proteins; decreased oxygen-sensitive enzyme inactivation as well as decreased accumulation of oxygen damaged DNA products; and reduced generation rate of oxidants in mitochondria. Recent studies have shown **lifespan increases of 40% in drosophila with abundant human superoxide dismutase gene expressions in motor neurons. I believe that this is directly due to the increased peroxide generation by SOD, which maintains an EMOD sufficiency.**

(Accessed 7-19-09 http://www.abcvitaminslife.com/HealthFacts/ Article428.aspx)

It has occurred to me that conditions such as hypothyroidism could be because of a peroxide deficiency (EMOD insufficiency). Since peroxide serves as a substrate for thyroxine synthesis, a low level of peroxide would result in low levels of thyroxine synthesis. This could be extrapolated to other peroxidases, in that deficiencies in peroxide would result in low levels of their respective reaction products and with the consequent manifestation of the associated symptoms or disease.

It appears to me that chronic disease syndrome is intimately related to energy metabolism, which is closely related to the electron transport chain and oxidative phosphorylation. This focuses attention to the EMODs being in a deficiency state.

Hyperoxia increases spontaneous regression

Pulmonary neuroendocrine cell (PNEC) hyperplasia is associated with chronic lung diseases in humans, where it is thought to play a role in reparative responses to lung injury. To investigate the kinetics of strongly induced PNEC hyperplasia in an animal model, we exposed hamsters to a combination of **hyperoxia (60% O2)** and diethylnitrosamine (DEN) for up to 20 weeks. We thus demonstrate not only **the induction but also spontaneous regression of intense PNEC differentiation and growth, which are much more intense than those observed with DEN alone.** (Sunday, Willett, 1992). **I believe that this illustrates the positive impact of hyperoxia on spontaneous regression.**

Spontaneous regression of cancer

Because most cancers that are detected are also treated, **there are only a few reports documenting spontaneous regression of breast cancer.** (Dussan et al, 2008) (Krutchik et al, 1978).

However, **spontaneous regression of advanced cancer has long been recognized in metastatic melanoma and metastatic renal cell carcinoma,** and, in fact, such observations have motivated the interest in immunotherapy in these settings. (Printz 2001) (Gleave et al, 1998) (de Gast et al, 2000).

Furthermore, **more systematic investigations of spontaneous regression are beginning to be reported in the context of screen-detected abnormalities.** There are data suggesting that **regression routinely occurs in colonic adenomas** (both from the National Polyp Study and others) (Loeve et al, 2004) (Hofstad et al, 1996).

There is a growing literature **documenting regression in precancerous lesions of the cervix.** (Schlecht et al, 2003) (Moscicki et al, 2004).

Documentation of regression in screen-detected cancer is limited to neuroblastoma, for which investigators have found that screening detects far more cancer than will ever become clinically apparent and that a substantial proportion regress. (Schilling et al, 2002) (Yamamoto et al, 1998).

Spontaneous regression has been seen in:

- **metastatic melanoma**
- **metastatic renal cell carcinoma**

- **precancerous lesions of the cervix**
- **neuroblastoma**
- **some prostate cancer**
- **some lung cancer**

Spontaneous regression of malignant breast cancer

Spontaneous regression of malignant tumors is a rare event. It is defined as partial or total disappearance of a proven malignant tumor without adequate medical treatment. The causes of this phenomenon are various. Nevertheless, **malignant tumors do regress occasionally for no apparent reason,** as evidenced by many clinical observations. We report a case of a 68-year-old woman, who was presented with a several-month history of a painless firm lump, initially of 1 cm in diameter and growing to a large solid regular tumor of 2.5 × 2.5 cm in size, in the upper outer quadrant of her right breast. Preoperative histopathological diagnosis revealed ductal invasive carcinoma. Later on, while awaiting surgical treatment, she suffered an arm injury requiring a 1-month delay of surgery. After recovery, on the date of surgery the tumor disappeared, and, in addition, it was not found in tissue specimens obtained from quadrantectomy. After 78 months of follow-up there was no evidence of relapse. In this report, we discuss clinical and histopathological findings, patient management and possible mechanisms of cancer regression. (Dussan et al, 2008). **I believe that the "trauma" of the biopsy could have stimulated a strong oxidative WBC response, which produced EMODs and caused the apoptosis.**

Some breast cancers may resolve without treatment

The following article was provided by: Canadian Press and written by: Helen Branswell on Nov. 24, 2008.

A significant portion of invasive breast cancers may regress on their own without treatment, a new study that is bound to provoke controversy suggests.

The study, published 11/24/08 in the journal Archives of Internal Medicine, suggested **breast cancer screening may be leading to over diagnosis of cancer,** with upwards of 22 per cent of cases likely to resolve themselves without treatment.

Once a breast cancer is found, however, it wouldn't currently be considered ethical not to treat. So - **if the theory is correct - large numbers of women may be having surgeries, radiation, chemotherapy and other treatments that would never have been needed if their cancers hadn't bee**"If we are right, then this is a kind of paradigm shift," said lead author Dr. Per-Henrik Zahl, a senior statistician with the Norwegian Institute of Public Health. Zahl, who admitted he has been trying to get the study published for about four years, said the risks of over diagnosis of breast cancer are real.

Radiation can do significant and permanent damage to the heart and coronary arteries. Chemotherapy can cause cognitive confusion. And surgery that involves the removal of lymph nodes can cause lymphedema, the painful swelling of the arm closest to the involved breast.

Dr. Patrick Remington has been studying the idea of self-limiting breast cancers since the early 1990s, when the introduction of breast screening programs showed a sharp and sustained increase in the incidence of the disease in the United States. **He is convinced some invasive breast cancers do regress**; they have become known as **LMPs or cancers of "limited malignant potential."**

"I would say a very good guess would be about one out of three women have cancers detected today that would not have progressed otherwise," said Remington, a professor of population health sciences at the University of Wisconsin. Remington was not involved in this study. He notes **some other types of cancers - prostate and recently lung - have been shown to spontaneously regress in some patients**.

In the case of prostate cancer, some physicians urge an approach known as watchful waiting, where patients are monitored to see if their disease is progressing; only then is it treated. That approach is not currently an option with breast cancer.

Zahl's findings are likely to spark heated debate. In fact, he acknowledged several journals refused to publish the study before it was accepted by Archives of Internal Medicine, a journal published by the American Medical Association.

But an editorial in the journal stressed that **the findings are consistent with several observations about breast cancer that have troubled investigators for years**.

And the editorial's authors, Dr. Robert Kaplan of the UCLA School of Public Health and Dr. Franz Porzsolt of Germany's Clinical Economics University of Ulm, said **the hypothesis of breast cancer regression, while counterintuitive, is "difficult to rule out."**

"We know from autopsy studies that a significant number of women die (from other causes) without knowing that they had breast cancer," they noted.

Dr. Steven Narod, a leading breast cancer researcher at Toronto's Sunnybrook Health Sciences Centre, agreed the findings are persuasive. "I do agree with them that the best explanation of the findings is that about 10 to 20 per cent of the breast cancers ... disappeared on their own," he said. "I'm still a bit skeptical and there's alternative explanations, but I think this one is worth paying attention to."

In what Narod described as an "elegant" study design, Zahl and his colleagues used the introduction of a breast cancer screening program in Norway to explore the question.

They compared breast cancer rates among nearly **120,000 women** who had three rounds of mammography between 1996 and 2001 to those among nearly 110,000 women of the same age range (50 to 64) in the five-year period preceding the start of the breast cancer screening program. Those women, known as the controls, had one mammogram.

In statistical terms, the two groups of women were identical. Their educational profile was closely matched, they had roughly the same average family income and the same average number of children. So the rates of cancers in the two groups should have been equal.

In fact, **the women who hadn't been regularly screened had 22 per cent fewer breast cancers.**

The authors explore a number of arguments about why that might be. They noted for instance that use of hormone replacement therapy in the part of Norway where the women lived increased substantially between 1996 and 2001, the period when the screened women were undergoing regular mammograms. **HRT use is linked to increased risk of breast cancer.**

But the authors conclude that none of the other explanations could account for such a large difference between the two groups.

"All the caveats that could be explored have been explored in terms of accounting for the things that people would call ... weaknesses" of the study, agreed Dr. Cornelia Baines, a professor in the University of Toronto's school of public health and co-principal investigator of a landmark study into mammography, the Canadian National Breast Screening Study.

Baines, who has been diagnosed with breast cancer which was earlier missed in a mammogram, said the findings are important. But she added that even if Zahl and his co-authors are correct, there's no way currently to put the findings into application. "The incontrovertible truth is that once you've screened a woman and you find an abnormality, you have to biopsy," she said.

"If you biopsy, you have to follow through with surgery if the biopsy reveals malignant tissue. You can't stop that. You can't say: 'Well, I've been screened and there is a chance that this is over diagnosis.' You can't do that."

Finding ways to answer the questions raised by the study will be difficult, experts said. And Remington noted even if doctors could differentiate, women and-or their health-care professionals might still opt for treatment to play it safe.

He suggested, though, **studying women whose cancers regress on their own could teach scientists how to trigger the same response in women whose cancers aren't self-limiting**, and maybe even to prevent breast cancer from developing.

And in the meantime, Baines said, this study may serve as an important reminder to women and the medical community.

"What is important and it seems to me it's been ignored for a long, long time is that ... screening doesn't only have upsides. It has downsides," she said.

"And if women want to accept the downsides and proceed with screening, then that's great. But I personally believe that they should only make that choice when they are fully informed. And a lot of them have not been fully informed about the over diagnosis scenario."

The natural history of invasive breast cancers detected by screening mammography

Background: The introduction of screening mammography has been associated with sustained increases in breast cancer incidence. The natural history of these screen-detected cancers is not well understood.

Methods: We compared cumulative breast cancer incidence in age-matched cohorts of women residing in 4 Norwegian counties before and after the initiation of biennial mammography. The screened group included all women who were invited for all 3 rounds of screening during the period 1996 through 2001 (age range in 1996, 50-64 years). The control group included all women who would have been invited for screening had there been a screening program during the period 1992 through 1997 (age range in 1992, 50-64 years). All women in the control group were invited to undergo a 1-time prevalence screen at the end of their observation period. Screening attendance was similar in both groups (screened, 78.3%, and controls, 79.5%). Counts of incident invasive breast cancers were obtained from the Norwegian Cancer Registry (in situ cancers were excluded).

Results: As expected, before the age-matched controls were invited to be screened at the end of their observation period, the cumulative incidence of invasive breast cancer was significantly higher in the screened group than in the controls. Even after prevalence screening in controls, however, the cumulative incidence of invasive breast cancer remained 22% higher in the screened group. Higher incidence was observed in screened women at each year of age.

Conclusions: Because the cumulative incidence among controls never reached that of the screened group, **it appears that some breast cancers detected by repeated mammographic screening would not persist to be detectable by a single mammogram at the end of 6 years.** This raises the possibility that **the natural course of some screen-detected invasive breast cancers is to spontaneously regress. (Abstract:** November 24, 2008 edition of the *Archives of Internal Medicine The Natural History of Invasive Breast Cancers Detected by Screening Mammography.* Per-Henrik Zahl, Jan Moehlen, H. Gilbert Welch).

SECTION THREE:

Antioxidants to avoid in cancer patients

CHAPTER SEVEN:

Vitamin Supplements

People should be informed of antioxidant harm

Dr. Gluud said these observations were "a huge disappointment," but added that at least it has been discovered. "We must see the positives in this. **The question has been thoroughly addressed and we now know the answer — these agents are harmful.** The companies selling these anti-oxidant vitamins have been able to dodge the issue for a long time, saying that any negative data has not been comprehensive. They cannot do this any longer. There are lessons to be learnt here. For example, the importance of conducting trials with these agents and publishing the results."

Dr. Gluud added that **food supplements should be regulated in the same way as medical products.** "The governments of the world now have the responsibility to inform people of these results. They have been too slow in the past in requesting that health supplements are properly evaluated, and allowing these products to be added to foods. People have been buying these supplements and foods advertised as having these supplements added under the impression that they are good for them, when in actual fact they are harmful. **Any potential health supplements should not be allowed to be added to foods unless they have been shown to be beneficial, or at least proven not to be harmful.**" (Bjelakovic et al, 2007).

People who take antioxidant vitamins such as A, C and E -- long touted as protecting against cancer, heart disease and other health problems - don't live any longer, new research shows.

Worse yet, **there is actually evidence that they die younger than people who don't take vitamins.**

"Our findings contradict the findings of observational studies claiming that antioxidants improve health," said Goran Bjelakovic, a researcher at the Centre for Clinical Intervention Research at Copenhagen University Hospital in Denmark.

The review examined the effects of beta carotene, vitamins A, E and C and selenium in the deaths of more than 230,000 adults involved in

trials. (Skibsted et al, 2006). When looking at both low and high-quality studies, they found no significant link between vitamin use and death.

But high quality results analyzed alone showed an average 5 per cent increase in mortality for the three supplements vitamins A and E and beta carotene.

Antioxidant vitamins are bad for your health

Antioxidant supplements have failed to decrease cardiovascular risk in extensive human clinical trials to date. Paradoxically, many well-established components of the heart-healthy lifestyle are prooxidant, including polyunsaturated fat, exercise and moderate alcohol consumption. Oxidation includes distinct biochemical reactions, and it is overly simplistic to gather them into a unitary process that affects all cell types and metabolic pathways adversely. Guidelines for diet should adhere closely to what has been clinically proved, and by this standard there is no basis to recommend antioxidant use, beyond what is inherent to the 'heart healthy' diet in order to benefit cardiovascular health. (Williams, Fisher, 2005).

Danish researchers warned that consumers should be cautious about taking supplements containing nutrients. Supplements that millions of North Americans take to stave off disease and slow the aging process do not boost longevity and appear to actually increase the risk of dying. Bjelakovic's analysis, which pooled data from 68 studies involving more than 232,000 people, found no evidence that taking beta-carotene, Vitamin A or Vitamin E extends life span. (Bjelakovic et al, 2007).

In fact, Bjelakovic's analysis found that beta carotene, vitamin A and vitamin E, taken singly or combined with other antioxidant supplements, were associated with increased all-cause mortality. The supplements increase the likelihood of dying by about 5 percent, as a conservative estimate. Vitamin C and selenium appeared to have no impact - either way - on longevity.

According to Bjelakovic's study, vitamin supplements taken by millions of people every day for their health could be increasing their risk of death. The international research team, led by Dr. Goran Bjelakovic, reviewed the published evidence on beta carotene, vitamin A, vitamin E, Vitamin C and selenium. These dietary supplements are marketed as antioxidants and people take them in the hope they will improve health and guard against diseases like cancer and heart disease by eliminating the oxgen free radicals that cause so-called "oxidative stress" and allegedly damage and/or kill cells.

Antioxidants are also marketed as anti-aging products because they are thought to slow down the aging process.

In this study, Dr. Bjelakovic and colleagues did a meta-analysis on research published before October 2005. The researchers followed a method established by the Cochrane Collaboration, a group of 6,000 health care specialists who review biomedical trials and other research projects. They started with 815 clinical trials of which 68 passed the first level of quality standard (68 randomized trials with 232,606 participants (385 publications). At this level the results were inconclusive. The supplements were found to have no effect on death risk one way or the other. They then went back and eliminated 21 of the trials, leaving only the "low-bias" ones. This was the next level of quality standard.

Results showed that when all trials of antioxidant supplements were pooled together, there was no significant effect on mortality, but Bjelakovic's analysis found that beta carotene, vitamin A and vitamin E, taken singly or combined with other antioxidant supplements, were associated with increased all-cause mortality. The supplements increase the likelihood of dying by about 5 percent, as a conservative estimate. Vitamin C and selenium had no significant effect on mortality.

Relative Risk for All-Cause Mortality With Antioxidant Vitamins

Trials/Agent	Relative Risk of Mortality With Antioxidant Vitamins	95% Confidence Interval
All trials — all agents	1.02	0.98 - 1.06
Low bias trials — all agents	1.05	1.02 - 1.08
Beta-carotene	1.07	1.02 - 1.11
Vitamin A	1.16	1.10 - 1.24
Vitamin E	1.04	1.01 - 1.07

Source: (Bjelakovic et al, 2007).

The researchers note that more than two thirds of the included trials fell into the category of low-bias risk trials, which they say highlights the validity of their results. "Antioxidant supplements not only seem to be one of the most researched topics in the world, they also seem to be one of the most adequately researched clinical questions," they say.

When looked at separately, they found that **Vitamin A increased death risk by 16 per cent, beta carotene by 7 per cent and Vitamin E by 4 per cent.** *The results for Vitamin C were not so clear, but by looking at the best quality trials there was a suggestion that it increased death risk by 6 per cent, either on its own or in combination with other supplements.* Duration of supplementation differed among the trials but duration had no significant effect on their results.

The figures from the best quality trials on **selenium however showed that it might reduce death risk by 10 per cent,** either on its own or in combination with other supplements, but this was not found to be statistically significant. The overall conclusion of the study was that on balance, the best quality research shows that beta carotene, vitamin A and vitamin E may increase mortality risk, but vitamin C and selenium need further study. Vitamin C can act as a prooxidant or an antioxidant in vivo. (Duarte, Lunec, 2005) (Podmore et al, 1998).

The researchers say there are several potential reasons for these results. One is that the free radicals that are thought to cause the oxidative stress are the byproduct rather than the cause of disease. Another is that they may play an important role in the immune system and eliminating them could be counterproductive. They added that this study is important for public health reasons because **between 10 and 20 per cent of people in Europe and North America take dietary supplements**.

Bjelakovic's findings contradicts the older findings of observational studies, which claimed that antioxidants improved health. (Machlin, Bendich, 1987) (Diplock, 1994) (van Poppel, vanden Berg, 1997) (Diplock et al, 1998).

Some prior studies have resulted in no beneficial or harmful effect of the antioxidant supplements. (Bjelakovic et al, 2006) (Caraballoso et al, 2003) (Vivekanagthan et al, 2003) (Davies et al, 2006) (Huang et al, 2006).

Whereas, other studies reported that antioxidant supplements significantly increased mortality and these findings bolster prior reports, which also showed increased mortality from antioxidants. (Bjelakovic et al. 2004) (Bjelakovic et al, Lancet 2004) (Miller et al, 2005).

Vitamin Supplements: A Word of Caution for Cancer Patients

The finding that vitamin C antagonized (offset) the cytotoxic effects of such a wide range of antineoplastic agents was unexpected.

Cancer patients should avoid the routine use of antioxidant supplements during radiation and chemotherapy because the supplements may reduce the anticancer benefits of therapy, researchers concluded in a commentary published online May 27, 2008 in the Journal of the National Cancer Institute.

Radiation and many chemotherapy agents work to kill cells by inducing free radicals that damage DNA and proteins. Therefore, there is a possibility that taking antioxidant supplements, such as vitamin E or -carotene, may interfere with the therapies and reduce their anticancer activity. On the other hand, some investigators hypothesize that antioxidant supplementation may protect healthy tissues and reduce the side effects of treatment. **Despite two decades of research into this question, no clear answer has appeared.**

To evaluate the potential harms or benefits of antioxidant supplementation, Brian D. Lawenda, M.D., of the Naval Medical Center San Diego and colleagues reviewed all of the randomized trials they could identify that tested the effect of antioxidant supplements on radiation therapy or chemotherapy. (Lawenda et al, 2008).

In the case of radiotherapy, they identified nine studies that addressed the question, including two meta-analyses. However, only three studies were randomized controlled trials designed to look at the clinical effect of antioxidant therapy on radiation. **In the largest of the randomized trials, antioxidant supplementation was associated with a reduction in overall survival.** One antioxidant agent, amifostine, which is already approved by the U.S. Food and Drug Administration to increase radioresistance in healthy salivary gland tissues, may protect normal tissues without increasing tumor radioresistance. Lawenda and colleagues caution that the question needs to be studied further before a solid conclusion can be made.

The authors identified 16 randomized controlled trials that examined the impact of antioxidant supplementation on chemotherapy. Six of the trials were placebo-controlled.

Of the studies that included information on response rates, **none reported a decrease in response in the antioxidant arm of the trial compared with the control arm**. However, Lawenda and colleagues caution that **none of the trials was large enough to reliably detect such differences.**

Despite some intriguing studies that have suggested the benefit of adjunctive antioxidant treatments in cancer patients, the totality of the available evidence is equivocal at best and **leaves us with serious concerns about the potential for harm**, the authors write.

Vit. C reduces benefits of cancer drugs

WASHINGTON -- **Vitamin C supplements may significantly reduce the effectiveness of several anti-cancer drugs**, according to a new study published 10/1/08.

"It is possible that vitamin C supplementation may alter the effectiveness of commonly used chemotherapeutic agents and adversely influence treatment outcome," the researchers write in the October 1, 2008 issue of *Cancer Research*.

In tests on isolated cancer cells in the laboratory, researchers found that **30 to 70 percent fewer of the cells were killed if pretreated with vitamin C.**

In studies of cancer cells in mice, studies found that tumors grew more rapidly if the animal was treated with chemotherapy and also given vitamin C supplements. (Agence France-Presse, First Posted 08:25:00 10/02/2008. Inquirer.net).

Researchers suggest that similar effects may occur in human patients.

"The use of vitamin C supplements could have the potential to reduce the ability of patients to respond to therapy," said Mark Heaney, an Associate Attending Physician at Memorial Sloan-Kettering Cancer Center, and lead author of the study.

Past studies have suggested vitamin C could be beneficial to cancer patients because it is an antioxidant. **In August, 2008, a study showed that injected high doses of vitamin C reduced the size of tumors and slowed cancerous growths by about 50 percent in laboratory mice.**

The new research shows that a number of chemotherapy drugs produce "oxygen free radicals." According to the study's theory, **vitamin C could "sop up the radicals," keeping cancer cells alive despite chemotherapy treatment.**

Heaney said that he suspects vitamin C is good for cells in normal tissue, and extends cell life by protecting the all-important mitochondria, the cell's "power plant" that keeps it running.

"But that isn't what you want when you are trying to eliminate cancer cells," said Heaney.

All cancer chemotherapy drugs work to disrupt the mitochondria, to push for cell death.

The study notes that cancer patients should eat a healthy diet, including foods rich in vitamin C. (Heaney et al, 2008).

Even though **vitamin C treatment led to a dose-dependent decrease in apoptosis in cells treated with the antineoplastic agents** that was not due to up-regulation of P-glycoprotein or vitamin C retention modulated by antineoplastics. Vitamin C had only modest effects on intracellular EMODs (ROS) and a more general cytoprotective profile than N-acetylcysteine, **suggesting a mechanism of action that is not mediated by EMODs (ROS).**

"The use of vitamin C supplements could have the potential to reduce the ability of patients to respond to therapy," said Dr Mark Heaney of Memorial Sloan-Kettering Cancer Center and **he advises his cancer patients to avoid supplemental vitamin C during chemotherapy.** "I recommend that my patients continue to eat a well-balanced diet that includes fruits and vegetables that contain vitamin C."

Oral vitamin C supplementation with doses as low as 250 mg over a 1-month period resulted in intracellular vitamin C concentrations in normal white blood cells that were close to those that we studied in white blood cell cancers," Dr. Heaney said.

"It was notable that the concentration of vitamin C measured in the tumors of the mice in this study was similar to what can be achieved in human leucocytes with oral vitamin C supplementation, suggesting that our study conditions were relevant to clinical conditions," the researchers write.

Does vitamin C kill cancer as an antioxidant or a prooxidant?

the emphasis of these studies in the potential antioxidant properties of vitamin C overlooks the capacity of ascorbate to act as a prooxidant. In our previous studies, we have shown that ascorbate induces apoptosis in B16F10 murine melanomas through mitochondrial dysfunction. (Hahm et al, 2007).

A high dose of ascorbate induced a decrease in mitochondrial membrane potential and a release of cytochrome c from mitochondria to cytosol, which acted to promote apoptosis. A low dose of ascorbate induced cell-cycle arrest of cancer cells. (Kang et al, 2003) (Kim et al, 2008).

Thus, the effect of ascorbate on cancer cells was mediated by an increase in intracellular ROS levels. In addition, we showed that ascorbate, acting as a prooxidant, inhibited cancer cell growth through other mechanisms, including induction of endoplasmic reticulum stress, suppression of insulin-like growth factor production, and inhibition of angiogenic factor production. (Lee et al, 2008) (Ashino et al, 2003).

Levine and colleagues have also reported anticancer activities of ascorbate that were attributable to its prooxidant properties, showing that ascorbate acts as a prooxidant and decreases tumor growth in mice. (Chen et al, 2008).

They also showed that ascorbate produced hydrogen peroxide-dependent cytotoxicity in various cancer cells without affecting normal cells. More importantly, Levine suggested that ascorbate-induced formation of hydrogen peroxide preferentially occurs in extracellular fluid compared with blood. (Chen et al, 2007).

These studies provide a mechanistic basis for applying ascorbate as a prooxidant therapeutic agent for cancer treatment.

More vitamin C confusion

Ascorbate is the reduced form of vitamin C, which also exists physiologically in the oxidized form, dehydroascorbic acid (DHA). DHA is taken up into cells by glucose transporters. (Vera et al, 1993) (Vera et al, 1994).

Inside the cell, it is reduced to ascorbic acid and decreases intracellular ROS levels, thus acting initially as an antioxidant. (Guaiquil et al, 1997) (Guaiquil et al, 2001) (Galleano et al, 2002).

In a recent study, Conner and colleagues reported that all antineoplastic drugs tested produced mitochondrial dysfunction, including loss of mitochondrial membrane potential and an increase in ROS levels, and showed that this phenomenon was inhibited by vitamin C. They postulated that vitamin C acts as an antioxidant to protect cells against mitochondrial dysfunction induced by antineoplastic agents, and thus antagonizes the cytotoxic effects of antineoplastic drugs. (Heaney et al, 2008).

In a similar vein, Blair cautioned that because vitamin C/d (200 mg) induced decomposition of lipid hydroperoxides to endogenous genotoxins, it might be counterproductive in cancer treatment. (Lee et al, 2001) (Lee et al, 2003).

This study was also unable to find support for the notion that vitamin C induced lipid peroxidation. (Levine et al, PNAS 2001).

Thus, the vitamin C controversy continues as to its redox identity. (Lee W, 2009)

More clinical and basic research studies are needed to clarify the scientific support for the clinical plausibility of using vitamin C in the treatment of cancer but **currently, it appears that its tumoricidal activity can be attributed to its prooxidant activity.**

Ascorbate generated H_2O_2 kills cancer cells (Human lymphoma cells)

Human pharmacokinetics data indicate that i.v. ascorbic acid (ascorbate) in pharmacologic concentrations could have an unanticipated role in cancer treatment. Our goals here were to test whether ascorbate killed cancer cells selectively, and if so, to determine mechanisms, using clinically relevant conditions. Cell death in 10 cancer and 4 normal cell types was measured by using 1-h exposures. Normal cells were unaffected by 20 mM ascorbate, whereas 5 cancer lines had EC(50) values of <4 mM, a concentration easily achievable i.v. **Human lymphoma cells** were studied in detail because of their sensitivity to ascorbate (EC(50) of 0.5 mM) and suitability for addressing mechanisms. Extracellular but not intracellular ascorbate mediated cell death, which occurred by apoptosis and pyknosis/necrosis. Cell death was independent of metal chelators and absolutely dependent on H_2O_2 formation. **Cell death from H_2O_2 added to cells was identical to that found when H_2O_2 was generated by ascorbate treatment.** H_2O_2 generation was dependent on ascorbate concentration, incubation time, and the presence of 0.5-10% serum, and displayed a linear relationship with ascorbate radical formation. Although ascorbate addition to medium generated H_2O_2, ascorbate addition to blood generated no detectable H_2O_2 and only trace detectable ascorbate radical. Taken together, these data indicate that **ascorbate at concentrations achieved only by i.v. administration may be a pro-drug for formation of H_2O_2,** and that blood can be a delivery system of the pro-drug to tissues. These findings give plausibility to i.v. ascorbic acid in cancer treatment, and have unexpected implications for treatment of infections where H_2O_2 may be beneficial. (Chen et al, 2005). **I believe that this shows that peroxide, either directly or by ascorbate generation, selectively kills human cancer cells. This is the basis of my singlet oxygen tumoricidal system.**

Many Cancer Patients Take Vitamin C

"Our study is a preclinical model that addresses only the situation when vitamin C is given in the setting of chemotherapy treatment," Dr. Heaney emphasized. There have been no clinical studies of this topic so far, he said.

However, **the finding could be of potential concern because "many people, cancer patients included, take supplemental vitamin C,"** Dr. Heaney pointed out. Clinical studies of vitamin C supplementation in patients with advanced cancers have had mixed results. There are conflicting hypotheses, he explained. One theory is that vitamin C supplementation protects the cancer and is therefore detrimental to the patient. But there is also the opposite view, that vitamin C supplementation enhances the immune system or prevents indolent cancers from mutating more and becoming aggressive, which would be beneficial for the patient.

Asked to comment on this study, Len Lichtenfeld, MACP, deputy chief medical officer at the American Cancer Society said: "Vitamin C has a long history in cancer prevention and treatment. Although there is no evidence to demonstrate that vitamin C improves the outlook for patients with cancer, there are still reported observations that cancer patients continue to believe in the potential benefits of vitamin C. Although oncologists do not routinely recommend that patients with cancer take excessive doses of vitamin C, there are reports that cancer patients are being treated with vitamin C by alternative practitioners."

"Recently, there have been research papers [indicating] that intravenous vitamin C may be beneficial in reducing the growth rates of cancers in laboratory animals. There are human clinical trials underway to determine whether or not this approach will be helpful in patients being treated for cancer," Dr. Lichtenfeld added.

However, he points out that **the current report suggests that in laboratory experiments, adding vitamin C to cancer cells may reduce the effectiveness of cancer chemotherapy drugs.**

"Clearly, there remains an open question as to whether or not vitamin C supplementation is helpful or harmful in the treatment of patients with cancer. Until those questions are resolved with further clinical studies, **it would be inappropriate to recommend that patients take large quantities of vitamin C if they have cancer**," Dr. Lichtenfeld told *Medscape Oncology*. (Heaney et al, 2008).

EMODs from As2O3 kill leukemia cells

Cancer cells are under intrinsic increased oxidative stress and vulnerable to free radical-induced apoptosis. Here, **Pelicano et al.** report a strategy to hinder mitochondrial electron transport and increase superoxide $O_2.-$ radical generation in human leukemia cells as a novel mechanism to enhance apoptosis induced by anticancer agents. This strategy was first tested in a proof-of-principle study using rotenone, a specific inhibitor of mitochondrial electron transport complex I. Partial inhibition of mitochondrial respiration enhances electron leakage from the transport chain, leading to an increase in $O_2.-$ generation and sensitization of the leukemia cells to anticancer agents whose action involve free radical generation. Using leukemia cells with genetic alterations in mitochondrial DNA and biochemical approaches, we further demonstrated **that As_2O_3, a clinically active anti-leukemia agent, inhibits mitochondrial respiratory function, increases free radical generation, and enhances the activity of another $O_2.-$ generating agent against cultured leukemia cells and primary leukemia cells isolated from patients. Pelicano et al.** study shows that interfering mitochondrial respiration is a novel mechanism by which As_2O_3 increases generation of free radicals. This novel mechanism of action provides a biochemical basis for developing new drug combination **strategies using As_2O_3 to enhance the activity of anticancer agents by promoting generation of free radicals.** (Pelicano et al, 2003).

Differential effect of ascorbic acid and NAC on As_2O_3-mediated oxidative stress in human leukemia (HL-60) cells: blocked by NAC

Arsenic trioxide (ATO) has been recommended for the treatment of refractory cases of acute promyelocytic leukemia (APL). Recent studies in our laboratory indicated that **oxidative stress plays a key role in ATO-induced cytotoxicity in human leukemia (HL-60) cells**. In the present investigation, we performed the MTT assay and trypan blue exclusion test for cell viability. We also performed the thiobarbituric acid test to determine the levels of malondialdehyde (MDA) production in HL-60 cells coexposed to either ascorbic acid (AA) and ATO or to n-acetyl-L-cysteine (NAC) and ATO. The results of MTT assay indicated that **AA exposure potentiates the cytotoxicity of ATO in HL-60 cells, as evidenced by a gradual increase in MDA levels with increasing doses** of AA. In contrary, **the addition of NAC to ATO-treated HL-60 cells resulted in a dose-dependent decrease of MDA production.** From these results, we conclude that **the addition of the AA to ATO-treated HL-60 cells enhances the formation of reactive oxygen species (ROS), whereas the addition of NAC under the same experimental condition significantly ($p < .05$) decreases the level of ROS formation.** On the basis of these direct in vitro findings, our studies provide evidence that AA may extend the therapeutic spectrum of ATO. **The coadministration of NAC with ATO shows a potential specificity for tumor cells, indicating that it may not enhance the clinical outcome associated with ATO monotherapy in vivo.** (Yedjou et al, 2008). I believe this shows that **NAC blocks EMOD induced apoptosis and AA enhances it, as I would have expected.**

Arsenic trioxide and ascorbic acid demonstrate promising activity against primary human CLL cells in vitro: blocked by NAC

The compromised antioxidant defense system in **chronic lymphocytic leukemia (CLL)** suggested a potential use for reactive oxygen species (ROS) generating arsenic trioxide (ATO) and ascorbic acid. While both ATO and ascorbic acid mediate cytotoxicity in CLL B cells as single agents, the efficacy of ATO is enhanced by ascorbic acid. This effect is dependent on increased ROS accumulation, as pretreatment of B-CLL cells with a glutathione reducing buthionine sulfoximine or catalase inhibiting aminotriazole, enhanced ATO/ascorbic acid-mediated cytotoxicity. **Pretreatment with reducing agents such as catalase, or thiol antioxidant, N-acetyl cysteine or GSH also abrogated ATO/ascorbic acid-mediated cytotoxicity.** Furthermore, HuID10-mediated cell death was enhanced with ATO and ascorbic acid, thus justifying potential combination of ATO/arsenic trioxide therapy with antibodies such as HuID10 that also cause accumulation of ROS. (Biswas et al, 2010).

Here is just a glimpse at vitamin C

Vitamin C may blunt cancer therapy

In 2008, it was shown that vitamin C supplements may substantially reduce the benefit from a wide range of anti-cancer drugs. Thirty to 70% less cancer cells in a lab were killed by a range of drugs, after pretreatment with vitamin C. **Follow-up chemotherapy tests found tumors grew more rapidly in mice given cancer pretreated with vitamin C.** (http://news.bbc.co.uk/2/hi/health/7643533.stm).

Scientists recently discovered that **cancer cells contain large amounts of vitamin C, which appears to protect them—just as it protects healthy cells—from oxygen damage to the genes. Cancer cells readily take up vitamin C *in vitro*.** (Baader et al, Anticancer Res. 1994) (Spielholz et al. 1997).

Studies have demonstrated high vitamin C concentrations in neoplasms compared with the adjacent normal tissue (Langemann et al, 1989).

As reported on 2-04-09 in the journal *Nature*, Stanford researcher, Robert Cho, found that breast cancer stem cells make much higher levels of protective antioxidants than other cancer cells. Use of a drug to block the antioxidant, glutathione, caused the cancer stem cells to become far more vulnerable to radiation. Using cells from mice and human breast cancer, the antioxidant glutathione protected the cancer cells from being killed by radiation EMOD-induced apoptosis.

I believe that this is why cancer cells have lower MnSOD levels and accumulate vitamin C, just as with glutathione and lactate. The antioxidants are protecting the cancer cells from EMOD induced apoptosis.

Incidentally, it may also be that since atheromatous plaques contain high levels of antioxidants, they are protected from oxidation and excretion.

To repeat, lactic acid is an antioxidant and it is in this capacity that it is advantageous for cancer cells to produce it, such that EMODs can be kept at sub-apoptotic levels. Salts of lactic acid are used in foods as a humecticant and an antioxidant which can increase the effect of other antioxidants.

Prior to these studies, **another mouse study suggested that tumor cells need high amounts of vitamin C to thrive.** Moreover, years ago, **two human studies found that smokers with high levels of beta-carotene in their blood had a higher risk of lung cancer (ATBC and CARET studies),** compared with smokers with low levels of the antioxidant. I believe that this supports my contention that antioxidants lower apoptosis-inducing EMOD levels and can protect cancer cells.

However, we must remember that mega-doses of intravenous vitamin C kill cancer, but it does so because it generates hydrogen peroxide. Ergo, vitamin C actually kills cancer cells in mega-doses "prooxidatively" (Howes R : Cancer Therapy, 2010) (Howes R : Hydrogen Peroxide: 2010).

The idea of using vitamin C to treat and prevent cancer was first proposed in 1949 and later supported by Cameron et al. who, in a controversial study, showed that administration of high-dose ascorbic acid improved the survival of patients with terminal cancer. Their results led to the proposal of using megadoses of vitamin C to combat degenerative diseases, including cancer and CVD.

The inconsistency of the vitamin C-cancer correlation and lack of validated mechanistic basis for its therapeutic action has critically undermined the feasibility of using vitamin C in clinical treatment or prevention of cancer.

Andrew W. Saul states that Linus Pauling took 18,000 mg/day of vitamin C. Pauling died from cancer in 1994. Dr. Charles Moertel of the Mayo Clinic, critic of vitamin C, died of cancer the same year. Moertel was 66. Pauling was 93. Did vitamin C fail to cure Pauling's cancer? If so, then not taking vitamin C failed to cure Moertel's. Pauling lived 27 years longer with ascorbate than Moertel lived without it. So? (Moertel, Creagan, 1980). **As I have said before, ascorbate at exceedingly high levels becomes a prooxidant.**

Failure of high-dose vitamin C (ascorbic acid) therapy to benefit patients with advanced cancer. A controlled trial

One hundred and fifty patients with advanced cancer participated in **a controlled double-blind study** to evaluate the effects of high-dose vitamin C on symptoms and survival. Patients were divided randomly into a group that received **vitamin C (10 g per day)** and one that received a comparably flavored lactose placebo. Sixty evaluable patients received vitamin C and 63 received a placebo. Both groups were similar in age, sex, site of primary tumor, performance score, tumor grade and previous chemotherapy. **The two groups showed no appreciable difference in changes in symptoms, performance status, appetite or weight. The median survival for all patients was about seven weeks, and the survival curves essentially overlapped**. In this selected group of patients, we were unable to show a therapeutic benefit of high-dose vitamin C treatment. (Creagan et al, 1979).

Vitamin C: intravenous use by complementary and alternative medicine practitioners and adverse effects

We surveyed attendees at annual CAM Conferences in 2006 and 2008, and determined sales of intravenous vitamin C by major U.S. manufacturers/distributors. We also queried practitioners for side effects, compiled published cases, and analyzed FDA's Adverse Events Database. Of 199 survey respondents (out of 550), 172 practitioners administered IV vitamin C to **11,233 patients** in 2006 and 8876 patients in 2008. Average dose was 28 grams every 4 days, with 22 total treatments per patient. Estimated yearly doses used (as 25 g/50 ml vials) were 318,539 in 2006 and 354,647 in 2008. Manufacturers' yearly sales were 750,000 and 855,000 vials, respectively. Common reasons for treatment included infection, cancer, and fatigue. **Of 9,328 patients for whom data is available, 101 had side effects, mostly minor, including lethargy/fatigue in 59 patients,** change in mental status in 21 patients and vein irritation/phlebitis in 6 patients. Publications documented serious adverse events, including **2 deaths** in patients known to be at risk for IV vitamin C. Due to confounding causes, the FDA Adverse Events Database was uninformative. Total numbers of patients treated in the US with high dose vitamin C cannot be accurately estimated from this study. **There are two more dead bodies caused by an antioxidant.**

CONCLUSIONS: High dose IV vitamin C is in unexpectedly wide use by CAM practitioners. Other than the known complications of IV vitamin C in those with renal impairment or glucose 6 phosphate dehydrogenase deficiency, high dose intravenous vitamin C appears to be remarkably safe. Physicians should inquire about IV vitamin C use in patients with cancer, chronic, untreatable, or intractable conditions and be observant of unexpected harm, drug interactions, or benefit. (Padayatty et al, 2010).

At physiological concentrations, vitamin C is a potent free radical scavenger in the plasma, protecting cells against oxidative damage caused by ROS. Paradoxically, ascorbic acid may also function as a pro-oxidant. When used at pharmacological concentrations (0.3–20 mmol/L), ascorbic acid displays transition metal-independent pro-oxidant activity, which is more profound in cancer cells and causes cell death. This tumor cell-killing response is dependent upon ascorbate incubation time and extracellular ascorbate concentration.

Several intrinsic properties of cancer cells, including reduced concentrations of antioxidant enzymes, such as catalase and superoxide dismutase, increased intracellular transitional metal availability, and better accumulation of DHA through GLUT transporter overexpression, **all contributing to the**

augmented intracellular **hydrogen peroxide** concentrations. Therefore, **a nutritional regimen resulting in increased generation of hydrogen peroxide in vivo may be exploited as a means for inducing tumor-specific cytotoxicity**.

In a mouse model, **vitamin C depletion significantly attenuated tumor growth by impairing angiogenesis.** This sounds similar to the work of Salganik.

Whether vitamin C functions as an antioxidant or pro-oxidant is determined by at least 3 factors: *1*) the redox potential of the cellular environment; *2*) the presence/absence of transition metals; and *3*) the local concentrations of ascorbate.

Vitamin C mega-doses and H_2O_2

Also, mega-doses given intravenously can generate anti-cancer hydrogen peroxide. Vitamin C (ascorbate, ascorbic acid) has had a controversial history in the prevention of cancer. Much of this work was based on the pioneering work of Dr. Hugh Riordan and there have been some significant recent developments.

One clinical case report by Drisko et al showed that vitamin C together with other oxidants, when added adjunctively to first-line chemotherapy, prevented recurrence in two ovarian cancer patients. (Drisko et al, 2003).

This high dose, intravenous vitamin C therapy was shown to operate through the generation of hydrogen peroxide. Ascorbate-mediated cell death was due to protein-dependent extracellular H_2O_2 generation (i.e., prooxidant EMOD generation). Ascorbate, an electron-donor in such reactions, ironically initiates prooxidant chemistry and H_2O_2 formation. It was concluded that **ascorbate at pharmacologic concentrations in blood is a pro-drug for H_2O_2 delivery to tissues.** (Buettner, Jurkiewicz, 1996) (Halliwell, 1990).

Mechanisms of ascorbate-induced cytotoxicity in pancreatic cancer

Pharmacologic concentrations of ascorbate may be effective in cancer therapeutics. Investigators hypothesized that ascorbate concentrations achievable with i.v. dosing would be cytotoxic in pancreatic cancer for which the 5-year survival is <3%.

Pancreatic cancer cell lines were treated with ascorbate (0, 5, or 10 mmol/L) for 1 hour, then viability and clonogenic survival were determined. Pancreatic tumor cells were delivered s.c. into the flank region of nude mice and allowed to grow at which time they were randomized to receive either ascorbate (4 g/kg) or osmotically equivalent saline (1 mol/L) i.p. for 2 weeks.

There was a time- and dose-dependent increase in measured H_2O_2 production with increased concentrations of ascorbate. Ascorbate decreased viability in all pancreatic cancer cell lines but had no effect on an immortalized pancreatic ductal epithelial cell line. Ascorbate decreased clonogenic survival of the pancreatic cancer cell lines, which was reversed by treatment of cells with scavengers of H_2O_2. Treatment with ascorbate induced a caspase-independent cell death that was associated with autophagy. In vivo, treatment with ascorbate inhibited tumor growth and prolonged survival.

CONCLUSIONS: These results show that pharmacologic doses of ascorbate, easily achievable in humans, may have potential for therapy in pancreatic cancer. (Du et , 2010).

–Albert Szent-Gyorgyi. "The medical profession itself took a very narrow and very wrong view. Lack of ascorbic acid caused scurvy, so if there was no scurvy there was no lack of ascorbic acid. Nothing could be clearer than this. The only trouble was that scurvy is not a first symptom of a lack but a final collapse, a premortal syndrome and there is a very wide gap between scurvy and full health."

The above quotation, taken from Szent-Gyorgyi's Nobel Prize acceptance speech, was remarkably prescient. Few nutritional issues have received as much attention or been as hotly debated as the dietary requirement for vitamin C since the discovery of this vitamin in 1932. The recognition that vitamin C may also be important in cancer and heart disease has spurred renewed interest in dietary vitamin C requirements with the view that amounts consumed should account for a potential therapeutic role in ameliorating chronic disease. However, RCTs have not clarified vitamin C' preventative or curative role thus far.

Caution: vitamin C may block anticancer activity

PS-341 (bortezomib, Velcade), the first proteasome inhibitor approved by the Food and Drug Administration for the treatment of patients with relapsed multiple myeloma, induces apoptosis in human cancer cell lines. Vitamin C (ascorbic acid) is an essential water-soluble vitamin required for many normal physiologic functions and has to be obtained through diet or supplemental tablets in humans. Vitamin C directly binds to PS-431, thus inactivating PS-341 independent of its antioxidant activity. **Zou** et al. findings suggest that vitamin C may have a negative effect on

PS-341-mediated anticancer activity (Zou et al, 2006). This was a cell culture in vitro study and has limited applicability.

H_2O_2 generated by ascorbate oxidation and exogenously added H_2O_2 produced cell death curves that were indistinguishable. **Sensitivity to direct exposure to H_2O_2 was greater in lymphoma cells compared with normal lymphocytes and normal monocytes**, consistent with the cytotoxicity pattern found above with pharmacologic ascorbate exposure. Taken together, these data are consistent with the conclusion that **extracellular ascorbate induced cell death by formation of H_2O_2.**

These data imply that ascorbate radical is a surrogate marker for H_2O_2 formation.

Ascorbate at pharmacologic concentrations is a pro-drug for H_2O_2

Intravenous ascorbate infusion is expected to drastically change extracellular but not intracellular concentrations. For i.v. ascorbate to be clinically useful in killing cancer cells, pharmacologic but not physiologic extracellular concentrations should be effective, independent of intracellular ascorbate concentrations. This was what was observed by Chen et al. The experiments here provide a cohesive explanation for ascorbate action in generating H_2O_2 outside cells, without H_2O_2 accumulation in blood, leading to the conclusion that **ascorbate at pharmacologic concentrations in blood is a pro-drug for H_2O_2 delivery to tissues**.

While chelators may marginally affect these metals, they could participate in the oxidation of ascorbate when it is at pharmacologic concentrations, with subsequent formation of superoxide and H_2O_2 (Halliwell, 1990).

It is also possible that in vivo, cell membranes and their associated proteins could harbor metals accessible to extracellular fluid and could react similarly. In either case, **ascorbate, an electron-donor in such reactions, ironically initiates pro-oxidant chemistry and H_2O_2 formation.** (Buettner, Jurkiewicz, 1996) (Halliwell, 1990).

Vitamin C blocks apoptosis of human colon cancer cells

Although a high alimentary intake of **antioxidant vitamins** such as ascorbic acid may play an important role in **cancer** prevention, a high level of **antioxidant**s may have quite different effects at different stages of the transformation process. In **cancer** development, the resistance of **cell**s to **apoptosis** is one of the most crucial steps. We have tested the effects of ascorbic acid on apoptosis in **HT-29 human colon carcinoma cells** when induced **by** two potent **apoptosis** inducers, the classical antitumor drug **c**amptothecin or the flavonoid flavone. **Apoptosis** was assessed based on **c**aspase-3-like activity, plasma membrane disintegration and finally nuclear fragmentation and chromatin condensation. Ascorbic acid dose-dependently inhibited the apoptotic response of cells to camptothecin and flavone. RT–PCR analysis and western blot analysis revealed that ascorbic acid specifically **blocked** the decrease of bcl-X$_L$ **by** camptothecin or flavone. **A**n increased generation of mitochondrial superoxide precedes the down-regulation of bcl-X$_L$ **by** camptothecin and flavone and ascorbic acid at a concentration of 1mM prevented the generation of this reactive oxygen species. In conclusion, **ascorbic acid functions as a potent antioxidant in mitochondria of human colon cancer cells and thereby blocks drug mediated apoptosis induction allowing cancer cells to become insensitive to chemotherapeutics.** (Wenzel et al, 2004).

Vitamin E blocks breast cancer cell apoptosis

Induction of apoptosis by tamoxifen has been postulated to involve oxidative stress. Tamoxifen (TAM) may act on estrogen receptors (ER) located in the plasma membrane. Supplemental antioxidant vitamin E (a-tocopherol) acts at the plasma membrane to alter the effectiveness of tamoxifen and vitamin E was tested in ER-positive breast cancer cell lines, MCF-7 and T47D. Studies suggest that supplemental vitamin E decreases the inhibitory effect of TAM on the proliferation of ER+ breast cancer cells and eliminates the rapid rise in intracellular calcium that leads to apoptosis stimulated by TAM. The use of vitamin E acetate supplements may be inadvisable for women taking tamoxifen. (Peralta et al, 2006).

Conclusions drawn from these studies suggest that there is a higher prevalence of antioxidant dietary supplement use among cancer survivors than among the general population, and that supplements being used are an increasingly complex mixture of ingredients.

I believe that this is a very dangerous practice, since it has repeatedly been shown that antioxidants block EMODs ability to kill cancer cells.

Vitamin E slows rate of free radical-mediated lipid peroxidation in cells

Much of what is known about the antioxidant mechanism of vitamin E has been learned from studies of lipid dispersions, solutions, or subcellular organelles. We have investigated the effect of vitamin E supplementation on intact live eucaryotic cells. **L1210 murine leukemia cells** were exposed to an oxidative stress induced by 20 microM Fe2+ and 100 microM ascorbic acid introduced immediately before oxidative measurements were begun, and the kinetics of the generation of lipid-derived free radicals, as measured by EPR spin trapping (a product) and O2 consumption (a reactant) were measured. Cells grown for 24 h with supplemental (5-100 microM) vitamin E in their media had a slower rate of lipid radical generation compared to cells grown without vitamin E supplementation; this inhibition in the rate of oxidation was generally dependent upon the amount of vitamin E supplementation. In complementary studies measuring O2 consumption, 5-100 microM vitamin E slowed the rate of oxidation (10-fold with 100 microM supplemental vitamin E) consistent with the EPR studies. The membrane active drug edelfosine accentuated the vitamin E effects; **vitamin E introduced a discernible lag phase (time delay) in both lipid radical generation and O2 consumption** that was not seen in the absence of edelfosine. Vitamin E supplementation of cells also altered the kinetics of ascorbate free radical formation. We conclude that **vitamin E inhibits lipid peroxidation in cells by slowing the rate of lipid peroxidation**; but with iron/ascorbate as the initiating system, vitamin E does not delay the onset of peroxidation. Of special interest is that these free radical peroxidation events parallel cell membrane damage as detected using trypan blue exclusion. These observations are consistent with the free radical events preceding and causing the observed membrane damage. (Wagner et al, 1996). **I believe that this argues that vitamin E will block EMOD-induced apoptosis.**

Antioxidants block the kill of human cancer cells

In 2009, I wrote a paper describing 20 different types of human cancer cell in which apoptosis was blocked by antioxidants. **In short, data has shown that antioxidants block the kill of the following 20 human cancer cell types:**

- **human metastatic melanoma**
- **human breast cancer**
- **human lymphoma**
- **human melanoma**
- **human leukemia**
- **human prostate cancer**
- **human hepatocellular liver carcinoma**
- **human colon adenocarcinoma**
- **human multiple myeloma**
- **Burkitt's lymphoma**
- **human chronic lymphocytic leukemia**
- **human acute myeloid leukemia**
- **human non-small cell lung cancer**

- **human hepatoma**
- **murine pheochromocytoma**
- **human pancreatic cancer**
- **human colon cancer**
- **human endometrial cancer**
- **human colorectal carcinoma**
- **human ovarian carcinoma**
- **murine retinoblastoma**

(Howes, Philica. Feb 7, 2009).

Now, in 2011, that number is 27 (Please see Introduction) and 9 murine cancer cell types.

Published data has shown that antioxidants blocked the killing of the following 27 human cancer cell types:

- **human breast cancer** (J. Nutr. 134, 2004) (Gundimeda et al, 1996) (Peralta et al, 2006) (Aykin-Burns et al, 2009) (Xiao et al, Mol Cancer Ther. 2006)
- **human prostate carcinoma** (Xiao et al, 2006) (Wu et al, 2005) (Singh et al, 2005) (Cho et al, 2005) (Milanesa et al, 2000)
- **human non-small cell lung cancer** (Ling et al, 2003) (Wu et al, 2006)
- **human colon adenocarcinoma** (Wenzel et al, 2005)
- **human colon cancer** (Wenzel et al, 2004) (Aykin-Burns et al, 2009)
- **human colorectal carcinoma** (Chen et al, 2004) (**Gali-Muhtasib** et al, 2008)
- **human ovarian cancer cells** (Pak et al, 2011)
- **human melanoma** (Marcin et al, 2005) (Okroj et al, 2006) (Nishikawa et al, 2004) (Grimm et al, 2011)
- **human metastatic melanoma** (Kirshner et al, 2008)
- **human head and neck cancer** (Mattson et al, 2009)
- **human lymphoma** (J. Nutr. 134, 2004) (Mansat-De Mas et al, 1999)
- **human leukemia** (Hileman et al, 2004) (McKallip et al, 2006) (Hou et al, 2005) (Feng et al, 2007) (Yedjou et al, 2008) (Hiraoka et al, 1998)
- **human hepatoma** (Wu et al, 2004) (Wu, Ng, Lin, 2004)
- **human hepatocellular liver carcinoma** (Shimoda et al, 2003)
- **human pancreatic cancer** (Maehara et al, 2004)
- **human multiple myeloma** (Grad et al, 2001) (Ahmad et al, 1997) (Gupta et al, 2000) (Nakazato et al, 2005) (Isham et al, 2007)
- **Burkitt's lymphoma** (Ahmad et al, 1997) (Gupta et al, 2000) (Nakazato et al, 2005) (Ahmad et al, 1997)

- **human chronic lymphocytic leukemia** (Kay, 2006) **(Chandra et al, 2003)** (Shanafelt et al, 2005) (Mow et al, 2002) (Biswas S, et al, 2010)
- **human acute myeloid leukemia** (Kay, 2006) **(Chandra et al, 2003)** (Shanafelt et al, 2005) (Mow et al, 2002)
- **human promyelocytic leukemia** (Hou et al, 2005)
- **human erythromyeloid leukemia** (Wagner et al, 2000)
- **human epithelial cancer cells** (breast and colon) (Aykin-Burns et al, 2009)
- **human endometrial cancer** (Llobet et al, 2008)
- **human bladder cancer cells** (Miyajima et al, 1999)
- **human invasive bladder cancer** (Miyajima et al, 1999 - human bladder cancer KU-1 cell line)
- **human glioblastoma cells** (Lee et al, 2004)
- **human osteosarcoma** (Ahmad et al, 2005)
- **murine pheochromocytoma** (Jang, Surh, 2001)
- **murine retinoblastoma** (Salganik et al, 2000)
- **murine thymoma** (Tome et al, 2001)
- **murine lymphoma- six cell types** (Nathan et al, vol 153, 1981)
- **murine leukemia** (Wagner et al, 1996)
- **murine fibrosarcoma** (Teicher et al, 1994)
- **murine neuroblastoma** (Prasad et al, PNAS. 1979)
- **murine mammary cancer** (Bracke et al, 1999)
- **murine brain cancer** (Zeisel (2), 2004)

There are twenty seven (27) types of human cancer cell types and nine (9) murine cancers that can be killed by EMODs and in which the killing can be blocked by antioxidants, thereby providing antioxidant protection and shielding of the cancer cells.

HUMAN CANCER CELL TYPES SHIELDED BY ANTIOXIDANTS: Expanded section to include cell types.

- **HUMAN _BREAST_ CANCER CELLS: T47D human mammary carcinoma, human breast cancer cells (MDA-MB-231 and MCF-7), human breast cancer cells - MCF-7 human breast cancer cells (Doroshow, 1986) (J. Nutr. 134, 2004) (Gundimeda et al, 1996) (Peralta et al, 2006) (Aykin-Burns et al, 2009) (Xiao et al, Mol Cancer Ther. 2006)**
- **HUMAN _PROSTATE_ CANCER CELLS: androgen-independent human prostate cancer PC-3 cells, (Xiao et al, 2006) (Wu et al, 2005) PC-3 and DU145 human prostate cancer cells (Singh et al, 2005),**

DU145 prostate cancer cells (Cho et al, 2005) (Milanesa et al, 2000)

- HUMAN *NON-SMALL CELL LUNG* CANCER CELLS: human H460 non-small cell lung cancer Cells (Ling et al, 2003) (Wu et al, 2006)
- HUMAN *COLON ADENOCARCINOMA* CELLS: HT-29 human colon cancer cells (Wenzel et al, 2005), SW480 human colon adenocarcinoma cell line (Aykin-Burns et al, 2009)
- HUMAN *COLON* CANCER CELLS: HT-29 human colon cancer cells (Wenzel et al, 2004), human colon and breast cancer cells (HT29 human colon cancer cells, HCT116 human colon cancer cells, SW480 human colon adenocarcinoma cells and MB231 human breast cancer cells) (Aykin-Burns et al, 2009)
- HUMAN *COLORECTAL* CARCINOMA CELLS: colon cancer cells HCT116 (Gali-Muhtasib et al, 2008), colorectal carcinoma cells (HT29, COLO205, COLO320-HSR) (Chen et al, 2004)
- HUMAN *OVARIAN* CANCER CELLS: SKOV-3 human ovarian carcinoma cells (Pak et al, 2011)
- HUMAN *MELANOMA* CELLS: (Marcin et al, 2005) (Okroj et al, 2006), MDA-MB-435S cells (originally a model for metastatic human breast cancer but now genetically tests more closely to human melanoma cell lines) (Nishikawa et al, 2004) (Grimm et al, 2011)
- HUMAN *METASTATIC MELANOMA*: actual human patients were used - not cell cultures (Kirshner et al, 2008)
- HUMAN *HEAD AND NECK* CANCER CELLS: FaDu, Cal-27, and SQ20B head and neck cancer cells (Mattson et al, 2009)
- HUMAN *LYMPHOMA* CELLS: U937 histiocytic lymphoma cells (Mansat-De Mas et al, 1999) (J. Nutr. 134, 2004)
- HUMAN *LEUKEMIA* CELLS: (Hileman et al, 2004) (McKallip et al, 2006) (Hou et al, 2005), HL-60 human leukemia cells (Feng et al, 2007) (Yedjou et al, 2008), PLB-985 human myeloid leukemia cells (Hiraoka et al, 1998)
- HUMAN *HEPATOMA* CELLS: PLC/PRF/5 human hepatoma cells (Wu et al, 2004), PLC/PRF/5 human hepatoma cells (Wu, Ng, Lin, 2004)
- HUMAN *HEPATOCELLULAR LIVER* CARCINOMA CELLS: human hepatocellular carcinoma (HCC) cell clone P1(0.5), derived from the PLC/PRF/5 cell line (P5) (Shimoda et al, 2003)
- HUMAN *PANCREATIC* CANCER CELLS: pancreatic PC-12 cancer cells (Maehara et al, 2004)
- HUMAN *MULTIPLE MYELOMA* CELLS: 4 human MM cell lines: 8226/S, 8226/Dox40, U266, and U266/Bcl-x(L) (Grad et al, 2001),

(Ahmad et al, 1997) (Gupta et al, 2000) (Nakazato et al, 2005), CD138+ myeloma cells (Isham et al, 2007)

- **BURKITT'S** *LYMPHOMA* **CELLS:** (Ahmad et al, 1997) (Gupta et al, 2000), Human malignant B-cell lines including myeloma cells (IM9, RPMI8226, and U266) and Burkitt's lymphoma cells (HS-sultan) (Nakazato et al, 2005), (Ahmad et al, 1997)
- **HUMAN** *CHRONIC LYMPHOCYTIC LEUKEMIA* **CELLS:** (Kay, 2006), CLL B-cells, K562 cells (Chandra et al, 2003) (Shanafelt et al, 2005) (Mow et al, 2002), Hu1D10 chronic lymphocytic leukemia cells (Biswas S, et al, 2010)
- **HUMAN** *ACUTE MYELOID LEUKEMIA* **CELLS:** (Kay, 2006) (Chandra et al, 2003) (Shanafelt et al, 2005), K562 cells and bcr/abl-transduced FDC-P1 cells and myeloid progenitors (Mow et al, 2002)
- **HUMAN** *PROMYELOCYTIC LEUKEMIA* **CANCER CELLS:** HL-60 human leukemia cells (Hou et al, 2005)
- **HUMAN** *ERYTHROMYELOID LEUKEMIA* **CELLS:** K562 human erythroleukemia cell line (Wagner et al, 2000) (acute nonlymphocytic leukemia cell line)
- **HUMAN** *EPITHELIAL* **CANCER CELLS:** (breast and colon): human colon and breast cancer cells (HT29 human colon cancer cells, HCT116 human colon cancer cells, SW480 human colon adenocarcinoma cells and MB231 human breast cancer cells) (Aykin-Burns et al, 2009)
- **HUMAN** *ENDOMETRIAL* **CANCER CELLS:** cell line not available unless purchase article (Llobet et al, 2008)
- **HUMAN** *BLADDER* **CANCER CELLS:** human bladder cancer KU-1 cell line (Miyajima et al, 1999)
- **HUMAN** *INVASIVE BLADDER* **CANCER CELLS:** (Miyajima et al, 1999 - human bladder cancer KU-1 cell line)
- **HUMAN** *GLIOBLASTOMA* **CELLS:** human glioblastoma cell line U251 (Lee et al, 2004)
- **HUMAN** *OSTEOSARCOMA* **CELLS:** several different human cancer cell lines, i.e., PC-3, DU145, MDA-MB231, and HT-29 and human osteosarcoma cells lacking functional mitochondrial electron transport chains (rho0) (Ahmad et al, 2005)

9 MURINE (mouse and rat family) CANCER and CELL LINES SHIELDED BY ANTIOXIDANTS

- **MURINE** *PHEOCHROMOCYTOMA* **CELLS:** rat pheochromocytoma (PC12) cells (Jang, Surh, 2001)

- **MURINE** *RETINOBLASTOMA*: The TgT121 transgenic line was previously referred to as **LST1137-5** (Salganik et al, 2000)
- **MURINE** *THYMOMA* **CELLS:** mouse thymoma cells WEHI7.2 (Tome et al, 2001)
- **MURINE** *LYMPHOMA* - **SIX CELL TYPES:** L5178Y mouse lymphoma cells (Agarwal et al, 1991), (Nathan et al, vol 153, 1981)
- **MURINE** *LEUKEMIA* **CELLS:** murine leukemia cells **L1210** (Wagner et al, 1996)
- **MURINE** *FIBROSARCOMA* **CELLS:** murine fibrosarcoma cells **FSaII** (Teicher et al, 1994)
- **MURINE** *NEUROBLASTOMA* **CELLS:** mouse neuroblastoma cells **NBP2 cells** (Prasad et al, PNAS. 1979)
- **MURINE** *MAMMARY* **CANCER:** female nude mice inoculated with human **MCF-7/6** mammary adenocarcinoma cells. (Bracke et al, 1999)
- **MURINE** *BRAIN* **CANCER:** TgT121 transgenic mouse model, which spontaneously develops brain cancer (Zeisel (2), 2004)

OTHER Human cancer cells killed by EMODs

- **human prostate cancer cells:** androgen-independent human prostate cancer **PC-3 (Wt)** cells (Venkataraman et al, 2004), (Venkataraman et al, 2005),
- **human diploid leukemia cells: PLB-985** myeloid leukemia cells (Hiraoka et al, 1998)
- **human leukemia cells isolated from patients:** human monoblastic **ML-1 and lymphoblastoid T-cell Jurkat** lines (Pelicano et al, 2003) (McKallip et al, 2006) Ahmad et al, 2003)
- **human colon cancer cells : HT-29** colon cancer cells (Malik et al, 2003).

MY remarks from my book, "Antioxidant Overkill"

The print and broadcast media have failed their primary mission of truthfully informing the general public about the potential dangers of the antioxidant vitamins and have betrayed the very audience they claim to serve. Big Pharma now owns a large portion of the supplement business and the media is afraid to upset their corporate string pullers, which might threaten their own financial survival. The truth about the antioxidant vitamins has been systematically hidden from the public and distortions of the so-called "wonders of the antioxidant vitamins" have been proclaimed everywhere. This represents one of the greatest media frauds ever perpetuated upon an unknowing public.

False glowing claims regarding the antioxidant vitamins are no longer about science, they are about marketing, pure and simple. Media coverage is about advertising dollars rather than legitimately informing hordes of unsuspecting victims of clever marketing campaigns. The public must know the truth and then they can decide if they are going to waste their money on ineffective or harmful products.

We must ask ourselves, "Why does the truth rarely make it into print or is seldom broadcast to the public?" Why isn't the public constantly informed about the serious and well documented side effects of the antioxidant vitamins? Mainstream media must do the right thing and not simply serve as a corporate mouthpiece, whoring itself out to the highest bidder. I believe that Big Pharma rules and controls the media outlets with a "gold-plated iron fist."

Perhaps the biggest offender of truth is the supplement industry itself. Study after scientific study points out the ineffectiveness and dangers of a wide variety of dietary supplements, including the antioxidant vitamins. Yet, those selling these potentially dangerous products forge full steam ahead. Many of their sales people know the truth but they ignore it. The truth would hurt sales.

TEN KEY LIES DOMINATE THE MAINSTREAM MEDIA

> **Lie #1 -** Antioxidant vitamins are completely safe and free from harm
> **Lie #2 -** There have never been any deaths attributable to any of the antioxidant vitamins
> **Lie #3 -** The antioxidant vitamins can cure, reverse or prevent cancer
> **Lie #4 -** The antioxidant vitamins can cure, reverse or prevent heart disease
> **Lie #5 -** The antioxidant vitamins can cure, reverse or prevent strokes
> **Lie #6 -** The antioxidant vitamins will increase your life span and prevent aging
> **Lie #7 -** The antioxidant vitamins can cure, reverse or prevent eye diseases, such as cataract formation or macular degeneration
> **Lie #8 -** Oxygen free radicals are toxic and lethal
> **Lie #9 -** Oxidation is destroying cells by blowing holes in them
> **Lie #10 - (and THE BIGGEST WHOPPER OF ALL):**
> Oxygen is killing all of us and will bring death to all humans!

Always get the facts and think for yourself.

Even though the antioxidant vitamins are not required to diagnose, treat, cure or prevent any disease, customers are lining up, like lemmings at a cliff, to buy them on a daily basis, absent any proof of safety or efficacy whatsoever. Health food stores and pharmacies are filled with "troughs of supplements" to feed the massive herds of human guinea pigs. The injudicious use of the antioxidant vitamins could be the beginning of a modern medical disaster, in which the federal authorities do not require safety data or large scale testing for efficacy.

Studies demonstrating the harmful side of the antioxidant vitamins is always referred to as being "disappointing, surprising or shocking." But, they should call it exactly what it is, "ANTIOXIDANT TOXICITY and POTENTIAL LETHALITY." They should refer to these results as being "deeply concerning, dangerous and potentially fatal." But they do not and the profits keep rolling in, the "sheeple" keep acting like guinea pigs.

TEN THINGS YOU ARE NOT SUPPOSED TO KNOW ABOUT ANTIOXIDANT VITAMINS

#1 - They are not tested by federal agencies for safety or efficacy
#2 - Many deaths are attributable to antioxidant vitamins
#3 - They can not prevent or cure cancer
#4 - They can not prevent or cure heart disease
#5 - They can not prevent or cure strokes
#6 - They can not prevent or cure eye diseases
#7 - They do not increase the life span or prevent aging and they may increase overall mortality
#8 - Over eighty scientific studies have shown their wide ranging harmful effects
#9 - Oxygen free radicals are of low toxicity and essential for normal metabolism
#10 - Oxygen is our most essential ally in sustaining a healthful condition, in fighting pathogens and in killing cancer cells

Basically, the antioxidant vitamins are today's snake oil. They have unknown benefits with known harmful effects. Patient safety, and not profits, should always be the priority.

Ultimately, the harm or safety of antioxidants will be determined by the evidence and I believe that current scientific evidence presents a convincing argument that the antioxidant vitamins are ineffective and harmful. Their use should be restricted until their safety is confirmed. If they are not proven to be safe, then they should be removed from the diet of humans. If they have the effects of drugs, then they should be regulated as drugs.

Common sense observations

Proponents for the daily use of the antioxidant vitamins espouse their wondrous effects upon normal cells (everything from preventing or reversing all manner of diseases, increasing immunity to prolonging the life span). Logically, one must assume that these same so-called beneficial effects will also be beneficial to the survival of cancerous cells. The data has proven that to be the case.

One, then, questions if EMODs also benefit cancer cells and the answer is likely "NO." Studies have proven that high EMOD levels cause EMOD-induced apoptosis and the death of cancer cells. In fact, antioxidants, such as vitamin E and NAC, have been proven to block the EMOD-induced killing of cancer cells.

Jack Chellam was told by Dr. Denham Harman that taking too many antioxidant vitamins would result in fatigue, due to the fact that these agents can block the electron transport chain and the production of ATP, our main energy source. That is a no-brainer because the electron transport chain, which generates superoxide anions, is our main energy source for ATP.

Four common antioxidant killers: uric acid, cholesterol, bilirubin and estrogen

Both uric acid and cholesterol are the two most common antioxidants in the body and elevated levels of both are associated with a high risk of associated diseases and increased mortality. The other two common antioxidants are estrogen and bilirubin, both of which can be quite harmful, if not lethal. Quite literally, these predominant, common antioxidants, when in excess, are killers. Lower levels of estrogen are known to reduce the risk for breast cancer.

These simple observations are an alarming indictment of the potential harm associated with prolonged and injudicious ingestion of antioxidant vitamins. Enough said!

Therefore, maintaining sufficient EMOD levels is protective; whereas, maintaining a state of good health and high antioxidant levels connotes potential problems and harm. Basically, it is that simple.

Thus, I have endeavored to find readily available, effective, safe and inexpensive means to increase one's oxidative capacity. But, according to Charles River Laboratories, "Estimates for bringing a new drug to market range between $500 million to $2 billion."

Antioxidants can have prolonged adverse effects after discontinuation of their use

The ATBC study, the CARET study and the SELECT studies were all shut down nearly two years early, due to the obvious fact that the antioxidant agents being tested were causing shocking and unexpected harmful adverse effects.

Please remember my previously quoted caveat concerning long time follow up on subjects in the CARET study: "A 6-year follow-up of a large, randomized trial in people with a history of smoking has found that the overall harm associated with beta-carotene supplementation on cardiovascular disease mortality disappeared quickly after participants stopped taking the supplements. However, **the risk of lung cancer may persist**, especially in females and former smokers, according to the study in the December 1, 2004 issue of the Journal of the National Cancer Institute. Gary E. Goodman, M.D., of the Fred Hutchinson Cancer Research Center in Seattle, and colleagues followed the more than 18,000 participants in CARET for 6 years after the trial was stopped, until the end of 2001. The increased risk of cardiovascular disease mortality quickly disappeared after participants stopped taking the supplements. **However, women had a higher risk of death from cardiovascular disease or from any cause than men.** In addition, the incidence of lung cancer and deaths from all causes decreased but **did not disappear completely after the supplementation ceased.** The excess risk of lung cancer was restricted primarily to females and former smokers. **The results of CARET and ATBC emphasize that chemoprevention trials require careful monitoring of all disease endpoints ... even after the study intervention is discontinued."** (Goodman et al, 2004).

Antioxidants can even kill you

First, please remember the work of Drisko et al with IV mega-doses of vitamin C which resulted in 2 deaths and other adverse effects. Then check out the deaths from clioquinol and of 38 infant deaths from vitamin E (E-ferol). (Padayatty et al, 2010).

Deaths in Japan: Clioquinol

In 1955 a mysterious disease, **resembling polio**, appeared in Japan and had symptoms of a **combination of diarrhea, internal bleeding and various signs of nerve degeneration. By 1959 the disease had become an epidemic.** The illness appeared to be **contagious**, but patients did not display the symptoms typically associated with infections. **By 1964 the epidemic had worsened and patients were exhibiting blindness, with some patients dying.**

During the 1960s thousands of Japanese users of the anti-diarrhea drug clioquinol were left crippled, blinded, or otherwise disabled (sometimes leading to death) by a nerve disease known as subacute myelo-optic neuropathy (SMON). Dozens of elderly women, and some men in their thirties, began filling the nearby hospitals, totaling almost 3 percent of the local population by 1971.

In May of 1964, the disease was given a formal name: **"Sub-acute Myelo-Optic Neuropathy" (SMON) and by 1971, the number of people hospitalized in the Okayama Province accounted for about three per cent of the province's population. SMON victims had received treatment for diarrhea with a number of drugs.** Upon investigation, **these different drugs turned out not to be different at all; they were all made of a substance called Clioquinol, an antioxidant, but marketed under different brand names and freely available.**

The antioxidant Clioquinol, a Ciba-Geigy product, was erroneously considered to be perfectly safe, because **its effects would be confined to the digestive tract where it was supposed to destroy germs associated with diarrhea without being absorbed into the bloodstream. But the evidence was irrefutable and** the SMON epidemic **lasted until just after the government finally banned the antioxidant drug in September 1970. But Ciba-Geigy nevertheless continued selling the drug worldwide.**

The Japanese government recognized about 11,000 SMON victims, 4,700 of whom had filed damage claims as of 1979 (Chapmann, 1979).

Curiously, overmedication is more common in Japan than elsewhere because doctors receive payment from the government health insurance for every drug they prescribe.

Clioquinol (5-chloro-7-iodo-8-hydroxyquinoline; CQ) belongs to the quinoline class of compounds and is structurally similar to 5,7-DiCl-8-OHQ. **This class of compound possesses an established toxicology profile with the US Pharmacopoeia**. During the 1950s to the 1970s, CQ was used as an **antibiotic**; however, **it was withdrawn due to association with subacute myelo-optic neuropathy** possibly due to overdose and/or a reversible vitamin B_{12} deficiency. Recently, interest in CQ has reemerged due to studies involving its use, in combination with B_{12}, for treatment of Alzheimer's disease. **It has a very controversial history.**

Clioquinol (5-chloro-7-iodo-8-quinolinol) chelates zinc and copper acts as an antioxidant. The main biochemical change induced in some studies by clioquinol was a marked reduction in lipid peroxidation at all time points. (Bareggi SR et al. 2009).

I believe that clioquinol is another example of dead bodies from antioxidant use.

One thousand and thirty-one longstanding patients with subacute myelo-optico-neuropathy (**SMON;** 275 males, 756 females) were examined in 2002, **32 years after banning of clioquinol.** About 41% of patients were still **difficult to walk** independently, including 15.8% of completely loss of locomotion. One point six percent of patients were in **complete blindness** and 5.8% had severe visual impairment. As for complications, a **high incidence was revealed with cataract (56.2%), hypertension (40.2%),** vertebral disease (35.5%), and limb articular disease (31.5%).

These results indicate the serious sequelae of clioquinol intoxication, SMON. (Konogaya et al. 2004).

I believe that this supports my view that an EMOD insufficiency is, in part, causative of cataract formation. This is the effect of the antioxidant clioquinol.

Tragic deaths of 38 infants by lethal IV antioxidant vitamin E

Also, please remember the **fatal syndrome characterized by progressive clinical deterioration with unexplained thrombocytopenia, renal dysfunction, cholestasis, and ascites developed in certain infants throughout the United States who had received E-Ferol, an intravenous vitamin E sup-**

plement. **(THE TRAGIC CASE HISTORY OF INTRAVENOUS VITAMIN E (The New York Times) May 27, 1984 By PHILIP M. BOFFEY).**

Prolonged exposure to E-Ferol was associated with progressive intra-lobular cholestasis, inflammation of hepatic venules, and extensive sinusoidal veno-occlusion by fibrosis. E-Ferol, contained 25 units per milliliter of dl-alpha-tocopheryl acetate solubilized with 9% polysorbate 80 and 1% polysorbate 20. They proposed that vasculocentric hepatotoxicity is the basis for the observed clinical syndrome that represents the cumulative effect of one or more of the constituents of E-Ferol. (Bove et al, 1985).

All affected infants received E-Ferol; some affected infants received up to 1 ml or more daily. **Both outbreaks ceased shortly after use of E-Ferol was discontinued. Three were jailed for selling the drug (vitamin E) that killed 38 babies.**

The **Center for Drug Evaluation and Research, Food and Drug Administration, Rockville, Maryland, concluded that the use of E-Ferol in these neonatal intensive care units was associated with increased morbidity and mortality among exposed infants.** (Arrowsmith et al, 1989).

Research has shown infants who received E-Ferol injections are at an increased lifetime risk for reproductive problems, cervical and vaginal cancer, and other health problems.

Here is another basic point: the increase in disease risk and mortality seen with the antioxidant vitamins can not be expected to increase the life span. Obviously, they would be expected to decrease the life span.

Additionally, for those that say that there have been only a "few" negative studies with the antioxidant vitamins, there are now hundreds (over 250) which I have compiled and reported on. That is, indeed, shocking!

**Every human body has a cure inside it
and it is my scientific task to discover it.**
R. M. Howes, M.D., Ph.D.
9/7/09

CHAPTER EIGHT:

Theoretical reason to avoid antioxidants in cancer patients

Induction of oxidative metabolism by mitochondrial frataxin inhibits cancer growth: Otto Warburg revisited

More than 80 years ago Otto Warburg suggested that cancer might be caused by a decrease in mitochondrial energy metabolism paralleled by an increase in glycolytic flux. In later years, it was shown that cancer cells exhibit multiple alterations in mitochondrial content, structure, function, and activity. We have stably overexpressed the Friedreich ataxia-associated protein frataxin in several colon cancer cell lines. These cells have increased oxidative metabolism, as shown by concurrent increases in aconitase activity, mitochondrial membrane potential, cellular respiration, and ATP content. Consistent with Warburg's hypothesis, we found that frataxin-overexpressing cells also have decreased growth rates and increased population doubling times, show inhibited colony formation capacity in soft agar assays, and exhibit a reduced capacity for tumor formation when injected into nude mice. Furthermore, overexpression of frataxin leads to an increased phosphorylation of the tumor suppressor p38 mitogen-activated protein kinase, as well as decreased phosphorylation of extracellular signal-regulated kinase. Taken together, **these results support the view that an increase in oxidative metabolism induced by mitochondrial frataxin may inhibit cancer growth in mammals**. (Schulz et al, 2006).

Oxidative metabolism in cancer growth

PURPOSE OF REVIEW: Recent evidence suggests that **oxidative metabolism may have a key role in controlling cancer growth.** This review will provide an overview of the evidence accumulated so far. More than 80 years ago, Otto Warburg suggested that impaired oxidative metabolism may cause malignant growth. This assumption, later known as Warburg's hypothesis, has been experimentally addressed for many decades. It employs multiple approaches including cell lines, implanted xenografts and other animal models, by biochemical methods to quantify glycolytic and mitochondrial fluxes and signaling pathways including the rates of intermediate metabolism, respiration and oxidative phosphorylation.

RECENT FINDINGS: The hallmarks of cancer growth, increased glycolysis and lactate production in tumors, have raised attention recently due to novel observations suggesting a wide spectrum of oxidative phosphorylation deficits and decreased availability of ATP associated with malignancies and tumor cell expansion. **The most recent findings suggest that forcing cancer cells into mitochondrial metabolism efficiently suppresses cancer growth, and that impaired mitochondrial respiration may even have a role in metastatic processes.**

SUMMARY: This review summarizes published evidence on the essential interaction of tumor growth and mitochondrial metabolism, implicating novel approaches for the prevention and treatment of malignant disease.

(Ristow, 2006). **Note that tumors also have high levels of other antioxidants such as ascorbic acid, lactic acid and glutathione, which interfere with EMOD induced apoptosis.**

And finally, as reported on 2-04-09 in the journal Nature, Stanford researcher, Robert Cho, found that breast cancer stem cells make much higher levels of protective antioxidants than other cancer cells. **Use of a drug to block the antioxidant, glutathione, caused the cancer stem cells to become far more vulnerable to radiation**. Using cells from mice and human breast cancer, the antioxidant glutathione protected the cancer cells from being killed by radiation EMOD-induced apoptosis.

I believe that it is apparent that cancer cells accumulate and produce high levels of protective antioxidants, such as lactate, ascorbic acid and glutathione.

Oxygen consumption can regulate the growth of tumors, a new perspective on the Warburg effect

BACKGROUND: The unique metabolism of tumors was described many years ago by Otto Warburg, who identified **tumor cells with increased glycolysis and decreased mitochondrial activity.** However, "aerobic glycolysis" generates fewer ATP per glucose molecule than mitochondrial oxidative phosphorylation, so in terms of energy production, it is unclear how increasing a less efficient process provides tumors with a growth advantage.

METHODS/FINDINGS: We carried out a screen for loss of genetic elements in pancreatic tumor cells that accelerated their growth as tumors, and identified mitochondrial ribosomal protein L28 (MRPL28). Knockdown of MRPL28 in these cells decreased mitochondrial activity, and increased glycolysis, but paradoxically, decreased cellular growth in vitro. Following Warburg's observations, this mutation causes decreased mitochondrial function, compensatory increase in glycolysis and accelerated growth in vivo. Likewise, knockdown of either mitochondrial ribosomal protein L12 (MRPL12) or cytochrome oxidase had a similar effect. Conversely, expression of the mitochondrial uncoupling protein 1 (UCP1) increased oxygen consumption and decreased tumor growth. Finally, **treatment of tumor bearing animals with dichloroacetate (DCA) increased pyruvate consumption in the mitochondria, increased total oxygen consumption, increased tumor hypoxia and slowed tumor growth**.

CONCLUSIONS: We interpret these findings to show that **non-oncogenic genetic changes that alter mitochondrial metabolism can regulate tumor growth through modulation of the consumption of oxygen, which appears to be a rate limiting substrate for tumor proliferation.** (Chen et al. PLoS 2009).

I believe that this is a valid concept, oxygen is a rate limiting substrate for cancer growth…the more oxygen, the slower growing the tumor.

In hypoxia, the O_2 sensor, is a prolyl hydroxylase. HIF-1, induces expression of more than 30 known genes, including EPO, VEGF, NOS2, Flt-1, GIUT-1 & 3, PK-M and IGF-2. Tumor hypoxia stimulates expressing of vascular endothelial growth factor (VEGF) and hypoxia-inducible factor-1a (HIF-1a).

FDA regulation of dietary supplements (or lack thereof)

In 1994, the Dietary Supplement Health and Education Act (DSHEA) defined dietary supplements as a category of food, which put them under different regulations than drugs. **They are considered safe until proven otherwise**. Under the DSHEA, **dietary supplements cannot contain any ingredients that may have "a significant or unreasonable risk of illness or injury"** when the supplement is used as directed on the label, or under normal conditions of use if there are no directions on the label. If a dietary supplement contains a new ingredient, the manufacturer must provide the FDA with adequate proof that the ingredient is safe before the supplement is marketed to the public.

But manufacturers are not required to test new ingredients or supplements in clinical trials, which would help find risks and potential interactions with drugs or other substances. The DSHEA gives the FDA permission to stop a company from making a dietary supplement, but **only when the FDA proves that the product poses a significant risk to the health of Americans. They are found unsafe only after they cause harm.** This approach is the reverse of the way over-the-counter and prescription medicines are treated. **Because dietary supplements are usually self-prescribed, there is no controlled system for reporting bad reactions and side effects.**

Structure or function claims are not reviewed by the FDA. In fact, labels that carry them must also include the disclaimer "This statement has not been evaluated by the Food and Drug Administration. This product is not intended to diagnose, treat, cure, or prevent any disease."

One must question, "Do EMODs benefit cancer cells?" and the answer is "NO." Study after study have proven that high EMOD levels cause EMOD induced apoptosis and the death of cancer cells. In fact, antioxidants, such as vitamin E and NAC, have been repeatedly proven to block the EMOD induced apoptotic killing of cancer cells.

These simple observations are an alarming indictment of the potential harm associated with prolonged and injudicious ingestion of antioxidant vitamins.

Keeping all antioxidant levels (cholesterol, uric acid, bilirubin and estrogen) levels low may help keep the oxidative capacity at an optimum, peak or prime level. Hyperuricemia, hyperbilirubinemia and hypercholesterolemia and elevated estrogen levels are well known risk factors for death and disease.

Death in Small Doses?: **observations and conclusions from my book as of 6-24-10**

Some authors speak of synergism of the antioxidants and use this point to discount antioxidant studies showing no effect or harmful effects. In reviewing the studies, it is apparent from the study results that the antioxidant vitamins alone have somewhat limited numbers of adverse effect such as follows:

- Vitamin A has 7 effects: **vitamin A could increase risk of lung cancer, heart disease, increased total mortality, osteoporosis and fractures, polyp recurrence and transfer of HIV.**

- Vitamin E has 8 effects: **vitamin E could increase the risk of mortality, increase hospitalizations and heart failure, decrease platelet function, increase blood vessel blockages, increase tuberculosis and pneumonia in smokers and falls in Alzheimer's patients.**

- Vitamin C has 3 effects: **vitamin C could increase the risk of cardiovascular disease in female diabetics, block the good effects of exercise and increase cataracts in women.**

- But the studies utilizing **combinations of A, C and E** have huge numbers (over 40) of harmful side effects. Thus, it appears that "antioxidant synergism" or "antioxidant networking" is seen in the production of a wide range of adverse effects. Unfortunately, the synergism has not proven to reduce adverse effects, but conversely, **the combined antioxidant vitamin interactions have been seen to increase the number of adverse effects dramatically.**

Additionally, this indicates that combinations of antioxidant vitamins such as C and E may aid in their recycling and further add to an EMOD insufficiency. Likewise, it indicates a dramatic "cumulative adverse effect" produced by adding more than one antioxidant. **This is, indeed, the height of "unintended consequences."**

Other conclusions from Death in small doses:

- Antioxidant vitamins cause harm...widespread harm
- They increase the risk of common cancers, such as breast, prostate and lung
- They increase total mortality
- They increase stroke mortality
- They increase risk of various forms of heart disease, i.e., heart failure, ischemia, non-fatal myocardial infarction
- They accelerate atherosclerosis and plaque formation
- They increase risk of bone fractures
- They increase disease risks for smokers, diabetics and those exposed to asbestos
- They increased the risk of falling
- They increased the risk of low-birth-weight babies
- They increased the risk of gestational hypertension
- They damage sperm DNA

- They do not perform as advertised in keeping disease at bay
- They do not prevent aging
- They shorten life span, due to increased mortality and disease incidence
- They are not recommended by the vast majority of major medical and scientific organizations

- They are an unnecessary expense, unless one has a proven vitamin deficiency
- They produce avoidable adverse effects
- Synthetic vitamin supplements do not replace those contained in a normal diet
- Selenium and multivitamins also carry risk of adverse effects

Apoptosis and cell death

Cell death is an essential phenomenon in normal development and homeostasis, but also plays a crucial role in various pathologies. **This means that generation of EMODs is essential also.** Our understanding of the molecular mechanisms involved has increased exponentially, although it is still far from complete. The morphological features of a cell dying either by <u>apoptosis</u> or by necrosis are remarkably conserved for quite different cell types derived from lower or higher organisms.

At the molecular level, several gene products play a similar, crucial role in a major <u>cell death</u> pathway in a worm and in man. However, one should not oversimplify. It is now evident that there are multiple pathways leading to <u>cell death</u>, and some cells may have the required components for one pathway, but not for another, or contain endogenous inhibitors which preclude a particular pathway. Furthermore, different pathways can co-exist in the same cell and are switched on by specific stimuli. Apoptotic <u>cell death</u>, reported to be non-inflammatory, and necrotic <u>cell death</u>, which may be inflammatory, are two extremes, while the real situation is usually more complex. The distinguishing features of the various <u>cell death</u> pathways are: <u>caspases</u> (cysteine proteases cleaving after particular aspartate residues), **mitochondria and/or reactive oxygen species are often, but not always, key components.** As these various <u>caspase</u>-dependent and <u>caspase</u>-independent <u>cell death</u> pathways are becoming better characterized, we may learn to differentiate them and perhaps exploit the knowledge acquired for clinical benefit (More than one way to die: apoptosis, necrosis and reactive oxygen damage. <u>W Fiers, R Beyaert, W Declercq, P Vandenabeele. Oncogene (1999) 18: 7719-30).</u>

Cannabidiol-induced apoptosis in human leukemia cells

Investigators examined the effects of the **nonpsychoactive cannabinoid, cannabidiol,** on the induction of apoptosis in leukemia cells. Exposure of leukemia cells to cannabidiol led to cannabinoid receptor 2 (CB2)-mediated reduction in cell viability and induction in apoptosis. Furthermore, **cannabidiol treatment led to a significant decrease in tumor burden and an increase in apoptotic tumors in vivo.** From a mechanistic standpoint, cannabidiol exposure resulted in activation of caspase-8, caspase-9, and caspase-3, cleavage of poly(ADP-ribose) polymerase, and a decrease in full-length Bid, suggesting possible cross-talk between the intrinsic and extrinsic apoptotic pathways. The role of the mitochondria was further suggested as exposure to cannabidiol led to loss of mitochondrial membrane potential and release of cytochrome c. It is noteworthy that **cannabidiol exposure led to an increase in EMODs (reactive oxygen species, ROS) production** as well as an increase in the expression of the NAD(P)H oxidases Nox4 and p22^{phox}. Furthermore, **cannabidiol-induced apoptosis and reactive oxygen species (ROS) levels could be blocked by treatment with the ROS scavengers or the NAD(P)H oxidase inhibitors**. Finally, cannabidiol exposure led to a decrease in the levels of p-p38 mitogen-activated protein kinase, which could be **blocked by treatment with a CB2-selective antagonist or ROS scavenger**. Together, the results from this study reveal that cannabidiol, acting through CB2 and regulation of Nox4 and p22^{phox} expression, may be a novel and highly selective treatment for leukemia. (McKallip et al, 2006). **I believe that this again emphasizes the significant role of EMODs in cancer apopt**According-ing to volume 24, 2006 of the Journal of Clinical Oncology, the eight most common malignancies are cancers of lung, breast, colon and rectum, stomach, prostate, liver, cervix, and esophagus. In 2002, an estimated 11 million new cancer cases and 7 million cancer deaths were reported worldwide; nearly 25 million persons were living with cancer. Among the eight most common cancers, global disparities in cancer incidence, mortality, and prevalence are evident, likely due to complex interactions of nonmodifiable (ie, genetic susceptibility and aging) and modifiable risk factors (ie, tobacco, infectious agents, diet, and physical activity). Indeed, when risk factors among populations are intertwined with differences in individual behaviors, cultural beliefs and practices, socioeconomic conditions, and health care systems, global cancer disparities are inevitable.

Polyphenols block angiogenesis, CVD and cancer

The next cancer drug might come straight from the grocery store, according to new research published in the **November 2007 issue of The FASEB Journal.** In the study, French scientists describe how high and low doses of polyphenols have different effects. Most notably, they found that **very high doses of antioxidant polyphenols shut down and prevent cancerous tumors by cutting off the formation of new blood vessels needed for tumor growth.** Polyphenols are commonly found in red wine, fruits, vegetables, and green tea. **(RMH Note: They missed the point that the polyphenols acts as prooxidants with the production of peroxide and that this may also be its mechanism of action.)**

At relatively low doses, the French researchers found that the same polyphenols play a beneficial role for those with diseased hearts and circulatory systems by facilitating blood vessel growth. **The amount of polyphenols necessary for this effect was found to be the equivalent of only one glass of red wine per day or simply sticking to a healthy diet of fruits and vegetables containing polyphenols. This diet is known as the "Mediterranean Diet."** This study also adds to a growing body of research showing dose-dependent relationships for many types of commonly used compounds. For instance, research published in the October 2006 issue of *The FASEB Journal* shows that aspirin, through different mechanisms, also has a dose-dependent relationship for heart disease and cancer.

"When it comes to finding treatments for complex diseases, the answers are sometimes right there waiting to be discovered in unexpected places like the produce aisles and wine racks of the nearest store," said Gerald Weissmann, M.D., Editor-in-Chief of *The FASEB Journal*. "But it takes modern science to isolate the pure compound, test it in the lab, and to go on from there to find new agents to fight disease." **I doubt that they have actually isolated "the compound" from the tens of thousands in fruits and vegetables.**

According to the authors, **the amount of polyphenols necessary to obtain an anti-cancer effect is the equivalent of drinking about a bottle of red wine each day.** This amount of daily alcohol consumption obviously is unhealthy, but the research suggests that polyphenols extracted from plants or red wine could be converted into a pill that is highly likely to be safe. Such a pill also would be relatively easy and inexpensive to create and deliver.

Polyphenols and flavonoids not encouraged by Halliwell

Flavonoids and other polyphenolic compounds have powerful antioxidant effects in vitro in many test systems, but **can act as pro-oxidants in some others**. Whether pro-oxidant, antioxidant, or any of the many other biological effects potentially exerted by flavonoids account for or contribute to **the health benefits of diets rich in plant-derived foods and beverages is uncertain.** Phenolic compounds may help to protect the gastrointestinal tract against damage by reactive species present in foods or generated within the stomach and intestines. The overall health benefit of **flavonoids is uncertain, and consumption of large quantities of them in fortified foods or supplements should not yet be encouraged.** (Halliwell et al, 2007).

Human breast cancer cells killed by EMODs induced byisothiocyanates

Epidemiologic studies have revealed **an inverse correlation between dietary intake of cruciferous vegetables and the risk of breast cancer**. Cruciferous vegetable constituent benzyl isothiocyanate (BITC) effectively suppresses growth of cultured human breast cancer cells (MDA-MB-231 and MCF-7) by causing G_2-M phase cell cycle arrest and apoptosis induction. On the other hand, a normal mammary epithelial cell line (MCF-10A) is significantly more resistant to growth arrest and apoptosis by BITC compared with breast cancer cells. **(RMH Note: This due to the fact that normal cells have lower levels of EMODs and need more than a neoplastic cell to induce apoptosis, which I have discussed in my other books.).** The BITC-mediated cell cycle arrest was associated with a decrease in levels of proteins involved in regulation of G_2-M transition, including cyclin B1, cyclin-dependent kinase 1, and cell division cycle 25C. The BITC-induced apoptosis correlated with induction of proapoptotic proteins Bax (MCF-7) and Bak (MDA-MB-231 and MCF-7) and down-regulation of antiapoptotic proteins Bcl-2 and Bcl-xL (MDA-MB-231). The SV40-immortalized mouse embryonic fibroblasts derived from Bax and Bak double knockout mice were significantly more resistant to BITC-induced DNA fragmentation compared with wild-type mouse embryonic fibroblasts. The BITC treatment caused rapid disruption of the mitochondrial membrane potential, leading to cytosolic release of apoptogenic molecules, which was accompanied by formation of autophagosome-like structures as revealed by transmission electron microscopy. **The BITC-mediated apoptosis was associated with generation of reactive oxygen species** and cleavage of caspase-9, caspase-8, and caspase-3. **Apoptosis induction by BITC was significantly attenuated in the presence of a combined superoxide dismutase and catalase mimetic EUK134** as well as caspase inhibitors. In conclusion, the present study reveals a complex signaling leading to growth arrest and apoptosis induction by BITC. (Xiao et al, Mol Cancer Ther. 2006).

Flavonoids and polyphenols are poorly absorbed, extensively metabolized, and possess only modest antioxidant activity in vitro so that they are not likely to make a significant contribution to the overall antioxidant defenses in humans. Over **4,000 flavonoids** have been identified. **Research has failed to demonstrate substantial cholesterol lowering with dietary isoflavones.**

Metallothionein is a potential negative regulator of apoptosis

Apoptotic resistance can either be desirable or undesirable, depending on the conditions. **In cancer chemotherapy, it is critical that tumor cells are selectively and effectively killed while leaving normal cells undamaged.** Since acquisition of apoptotic resistance appears to be a common occurrence during malignant transformation, elucidating the mechanisms underlying apoptotic resistance is an area of intense study. Previous studies have revealed that **metallothionein (MT) can protect cells from apoptosis induced by oxidative stress and metals**. In the present study, we tested the hypothesis that the presence of MT may somehow modulate apoptosis. Their results revealed a strong linear negative correlation between basal MT levels and etoposide-induced apoptosis in the human tumor cell lines PLC/PRF/5, H460, and HepG2 (r = -0.991). In HepG2 cells, 24 h pretreatment with cadmium resulted in concentration-dependent increases in MT levels and marked decreases in etoposide-induced apoptosis. **Zinc pretreatment also resulted in increased MT synthesis and decreased etoposide-induced apoptosis**. More importantly, induced MT levels were negatively correlated with sensitivity to etoposide-induced apoptosis (r = -0.965). These suggest that MT may play a role in regulating apoptosis and that modulating MT expression may provide a strategy for altering cellular resistance to chemotherapeutic compounds. (Shimoda et al, 2003). **Again, I believe that this indicates that antioxidants may block cancer cell apoptosis and lead to proliferation of cancerous growths.**

Tumor cells have relatively low amounts of superoxide dismutase (SOD), which quenches superoxide anion $O_2^{\cdot-}$, and as a result of a higher level of aerobic metabolism, higher concentrations of $O_2^{\cdot-}$, compared to normal cells. But this may not be true of all tumor cells. **Some tumor cells have relatively higher amounts of vitamin E, a potent anti-oxidant, and a higher level of anaerobic metabolism, resulting in a balance that is tilted more towards higher antioxidant capacity.**

In both instances of higher aerobic and anaerobic metabolism **methods designed to augment free radical generation in tumor cells can cause their death. It is suggested that free radicals and lipid peroxides suppress the expression of Bcl-2, activate caspases and shorten telomeres, and thus inducing apoptosis of tumor cells.**

Ionizing radiation, anthracyclines, bleomycin and cytokines produce free radicals and thus are useful as anti-cancer agents. But they also produce many side-effects.

Arsenic trioxide (As_2O_3) inhibited multiple myeloma cells

Recently, **arsenic trioxide (As_2O_3) was reported to inhibit the proliferation of human myeloma cells by induction of apoptosis via intracellular production of ROS (EMODs).** (Miller et al, 2002).

Medicinal use of arsenic and its derivatives dates back more than 2400 years to ancient Greece and Rome. Arsenic was viewed as both a therapeutic agent and a poison. Hippocrates administered orpiment (As_2S_3) and realgar (As_2S_2) as an ulcer remedy; Dioscorides used orpiment as a depilatory. Arsenic has also been used to treat the plague, malaria, and cancer and to promote sweating. Physicians prescribed arsenic for both external and internal use throughout the 18th century. Arsenides and arsenic salts were key ingredients in antiseptics, antispasmodics, antiperiodics, caustics, cholagogues, hematinics, sedatives, and tonics. Approximately 60 different arsenic preparations have been developed and distributed during the lengthy history of this agent. More than 20 of these preparations were still in use at the end of the 19th century, including Aiken's Tonic Pills, Andrew's Tonic, and Arsenauro. (Miller et al, 2002).

It has also been reported that GSH is an inhibitor of As_2O_3-induced cell death either through conjugating As_2O_3 or **sequestering ROS induced by As_2O_3** (Dai et al, 1999) (Green, Reed, 1998).

Several investigations suggested that **ascorbic acid decreases cellular GSH levels and potentiates As_2O_3-induced cell death of As_2O_3-resistant myeloma cells.** This implies that ascorbate is working as a prooxidant. (Miller et al, 2002).

Therefore, **I believe that (–)-epigallocatechin-3-gallate-induced apoptosis in myeloma cells is enhanced by As_2O_3 via production of intracellular EMODs. The same is true for arsenic trioxide and ascorbic acid. It is also important to point out the fact that antioxidants block the killing ability of EMODs.**

If our current concepts are accurate, development of neoplasia is potentially constantly present and our apoptotic abilities are responsible for the killing of these continually forming entities. I believe that EMODs serve as the basis for the apoptotic execution system. Agents which block or nullify EMODs, such as antioxidants, or agents which result in an EMOD insufficiency will create conditions which "allow" tumorous growth and proliferation.

CHAPTER NINE:

Inorganic selenium compounds and Tea

All inorganic selenium compounds that express carcinostatic activity against cancer cells *in vivo* do so by interaction with thiol compounds and generation of free radical species. **In 1988, the observation was made that oxidation of glutathione by selenite produced superoxide. Even a small dose of selenite and selenium dioxide prevent tumor growth.** Elemental selenium is a prooxidant.

I believe that this is the same tumoricidal pattern that I have seen over and over again with EMOD producing compounds. In short, EMODs (prooxidants) kill cancer and antioxidants block this activity.

Can selenium protect against cancer in women?

Investigators studied the Nurses' Health Study which began in 1976 with **121,700 female nureses.** In 1982, they requested toenail clippings from members and 62,641 with no history of cancer returned these clippings. Toenail selenium levels were not inversely associated with cancer risk in this study. Implications: These data, in conjunction with previous findings of no association between toenail selenium status and breast cancer risk, strongly suggest that higher **selenium intake within the range consumed by most U.S. women (as reflected by toenail selenium levels) is not protective against overall cancer incidence in women. Toenail selenium level was not inversely associated with cancer at any major site, including uterine cancer, colorectal cancer, melanoma, ovarian cancer, or lung cancer (after adjusting for smoking); in fact, nonsignificant positive associations were observed at several sites**. (Garland et al, 1995).

The production of reactive oxygen species (ROS) is a common mechanism in one of the representative pathways of apoptosis. (Troyano et al, 2001).

Oxidants are capable of depleting reduced glutathione (GSH) or damaging the cellular antioxidant defense system and can directly induce apoptosis. (Sergediene et al, 1999).

Tea EGCG can produce H_2O_2

There is a presumption that the active ingredient in tea is EGCG. **EGCG can be oxidized to form dimers and produce H_2O_2.** EGCG can induce apoptosis at concentrations of 10 μmol/L (micromolar), and this activity becomes more prominent at 30 and 100 μmol/L. **I believe that the production of peroxide explains the salutary effects of EGCG.**

EGCG can be a prooxidant

(–)-Epigallocatechin-3-gallate is generally well known as an antioxidant; however, it can also behave as a pro-oxidant under certain conditions. (Ahmed et al, 1997) (Grad et al, 2001).

Several investigators have reported that (–)-epigallocatechin-3-gallate-induced apoptosis is often associated with the generation of ROS, EMODs. (Ahmed et al,) (Nam et al, 2001).

Green tea EGCG activates prooxidant-induced apoptosis and is blocked by antioxidants

Green tea, obtained from the dried leaves of the plant C. sinensis, is a popularly consumed beverage throughout the world. All true teas may be broadly classified as either green tea or black tea. **Extensive in vitro cell culture studies, as well as in vivo studies in animal models, have verified the cancer chemopreventive effects of green tea, and specifically, of its individual polyphenols.** (Ahmad et al, 2000).

Epidemiologic studies, although inconclusive, have suggested that **green tea may reduce the risks associated with many cancers including bladder, prostate, esophagus, and gastric carcinomas.** (Ahmad et al, 1997).

Green tea extract, especially its major polyphenolic component (–)-epigallocatechin-3-gallate, is capable of inhibiting the growth of a variety of mouse and human cancer cells **via the induction of apoptosis in vitro.** (Yang et al, 1993) (Gupta et al, 2000) (Barthleman et al, 1998). **I believe that this is EMOD-induced apoptosis.**

Green tea polyphenol, (–)-epigallocatechin-3-gallate **(EGCG), has been shown to inhibit cellular proliferation and induce apoptosis of various cancer cells.** The aim of this study was to investigate the possibility of (–)-epigallocatechin-3-gallate as a novel therapeutic agent for the patients with B-cell malignancies including multiple myeloma.

They investigated the effects of (–)-epigallocatechin-3-gallate on the induction of apoptosis in HS-sultan as well as **myeloma cells** in vitro and further examined the molecular mechanisms of (–)-epigallocatechin-3-gallate-induced apoptosis.

Results: (–)-**Epigallocatechin-3-gallate rapidly induced apoptotic cell death in various malignant B-cell lines in a dose- and time-dependent manner.** (–)-Epigallocatechin-3-gallate-induced apoptosis was in association with the loss of mitochondrial transmembrane potentials (Δc_m); the release of cytochrome c, Smac/DIABLO, and AIF from mitochondria into the cytosol; and the activation of caspase-3 and caspase-9. **Elevation of intracellular reactive oxygen species (ROS) production was also shown during (–)-epigallocatechin-3-gallate-induced apoptosis of HS-sultan and RPMI8226 cells as well as fresh myeloma cells. Antioxidant, catalase, and Mn superoxide dismutase significantly reduced ROS production and (–)-epigallocatechin-3-gallate-induced apoptosis, suggesting that ROS plays a key role in (–)-epigallocatechin-3-gallate-induced apoptosis in B cells.**

Furthermore, **a combination with arsenic trioxide (As_2O_3) and (–)-epigallocatechin-3-gallate significantly enhanced induction of apoptosis** compared with As_2O_3 alone via decreased intracellular reduced glutathione levels and increased production of ROS. **This is an obvious EMOD-induced form of apoptosis.**

Conclusions: (–)-Epigallocatechin-3-gallate has potential as a novel therapeutic agent for patients with B-cell malignancies including multiple myeloma **via (EMOD) induction** of apoptosis mediated by modification of the redox system. In addition, (–)-epigallocatechin-3-gallate enhanced As_2O_3-induced apoptosis in human multiple myeloma cells. (Nakazato et al, 2005).

To me, the evidence is clear that these so-called antioxidants of green tea are functioning as prooxidants and EMOD-induced apoptosis of malignant cells and antioxidants are counter to this important event.

In fact, epidemiologic studies have shown that **green tea consumption can reduce the incidence of cancer and metastases.** (Ahmad et al, 1997).

Green tea has unique characteristics as an agent, possessing few adverse effects. In addition, it is inexpensive, can be orally consumed, and has a long history as a beverage of general tolerance among all races. Therefore, **green tea seems to have the potential of becoming an ideal agent for chemoprevention.** (Lepley et al, 1996).

CHAPTER TEN:

Antioxidant Supplements and Cancer

**I have a burning combustive love of oxygen
deep inside of me.
Honestly, I do....
and so do you.**
R. M. Howes, M.D., Ph.D.
9/10/09

Antioxidant supplements have no effect on cardiovascular risk

Not only are the antioxidants controversial in cancer patients, **the American Heart Association** (AHA) says "there is no good reason for people to take them."

An advisory statement published by the American Heart Association in the August 3, 2009 issue of *Circulation* says that there is no good reason for people to take antioxidant supplements. This conclusion was reached by the AHA's nutrition committee after an extensive review of the medical literature.

The committee reviewed 20 separate clinical trials, conducted between 1994 and 2002, that examined whether taking antioxidant supplements (specifically, vitamin E, beta-carotene, antioxidant cocktails, or the combination of vitamins E and C) would reduce the risk of cardiovascular disease. Most of these studies showed no effect at all on the risk of cardiovascular disease. A few of the studies (generally the smaller ones) did show some effect - but the effect was just as likely to be adverse (that is, to increase risk) as beneficial. **Taken together, the conclusion was clear and straightforward: these studies indicate that antioxidant supplements have no effect on cardiovascular risk, either one way or the other.**

Also, researchers from the University of Washington have reported that **patients taking antioxidant vitamins in addition to statin and niacin therapy failed to increase their HDL cholesterol (the "good" cholesterol) as much as patients not taking antioxidants**. These results, reported in the August 9, 2001 issue of Arteriosclerosis, Thorombosis, and Vascular Biology, are but the latest in a series of disappointing results in trials examining the ability of antioxidants to prevent heart disease.

The study results showed that the increase in HDL levels seen in patients receiving statin-niacin therapy was eliminated when they also received the antioxidants. That is, in these patients the antioxidants were potentially harmful.

The primary endpoints of the study also suggest that antioxidants blunt the benefits seen with statin-niacin therapy. (While patients receiving statin-niacin had a 4% reduction in coronary artery blockage, those who received antioxidants in addition to statin-niacin had a 7% increase in blockage.

This new study validates the unpopular stance on antioxidant supplements taken by both the American Heart Association and the Institute of Medicine, i.e., they do not prevent or reverse heart disease.

During the last few years, a number of randomized trials using antioxidant vitamin supplements have finally been reported, and the results have generally been failures. Because of the failure of randomized trials to demonstrate a benefit from taking antioxidants, both the **American Heart Association and the Institute of Medicine** have released recent statements saying that, while a diet rich in antioxidant vitamins seems prudent, **there is insufficient evidence to recommend using supplements of vitamin C, vitamin E, beta-carotene, selenium, or other antioxidants to prevent heart disease**.

Dietary supplement use and prostate cancer risk in the CARET study

They investigated dietary supplement use and prostate cancer risk in the Carotene and Retinol Efficacy Trial (CARET). CARET was a **randomized, double-blinded, placebo-controlled trial** testing a **daily dose of 30 mg beta-carotene + 25,000 IU retinyl palmitate** for lung cancer prevention (1985-1996; active follow-up occurred through 2005). Secondary outcomes, including prostate cancer, were also assessed. Participants were queried about dietary supplements, health history, family history of cancer, smoking, and lifestyle habits. Cox proportional hazards regression estimated multivariate-adjusted relative risk [and 95% confidence intervals (95% CI)] of prostate cancer for dietary supplement users and nonusers with or without the high-dose CARET vitamins during the intervention and post-intervention phases. After an average of 11 years of follow-up, 890 prostate cancer cases were reported. Neither the CARET nor other supplements were associated with total prostate cancer risk. **For aggressive prostate cancer, men in the**

CARET intervention arm who used additional supplements had a relative risk for aggressive prostate cancer (Gleason >or=7 or stage III/IV) of 1.52, **relative to all others.** These associations disappeared in the post-intervention period. Conversely, there was no association of CARET + other supplements with non-aggressive disease, relative to all others. There was no effect modification by smoking or time on CARET intervention in any analyses. **CARET only included smokers,** so findings reported here may not apply to nonsmokers. **Our results are consistent with other studies suggesting that dietary supplements may influence prostate cancer risk.** (Neuhouser et al, 2009).

Reactive oxygen species may be essential as activators of apoptosis to remove cells that have accumulated mutations. (Tsang et al, 2003) (Liu et al, 2003) (Djavaheri-Mergny et al, 2003).

We have shown previously that **nitric oxide (NO) scavenges mitochondrial superoxide and thereby prevents the down-regulation of bcl-Xl that is crucial for the occurrence of apoptosis in HT-29 cells.** (Wenzel et al, 2003).

One of the major goals in **cancer** therapy is to restore the sensitivity of transformed **cells** towards apoptotic signals and to allow the execution of apoptotic **cell** death. (Nicholson, 297–301. 1996) (Nicholson, 810-816. 1996).

Apoptosis is a crucial parameter in the carcinogenesis process as genetically damaged or mutated cells can be eliminated by apoptosis. (White, McCubrey, 2001). High vitamin **C** intake, however, was associated with reduced colorectal **apoptosis** rates among individuals with adenomas and it was suggested therefore, that vitamin **C** supplements might be contraindicated in patients with a history of adenomas. (Connelly et al, 2003).

Resveratrol

Unsubstantiated anti-aging claims had caused a meteoric rise in the popularity of the antioxidant, resveratrol. **Resveratrol was thought to work in humans by activating a protein called SIRT1, but at some doses it actually inhibits SIRT1. As reported by Zachary Knight, the originally reported activation of SIRT1 by resveratrol was shown to be an assay artifact by two independent studies published in 2005, one from Brian Kennedy's lab and the other from John Denu's lab. This finding was confirmed in 2009 by scientists from Amgen. It was confirmed again in March 2010 by scientists from Pfizer. It was confirmed again in August 2010 by scientists from Sirtris itself.**

Thus, the so-called "miracle drug" has been another failure. In fact, resveratrol is neither safe nor effective, which is why GSK is abandoning it (along with IP issues). **According to a GlaxoSmithKline spokesperson, an internal analysis of the kidney failure cases has concluded that they "most likely were due to the underlying disease ... However, the formulation of SRT501 was not well tolerated, and side effects of nausea / vomiting / diarrhea may have indirectly led to dehydration, which exacerbated the development of the acute [kidney] failure."**

Resveratrol can have prooxidant activity and EMODs needed for apoptosis

Investigators have recently shown that efficient apoptotic signaling is a function of a permissive intracellular milieu created by a decrease in **the ratio of superoxide to hydrogen peroxide and cytosolic acidification. Resveratrol, a phyto-alexin found in grapes and wines, triggers apoptosis in some systems and inhibits the death signal in others.** In this regard, **the reported inhibitory effect on hydrogen peroxide-induced apoptosis has been attributed to its antioxidant property**. Here, **Ahmad** provides evidence that exposure of human leukemia cells to low concentrations of resveratrol (4-8 µM) inhibits caspase activation and DNA fragmentation induced by incubation with hydrogen peroxide or upon triggering apoptosis with a novel compound that kills via intracellular hydrogen peroxide production. At these concentrations, **resveratrol elicits pro-oxidant properties** as evidenced by an increase in intracellular superoxide concentration. This pro-oxidant effect is further supported by our observations that the drop in intracellular superoxide and cytosolic acidification induced by hydrogen peroxide is completely blocked in cells preincubated with resveratrol. Thus, the inhibitory effect of resveratrol on hydrogen peroxide-induced apoptosis is not due to its antioxidant activity, but contrarily via a pro-oxidant effect that creates an intracellular environment nonconducive for apoptotic execution. (Ahmad et al, 2003). **This emphasizes the point that EMODs are essential for apoptosis and that this can be blocked by antioxidants. It also shows that resveratrol can have prooxidant activity. Again, this makes the data difficult to interpret because it resveratrol is usually thought of as an antioxidant.**

Resveratrol blocks cancer kill of H_2O_2

Oxidative stress has been considered as a major cause of cellular injuries in a variety of clinical abnormalities. One of the plausible ways to prevent the reactive oxygen species (ROS)-mediated cellular injury is dietary or pharmaceutical augmentation of endogenous antioxidant defense capacity. **Resveratrol**

(3,5,4'-trihydroxy-trans-stilbene), one of the major antioxidative constituents found in the skin of grapes, has been considered to be responsible in part for the protective effects of red wine consumption against
coronary heart disease ('French Pardox').** In this study, they investigated the
effects of resveratrol on hydrogen peroxide-induced oxidative stress and apoptotic
death in cultured rat pheochromocytoma (PC12) cells. PC12 cells treated with
hydrogen peroxide (H_2O_2) underwent apoptotic death as determined by
characteristic morphological features, internucleosomal DNA fragmentation and
positive in situ end-labeling by terminal transferase (TUNEL staining). **Resveratrol
pretreatment attenuated hydrogen peroxide-induced cytotoxicity, DNA
fragmentation, and intracellular accumulation of ROS.** Hydrogen peroxide
transiently induced activation of NF-kappaB in PC12 cells, which was **mitigated
by resveratrol pretreatment.** These results suggest that resveratrol has the
potential to prevent oxidative stress-induced <u>cell death</u>. (Jang, Surh, 2001). **Again,
this illustrates the fact that antioxidants will block the protective apoptotic effect of H_2O_2 and that antioxidants could allow for rapid neoplastic
growth.**

Resveratrol blocks EMOD-induced apoptosis

Epidemiological studies suggest that **Mediterranean diets rich in resveratrol
are associated with reduced risk of coronary artery disease.** However,
the mechanisms by which resveratrol exerts its vasculoprotective effects are not
completely understood. Because oxidative stress and endothelial cell injury play a
critical role in vascular aging and atherogenesis, we evaluated whether resveratrol
inhibits oxidative stress-induced endothelial apoptosis. We found that oxidized
LDL and TNF-a elicited significant increases in caspase-3/7 activity in endothelial
cells and cultured rat aortas, which were prevented by resveratrol pretreatment
(10^{-6}–10^{-4} mol/l). The protective effect of resveratrol was attenuated by inhibition
of glutathione peroxidase and heme oxygenase-1, suggesting a role for antioxidant
systems in the antiapoptotic action of resveratrol. Indeed, **resveratrol treatment
protected cultured aortic segments and/or endothelial cells against increases in intracellular H_2O_2 levels and H_2O_2-mediated apoptotic cell
death induced by oxidative stressors (exogenous H_2O_2, paraquat, and UV
light).** Resveratrol treatment also attenuated UV-induced DNA damage (comet assay). Resveratrol treatment upregulated the expression of glutathione peroxidase,
catalase, and heme oxygenase-1 in cultured arteries, whereas it had no significant
effect on the expression of SOD isoforms. Resveratrol also effectively scavenged
H_2O_2 in vitro. Thus **resveratrol seems to increase vascular oxidative stress
resistance by scavenging H_2O_2 and preventing oxidative stress-induced
endothelial cell death.** We propose that the antioxidant and antiapoptotic effects

of resveratrol, together with its previously described anti-inflammatory actions, are responsible, at least in part, for its cardioprotective effects. (Ungvari, 2007).

Resveratrol prooxidant activity

Investigators recently showed that efficient apoptotic signaling is a function of a permissive intracellular milieu created by a decrease in the ratio of superoxide to hydrogen peroxide and cytosolic acidification. **Resveratrol, a phytoalexin found in grapes and wines, triggers apoptosis in some systems and inhibits the death signal in others**. In this regard, **the reported inhibitory effect on hydrogen peroxide-induced apoptosis has been attributed to its antioxidant property**. Here, we provide evidence that exposure of human leukemia cells to low concentrations of resveratrol (4-8 micro M) **inhibits** caspase activation and DNA fragmentation induced by incubation with hydrogen peroxide or upon triggering apoptosis with a novel compound **that kills via intracellular hydrogen peroxide production**. At these concentrations, **resveratrol elicits pro-oxidant properties as evidenced by an increase in intracellular superoxide concentration**. This pro-oxidant effect is further supported by our observations that the drop in intracellular superoxide and cytosolic acidification induced by hydrogen peroxide is completely blocked in cells preincubated with resveratrol. Thus, **the inhibitory effect of resveratrol on hydrogen peroxide-induced apoptosis is not due to its antioxidant activity, but contrarily via a pro-oxidant effect that creates an intracellular environment nonconducive for apoptotic execution.** (Ahmad et al, 2003).

The prooxidant activity is well documented but not well known. I believe that its benefits, if any, are due to this prooxidant activity, including those with anti-aging. However, the above study is conflicted regarding the mechanism of action of resveratrol. Yet, it appears that prooxidants lead to EMOD activated apoptosis and antioxidant activity blocks it.

Garlic (ajoene) induces apoptosis and EMODs

Investigators tried to determine the biochemical pathways involved in induction of apoptosis by **ajoene, an organosulfur compound from garlic**. Ajoene induced apoptosis of 3T3-L1 adipocytes in a dose- and time-dependent manner. Ajoene treatment resulted in activation of JNK and ERK, translocation of AIF from mitochondria to nucleus, and cleavage of 116-kDa PARP-1 in a caspase-independent manner. **Ajoene treatment also induced an increase in intracellular ROS level.** Furthermore, the **antioxidant N-acetyl-l-cysteine effectively blocked ajoene-mediated ROS generation**, activation of JNK and ERK, translocation of AIF, and degradation of PARP-1. DISCUSSION: These results indicate that ajoene-induced **apoptosis in 3T3-L1 adipocytes is initiated by the generation of hydrogen peroxide,** which leads to activation of mitogen-activated protein kinases, degradation of PARP-1, translocation of AIF, and fragmentation of DNA. **Ajoene can, thus, influence the regulation of fat cell number through the induction of apoptosis and may be a new therapeutic agent for the treatment of obesity.** (Yang et al, 2996). **I believe that the blockage of apoptosis by NAC indicates the potential danger of antioxidants of this variety, in that they may block tumoricidal EMODs and also lead to more vulnerability to pathogens.**

Prooxidant Role for the Tumor Suppressor p53: blocked by NAC

The tumor suppressor p53 exerts its activity by preventing DNA-damaged cells from dividing until either the chromosomal repair is effected or the cell undergoes apoptosis. EMODs **(reactive oxygen species, ROS) are enhanced through the action of p53-mediated transcription of apoptosis-promoting genes; however, p53 also can promote the expression of many antioxidant genes that prevent apoptosis.** New research indicates that in **low cellular stress, low concentrations of p53 induce the expression of antioxidant genes,** whereas in severe cellular stress, **high concentrations of p53 promote the expression of genes that contribute to ROS formation and p53-mediated apoptosis.** p53-depleted cells injected into athymic mice increased significantly in tumor volume, whereas injected p53$^{+/+}$ cells did not grow to the same degree. **Interestingly, administration of the antioxidant compound N-acetylcysteine (NAC) inhibited the growth of tumor volume in p53-depleted injected cells,** and NAC supplementation of p53$^{-/-}$ mice from birth greatly decreased the number of karyotype abnormalities and tumors formed in these mice by six months of age. Thus, under normal (or low stress) conditions, p53 appears to have an antioxidant role that protects cells from oxidative DNA damage and although this effect might depend on the concentration of p53, other cellular factors likely participate in a cell's final fate. (Tomko et al, 2006). **I believe that low p53 levels "allow" the action of antioxidant enzymes and block apoptosis of cancer cells. High p53 levels and high EMOD levels promote apoptosis and tumoricidal activity.**

Antioxidants block the apoptotic effect of EMODs in multiple myeloma

Multiple myeloma (MM) is a clonal B-cell malignancy characterized by slow-growing plasma cells in the bone marrow (BM). Patients with MM typically respond to initial chemotherapies; however, essentially all progress to a chemoresistant state. Factors that contribute to the chemorefractory phenotype include modulation of free radical scavenging, increased expression of drug efflux pumps, and changes in gene expression that allow escape from apoptotic signaling. Recent data indicate that arsenic trioxide As$_2$O$_3$ induces remission of refractory acute promyelocytic leukemia and <u>apoptosis</u> of cell lines overexpressing Bcl-2 family members; therefore, it was hypothesized that chemorefractory MM cells would be sensitive to As$_2$O$_3$. **As$_2$O$_3$ induced apoptosis in 4 human MM cell lines: 8226/S, 8226/Dox40, U266, and U266/Bcl-x(L).** The addition of interleukin-6 had no effect on <u>cell death</u>. **Glutathione (GSH) has been implicated as an inhibitor of As$_2$O$_3$-induced cell death either through conjugating As$_2$O$_3$ or by sequestering reactive oxygen induced by As$_2$O$_3$.** Consistent with this possibility, **increasing GSH levels with N-acetylcysteine attenuated As$_2$O$_3$ cytotoxicity**. Decreases in GSH have been associated with ascorbic acid (AA) metabolism. **Clinically relevant doses of AA decreased GSH levels and potentiated As$_2$O$_3$-mediated cell death of all 4 MM cell lines. I believe this is due to the prooxidant character of AA.** Similar results were obtained in freshly isolated human MM cells. In contrast, normal BM cells displayed little sensitivity to As$_2$O$_3$ alone or in combination with AA. Together, these data suggest that As$_2$O$_3$ and AA may be effective antineoplastic agents in refractory MM and that AA might be a useful adjuvant in GSH-sensitive therapies. (Grad et al, 2001).

I believe that this indicates that antioxidants are counter productive in the treatment of neoplasia and may increase the rate of proliferation of tumors by blocking the apoptotic effect of EMODs.

Tamoxifen blocks estrogen, which can help fuel the growth of tumors

Tamoxifen is a drug that is taken daily as a pill. It has been used for more than 25 years to help treat women with breast cancer. Tamoxifen works against breast cancer, in part, by interfering with the activity of estrogen. Estrogen is a female hormone that can fuel the growth of breast cancer cells. Tamoxifen works by blocking estrogen from attaching to receptors on the surface of breast cells. For this reason, it is often called an **"anti-estrogen."** and is used as a treatment for estrogen receptor positive breast cancer. (Estrogen receptor positive breast cancer responds to estrogen, estrogen receptor negative breast cancer does not.).

Prooxidant role of tamoxifen

A prooxidant role of Tam or OH-Tam has been presented and I believe that the prooxidant activity of tamoxifen is of most importance. (Gundimeda et al, 1996).

Antioxidants block antineoplasic effects of tamoxifen

Various antioxidants (vitamin E, vitamin C, beta-carotene, catalase, and superoxide dismutase) inhibited all these cellular effects of Tam. Moreover, vitamin E strikingly blocked Tam-induced growth inhibition. (Gundimeda et al, 1996).

Autophagy regulated by EMODs and caspase

Autophagy is the process of self-digestion by a cell through the action of enzymes originating within the same cell. Autophagy plays a central role in regulating important cellular functions such as cell survival during starvation and control of infectious pathogens. Recently, it has been shown that autophagy can induce cells to die; however, the mechanism of the autophagic cell death program is unclear. Investigators show that **caspase inhibition leading to cell death by means of autophagy involves reactive oxygen species (ROS) accumulation, membrane lipid oxidation, and loss of plasma membrane integrity**. Inhibition of autophagy by chemical compounds or knocking down the expression of key autophagy proteins such as ATG7, ATG8, and receptor interacting protein (RIP) blocks ROS accumulation and cell death. The cause of abnormal ROS accumulation is the selective autophagic degradation of the major enzymatic ROS scavenger, catalase. **Caspase inhibition directly induces catalase degradation and ROS accumulation,** which can be blocked by autophagy inhibitors. These findings unveil a molecular mechanism for the role of autophagy in cell death and provide insight into the complex relationship between ROS and nonapoptotic programmed cell death. (Yu et al, 2006).

Gemcitabine-EMOD-tumoricidal activity blocked by selenoprotein P

Gemcitabine is a new standard chemotherapeutic agent used in the treatment of pancreatic cancer, but the mechanisms of gemcitabine sensitivity are still controversial. In their study to determine a mechanism that regulates gemcitabine sensitivity, they carried out molecular analysis on the susceptibility of the pancreatic cancer cells. Using a gemcitabine-sensitive pancreatic cancer cell line KLM1, they established a resistant cell line KLM1-R exhibiting a 20-fold IC50-value (the concentration of gemcitabine causing 50% growth inhibition). Microarray analysis of genes showed specific expression of **selenoprotein P, one of the antioxidants**, in the KLM1-R cell line but not in the KLM1 cell line. Administration of selenoprotein P inhibited the gemcitabine-induced cytotoxicity in the pancreatic cell lines. The levels of intracellular reactive oxygen species (ROS) were increased

219

in the KLM1 cells by gemcitabine, but **selenoprotein P suppressed the gem-citabine-induced ROS levels**. Furthermore interferon-gamma suppressed the expression of selenoprotein P mRNA and increased intracellular ROS level, leading to the recovery of the gemcitabine sensitivity in KLM1-R. These results suggest a novel mechanism that **selenoprotein P reduces the intracellular ROS levels, resulting in the insusceptibility to gemcitabine.** (Maehara et al, 2004). **This paper demonstrates that the tumoricidal activity of Gemcitabine increases EMODs, and this effect is blocked by selenoprotein P.**

CHAPTER ELEVEN:

More prooxidant straws on the cancer's back

Sulforaphane (SFN) EMOD induced apoptosis: blocked by NAC

Sulforaphane (SFN) is a major isothiocyanate compound in cruciferous vegetables such as broccoli, cauliflower, and Brussels sprouts. Preclinical animal models have recently shown that SFN and other isothiocyanates may be useful for **prostrate cancer** (PCa) chemoprevention. **Pretreatment of cells with N-acetylcysteine to enrich intracellular glutathione blocked SFN-induced ROS and apoptotic cell death.** Taken together, the data indicate that SFN decreased viable **DU145 cell** number in large part **through the generation of ROS** and JNK-mediated signaling to G2/M arrest and caspase-dependent apoptosis. **Selenium in the form of inorganic sodium selenite salt or methylseleninic acid did not enhance SFN-induced apoptosis** in this cell culture model. (Cho et al, 2005). **Again, we see that an antioxidant blocks neoplasia kill. I believe that this has significant clinical importance and relevance and that these antioxidants should be avoided in patients undergoing cancer treatment.**

EMODs induced apoptosis of prostate cancer: blocked by NAC

Investigators have shown previously that **sulforaphane (SFN), a constituent of many edible cruciferous vegetables including broccoli, suppresses growth of prostate cancer** cells in culture as well as in vivo by causing apoptosis, but the sequence of events leading to cell death is poorly defined. Using **PC-3 and DU145 human prostate cancer** cells as a model, **they demonstrate, for the first time, that the initial signal for SFN-induced apoptosis is derived from reactive oxygen species (ROS).** Exposure of PC-3 cells to growth-suppressive concentrations of SFN resulted in ROS generation, which was accompanied by disruption of mitochondrial membrane potential, cytosolic release of cytochrome c, and apoptosis. **All these effects were significantly blocked on pretreatment with N-acetylcysteine and overexpression of catalase.** The SFN-induced ROS generation was significantly attenuated on pretreatment with mitochondrial respiratory chain complex I inhibitors, including diphenyleneiodonium chloride and **rotenone**. SFN treatment also caused a rapid and significant depletion of GSH levels. Collectively, these observations indicate that SFN-induced ROS generation is probably mediated by a nonmitochondrial mechanism involving GSH depletion as well as a mitochondrial component. Ectopic expression of Bcl-xL, but not Bcl-2, in PC-3 cells offered significant protection against the cell death caused by SFN. In addition, SFN treatment resulted in an increase in the level of Fas, activation of caspase-8, and cleavage of Bid. Furthermore, SV40-immortalized mouse embryonic fibroblasts (MEFs) derived from Bid knock-out mice displayed significant resistance toward SFN-induced apoptosis compared with wild-type MEFs. In conclusion, the results of the present study indicate that SFN-induced apoptosis in prostate cancer cells is initiated by ROS generation and that both intrinsic and extrinsic caspase cascades contribute to the cell death caused by this highly promising cancer chemopreventive agent. (Singh et al, 2005). **This important study shows that the apoptosis was induced by H_2O_2 and blocked by the antioxidant NAC. Again, EMODs kill cancer and antioxidants protect cancerous cells and allow them to proliferate.**

To me, this data augments my Unified theory and the data indicating the significance of EMODs as tumoricidal agents.

Nicotine suppresses oxidative burst

Now new research published in the open access April 2008 issue of the journal *BMC Cell Biology* shows that **nicotine affects neutrophils, the short-lived white blood cells that defend against infection, by reducing their ability to seek and destroy bacteria.**

Neutrophils are generated by our bone marrow, which they leave as terminally differentiated cells. Although nicotine is known to affect neutrophils, there has been no study until now of the mechanisms at work when nicotine is present during neutrophil differentiation. David Scott from the Oral Health and Systemic Disease Research Group at the University of Louisville School of Dentistry, Kentucky, USA, along with a team of international colleagues decided to investigate how nicotine influenced the differentiation process.

The authors suggest **the processes they observed as contributing to impaired neutrophil function partially explain chronic tobacco users' increased susceptibility to bacterial infection and inflammatory diseases.** A better understanding of this relationship could pave the way for specific therapeutic strategies to treat a number of important tobacco-associated inflammatory diseases and conditions. The team modeled the neutrophil differentiation process beginning with promyelocytic HL-60 cells, which differentiated into neutrophils following dimethylsulfoxide (DMSO) treatment both with and without nicotine. The researchers found that nicotine increased the percentage of cells in late differentiation phases (metamyelo-cytes, banded neutrophils and segmented neutrophils) compared to DMSO alone, but did not affect other neutrophil differentiation markers that they examined.

However, the nicotine treated neutrophils were less able to seek and destroy bacteria than nicotine-free neutrophils. **The nicotine suppressed the oxidative burst in HL-60 cells, a function that helps kill invading bacteria**. Nicotine also increased MMP-9 release, a factor involved in tissue degradation.

"It must be acknowledged that our study model, DMSO-differentiated HL-60 cells, are not entirely similar to normal neutrophils," says Scott. "However, this leukemic human cell line does permit the reproducible study of differentiation while retaining many of the key effector functions of primary neutrophils." (Xu et al,).

I believe that the suppression of the oxidative burst, in combination with the effects of carbon monoxide, account for the increased association of diseases in smokers and the clustering of diseases, ROSI syndrome.

Phenylethyl isothiocyanate (PEITC) apoptosis: blocked by NAC and vitamin E

Phenylethyl isothiocyanate (PEITC) is a well recognized potential chemopreventive compound against human cancers. In this study, the molecular mechanism of PEITC-induced apoptosis was examined with two antioxidants (N-acetyl-cysteine and vitamin E) and a caspase-3 inhibitor (z-DEVD-fmk). Results demonstrated that PEITC significantly induced **human hepatoma PLC/PRF/5** (CD95-negative) cells undergoing apoptosis. Treatment with 0 approximately 10 microM PEITC-triggered cell apoptosis as revealed by the externalization of annexin V-targeted phosphatidylserine and the subsequent appearance of sub-G1 population. Results also displayed that PEITC-induced apoptosis involves the up-regulation of p53 and Bax protein, down-regulation of the XIAP, Bcl-2, Bcl-(XL) and Mcl-1 proteins, cleavage of Bid, and the release of cytochrome c and Smac/Diablo, which were accompanied by the activation of caspases -9, -3 and -8. **PEITC-induced the generation of reactive oxygen species** and the decrease of mitochondrial membrane potential (Deltapsim) in a time-dependent pattern. **N-acetyl-cysteine and vitamin E at 100 microM, and z-DEVD-fmk at 50 microM markedly blocked PEITC-induced apoptosis, which was demonstrated by a decline in the reactive oxygen species generation** and the release of the cytochrome c and Smac/Diablo from mitochondria to the cytosol. N-acetyl-cysteine, vitamin E and z-DEVD-fmk also prevented the PEITC in inducing the loss of Deltapsim. They also affected the activity of XIAP and Bax proteins. Taken together, these studies suggest that PEITC is an apoptotic inducer that acts on the mitochondria and the feedback amplification loop of caspase-8/Bid pathways in PLC/PRF/5 cells. (Wu et al, 2005). **Clearly, human cancer cells will be allowed to proliferate by the use of NAC and vitamin E.**

EMOD selective kill of cancer cells with beta-phenylethyl isothiocyanate (PEITC)

Oncogenic transformation usually leads to increase of cellular reactive oxygen species (ROS) level that **renders the cells vulnerable to additional ROS production**. By targeting ROS, a naturally occurring ROS-inducing compound, beta-phenylethyl isothiocyanate (PEITC), **selectively kills the transformed cells but not normal cells** (Wu, Hua, 2007).

Doxorubicin blocked by N-acetylcysteine

The cardiotoxicity induced by the **anticancer anthracycline doxorubicin (DOX)** is attributed to reactions between iron and reactive oxygen species (ROS) that lead to oxidative damage. They found that DOX forms ROS in **H9c2 cardiomyocytes**, as shown by dichlorodihydrofluorescein oxidation and the expression of stress-responsive genes such as catalase or aldose reductase. DOX also increased ferritin levels in these cells, particularly the H subunit. A considerable increase in ferritin mRNA levels showed that DOX acted at transcriptional level, but an additional potential mechanism was identified as the down-regulation of iron regulatory protein-2, post-transcriptional inhibitor of ferritin synthesis. Pretreatment with DOX protected H9c2 cells against the damage induced by subsequent exposure to ferric ammonium citrate, and experiments with [5][5]Fe revealed that the protection was due to the deposition of iron in ferritin. Cytoprotection was also observed when DOX was replaced by glucose/glucose oxidase, a source of H_2O_2, thus suggesting that DOX increases ferritin synthesis through the action of ROS. This concept was supported by three more lines of evidence. (i) **DOX-induced ferritin synthesis was blocked by N-acetylcysteine, a scavenger of ROS**. (ii) Mitoxantrone, a ROS-forming analogue, similarly induced ferritin expression and protected the cells against iron toxicity. (iii) 5-Iminodaunorubicin, an analogue lacking ROS-forming activity, did not induce ferritin synthesis or protect the cells against iron toxicity.

These results characterize a paradoxically beneficial link between anthracycline-derived ROS, increased ferritin synthesis, and resistance to iron-mediated damage. The role of iron and ROS in anthracycline-induced cardiotoxicity may, therefore, be more complex than previously believed. (Gianfranco et al, 2004).

CHAPTER TWELVE:

Quinones

Many naturally occurring quinones can be isolated from biological tissues. (O'Brien, 1991).

Also, chemotherapeutic drugs (adriamycine, daunorubicin, and mitomycine), acetaminophen (Tylenol), and air pollutants (cigarette smoke and automobile exhaust) are common source of quinones. Some quinones have potential to markedly induce the generation of prooxidant EMODs.

Lapacho (naphthoquinone) generates tumoricidal EMODs

The highly active, quinone-containing anticancer drugs, Adriamycin, daunorubicin, carminomycin, rubidazone, nogalamycin, aclacinomycin A, and steffimycin (benzanthraquinones); mitomycin C and streptonigrin (/V-heterocyclic quiÃ±tones); and lapacho (naphthoquinone) interact with mammalian microsomes and function as free radical carriers. These quinone drugs augment the flow of electrons from reduced nicotinamide adenine dinucleotide phosphate to molecular oxygen as measured by enhanced reduced nicotinamide adenine dinucleotide phosphate oxidation and oxygen consumption. This reaction is catalyzed by microsomal protein and **produces a free radical intermediate form of the drugs** as determined by electron paramagnetic resonance spectroscopy. Microsomes from mouse and rat liver, heart, lung, and spleen and mouse L1210 and P388 tumors all catalyze the augmented oxygen consumption. Apparent Km values determined with normal rat liver microsomes range from 0.49 x 10~"Mfor steffimycin to 13.4 x 10~"M for lapacho. Since SKF 525A and carbon monoxide have little effect on this reaction, cytochrome P-450 is probably not involved. Several nonquinone anticancer agents were tested and were found inactive in the system. Since quinone anticancer drugs are associated with chromosomal damage that appears to be dependent on metabolic activation of these drugs, **we propose that the intracellular activation of these drugs to a free radical state may be primary to their cytotoxic activity.** As free radicals, these drugs, because of their high affinity and selective binding to nucleic acids, have the potential to be "site-specific free radicals" that bind to DNA or RNA and either react directly or **generate oxygen-dependent free radicals such as superoxide radical or hydroxyl radical to cause the damage associated with their cytotoxic actions.** (Bachur et al, 1978).

Oysters contain EMOD-apoptosis-inducing ceramides: blocked by NAC

Ceramide is one of the major sphingosine-based lipid second messengers that is generated in response to various extracellular agents. However, while widespread attention has focused on ceramide as a second messenger involved in the induction of apoptosis, important issues with regard to the mechanisms of ceramide formation and mode of action remain to be addressed. Several lines of evidence suggest that **ceramide and oxidative stress are intimately related in cell death induction.** This review focuses on the putative relationships between oxidative stress and sphingolipid metabolism in the apoptotic process and discusses the potential mechanisms that connect and regulate the two phenomena. (Andrieu-Abadie et al, 2001).

Anthracyclines such as daunorubicin (DNR) generate radical oxygen species (ROS), which account, at least in part, for their cytotoxic effect. We observed that early ceramide generation (within 6–10 min) through neutral sphingomyelinase stimulation was **inhibitable by the antioxidants N-acetylcysteine and pyrrolidine dithiocarbamate, which led to a decrease in apoptosis** (.95% decrease in DNA fragmentation after 6 h). Furthermore, we observed that DNR triggers the c-Jun N-terminal kinase (JNK) and the transcription factor activated protein-1 through an antioxidant-inhibitable mechanism. **Treatment of U937 cells (**isolated from the histiocytic lymphoma of a 37 year old male patient**) with cell-permeant ceramides induced both an increase in EMOD generation and JNK activation, and apoptosis, all of which were antioxidant-sensitive.** In conclusion, DNR-triggered apoptosis implicates a ceramide-mediated, ROS-dependent JNK and activated protein-1 activation. (Mansat-De Mas et al, 1999).

Onion oil EMOD-induced apoptosis: blocked by NAC and glutathione

Protective effects of Allium vegetables against cancers have been shown extensively in experimental animals and epidemiologic studies. We investigated cell proliferation and the induction of apoptosis by onion oil extracted from Allium cepa, a widely consumed Allium vegetable, in **human non small cell lung cancer A549 cells**. GC/MS analysis suggested that propyl sulfides but not allyl sulfides are major sulfur-containing constituents of onion oil. Onion oil at 12.5 mg/L significantly induced apoptosis (13% increase of apoptotic cells) as indicated by sub-G1 DNA content. It also caused cell cycle arrest at the G2/M phase; 25 mg/L onion oil increased the percentage of G2/M cells almost 6-fold compared with the dimethyl sulfoxide control. The action of onion oil may occur via a reactive oxygen species–dependent pathway because **cell cycle arrest and apoptosis were blocked by the antioxidants N-acetylcysteine and exogenous glutathione.** Marked collapse of the mitochondrial membrane potential suggested that dysfunction of the mitochondria may be involved in the oxidative burst and apoptosis induced by onion oil. Expression of phospho-cdc2 and phospho-cyclin B1 were downregulated by onion oil, perhaps accounting for the G2/M arrest. Overall, these results suggest that onion oil may exert chemopreventive action by inducing cell cycle arrest and apoptosis in tumor cells. (Wu et al, 2006).

SECTION FOUR:

Vitamins, Chemo, radiation, PDT & HBO

CHAPTER THIRTEEN:

Chemotherapy

Summary of chemotherapeutic agents which generate EMODs:

Oxygen dependence has also been established for a number of chemo-therapeutic agents such as cyclophosphamide, carboplatin, doxorubicin, etc. and levels are different for each agent. Hypoxia can impart resistance to many chemotherapeutic agents (Teicher et al, 1990).

The chemotherapeutic agents doxorubicin, mitomycin C, etoposide and cisplatin are superoxide generating agents. (Yokomizo et al, 1995).

Many antitumor agents, such as vinblastine, cisplatin, mitomycin C, doxorubicin, camptothecin, inostamycin, neocarzinostatin and many others exhibit antitumor activity via EMOD induced apoptotic (ROS-dependent apoptosis activation) cell death, suggesting use of EMODs as an antitumor principle. (Fang, Nakamura, Iyer, 2007). In fact, some experts now believe that all chemotherapeutic agents generate some level of apoptosis activating EMODs.

Chemotherapeutic agents can **act solely via the production of reactive oxygen species and induction of apoptosis** (Ratnam et al, 2006). These agents include the **anthracyclines (e.g., doxorubicin), platinum-containing complexes (e.g., cisplatin, carboplatin), alkylating agents (e.g., cyclophosphamide, ifosfamide), and cytotoxic antibiotics (e.g., bleomycin, mitomycin-C).**

Although some classes of antineoplastic agents generate high levels of oxidative stress, others, including the taxanes, vinca alkaloids, antifolates, and nucleoside and nucleotide analogues, generate only low levels. Nevertheless, all drugs generate some free radicals as they induce apoptosis in cancer cells.

The highly active, quinone-containing anticancer drugs, Adriamycin, daunorubicin, carminomycin, rubidazone, nogalamycin, aclacinomycin A, and steffimycin (benzanthraquinones); mitomycin C and streptonigrin (/V-heterocyclic quiÃ±ones); and lapacho (naphthoquinone) interact with mammalian microsomes and function as free radical carriers. As free radicals, these drugs, because of their high affinity and selective binding to nucleic acids, have the potential to be "site-specific free radicals" that bind to DNA or RNA and either react directly or **generate oxygen-dependent free radicals such as superoxide radical or hydroxyl radical to cause the damage associated with their cytotoxic actions.** (Bachur et al, 1978).

Many antitumor agents, such as vinblastine, cisplatin, mitomycin C, doxorubicin, camptothecin, inostamycin, neocarzinostatin and many others exhibit antitumor activity via (EMOD) ROS-dependent activation of apoptotic cell death, suggesting potential use of ROS as an antitumor principle. (Fang, Nakamura, Iyer, 2007).

The basis of EMOD induced apoptosis cancer therapies

Chemotherapy-induced formation of EMODs is well demonstrated most notably with alkylating agents, anthracyclines, epipdophyllotoxins (e.g., etoposide and teniposide), and antitumor antibiotics (mitomycin, bleomycin). (Black and Livingston, I, 1990) (Black and Livingston, II, 1990).

Thus, theoretically, antioxidant vitamins may protect normal cells and shield cancer cells against free radicals that are generated by chemotherapy and radiation therapy. Obviously, agents not involving EMOD production pose less concern and may include hormonal therapy, biological agents, antimetabolites, vinca alkaloids, and taxanes. (Labriola and Livingston, 1999).

There has been some evidence supporting the concomitant use of antioxidants and chemotherapy. Administration of vitamin E enhanced antitumor activity of cisplatin *in vivo* in a murine neuroblastoma model. (Sue et al, 1998).

In vitro studies with neuroblastoma, melanoma and non-small cell lung cancer cell lines have also shown that antioxidants can enhance the antitumor effects of 5-FU, cisplatin, doxorubicin and dacarbazine. (Prasad KN, et al, 1979) (Prasad et al, 1994) (Chiang et al, 1994).

And, **paradoxically**, *in vitro*, **vitamin C is reported to improve the antineoplastic activity** of doxorubicin, cisplatin, and paclitaxil in human breast carcinoma cells. (Kurbacher, 1996).

This type of data emphasizes the fact that most antioxidants can have prooxidant activity under the right circumstances. I have found that when antioxidants are effective cancer cell killers, they are usually acting as prooxidants. The interactions between antioxidants and chemotherapy are more complex than might be predicted solely on the basis of oxidative mechanisms. As I have said many times, **antioxidants and prooxidants are flip sides of the same redox coin!** Such may be the case in which vitamin E induced apoptosis in colorectal cancer cells, and significantly enhanced tumor growth inhibition by 5-FU and doxorubicin. (Chinery et al, 1997).

This prooxidant stimulation of apoptotic pathways may explain the synergistic effects of chemotherapy and radiation with antioxidant therapy.

Even though chemotherapy-induced formation of free radicals is well documented, both **in vitro and animal studies** have shown that the co-administration of antioxidants did not reduce the antitumor effect of cytostatic agents such as doxorubicicn and cisplatin in some studies. Also, the survival of animals co-administered antioxidants was increased compared to the survival of animals that received chemotherapy alone. (Satoh et al, 1992) (Shimpo et al, 1991) (Saldew et al, 1990) (Siveski-Iliskovic et al, 1995).

Apparently, vitamin E pre-treatment did not interfere with the action of doxorubicin in rats with myeloid leukemia, but it seemingly did reduce cardiotoxicity. (Sonnevald, 1976).

In another study, a combination of vitamins A, C, and E, enhanced antitumor effects of doxorubicin on transplanted tumors in mice. (Mosienko et al, 1990).

Of great interest is the fact that the conclusions of these **old studies** (*in vitro* and animal studies) **have not been duplicated or confirmed by RCTs in humans over the past decade**.

In some older clinical studies, synthetic antioxidants did not alter the antitumor effect of chemotherapy. (Kemp et al, 1996) (Venturini et al, 1996) (Gandara et al, 1995).

In a randomized trial evaluating 100 breast cancer patients taking cyclophosphamide or doxorubicin, supplementation with vitamin A improved response rate to chemotherapy. (Israel et al, 1985). **Beta carotene has been shown to have significant prooxidant activity.**

Other older studies added to the mystic of antioxidants. (Jaakola et al, 1992).

Prof Randolph M. Howes MD, PhD

A review by Weijl et al. reports on numerous in vitro, animal and clinical studies (264 references) demonstrating a reduction in adverse effects from these chemotherapeutic agents with co-administration of various antioxidants. (Weijl et al, 1997).

Some believe that synthetic antioxidant cytoprotectants can be routinely used by to attenuate the toxicity of chemotherapeutic agents and radiation therapy while preserving its effectiveness, such as mesna or ifosfamide induced hemorrhagic cystitis, dexrazoxane for adriamycin cardiotoxicity and amifostine for cisplatin nephrotoxicity. This tends to indicate that natural antioxidant supplementation can safely be combined with chemotherapy and radiation therapy.

If only it were that simple.

EMODs, antioxidants and apoptosis: all antineoplastic drugs yield EMODs

The drugs of many classes of antineoplastic agents are known to generate a high level of oxidative stress in biological systems. These classes of drugs include the anthracyclines, most alkylating agents, platinum-coordination complexes, epipodophyllotoxins, and camptothecins. For these drugs, the hepatic microsomal monooxygenase system is a primary site where ROS are generated, although other enzymatic (e.g., xanthine oxidase) and nonenzymatic (Fenton and Haber-Weiss reactions) mechanisms also play a role. The electron transport system of cardiac mitochondria is another site where significant levels of ROS are generated by anthracyclines.

Although some classes of antineoplastic agents generate high levels of oxidative stress, others, including the taxanes, vinca alkaloids, antifolates, and nucleoside and nucleotide analogues, generate only low levels. Nevertheless, all drugs generate some free radicals as they induce apoptosis in cancer cells.

Although superoxide is not highly toxic, mitochondrial superoxide dismutase generates hydrogen peroxide from superoxide and, in the presence of reduced iron that is abundant in mitochondria, highly toxic hydroxyl radicals are formed via Fenton and Haber-Weiss reactions. Thus, **all drugs that induce apoptosis by this mechanism generate some degree of oxidative stress**, although this does not imply that free radical generation is necessary for a drug to exert its cytotoxic effect on neoplastic cells, because the apoptotic process is initiated by cytochrome c release and superoxide generation may occur secondarily. (Conklin, 2004).

Evidence supporting the avoidance of antioxidants with chemotherapy

There is considerable **evidence supporting the avoidance of antioxidants with chemotherapy.**

Some *in vitro* studies, however, have shown a **reduction in antitumor effect when antioxidants (N-acetylcysteine, selenium, superoxide dismutase and catalase) and iron chelating agents were co-administered with doxorubicin.** (Doroshow, 1986).

And a similar in vitro effect was shown with vitamin A and doxorubicin. (Doyle et al, 1989).

Further, **beta carotene has been shown to reduce the effect of 5-FU in a murine fibrosarcoma model.** (Teicher et al, 1994).

Vitamin C was shown to enhance doxorubicin resistance in human breast cancer cell lines. (Wells et al, 1995).

And vitamin C reduced the cytotoxic effects of methotrexate and DTIC on neuroblastoma cell lines. (Prasad et al, PNAS. 1979).

N-acetylcysteine has been shown to reduce the effect of doxoxrubicin in one animal study and reduce the effect of cisplatin in vitro. (Schmitt-Graff and Schuelen, 1986) and **to reduce the effects of sic-dichlorodiamineplatinum in human invasive bladder cancer cell line, KU1.** (Miyajima et al, 1999 - human bladder cancer KU-1 cell line).

And **the bioflavinoid tangeretin, has been shown to inhibit the effect of tamoxifen on mammary cancer in a mouse model.** (Bracke et al, 1999).

Chemotherapeutic agent categories

Based on their specificity, chemotherapy drugs can be classified as cell-specific agents (effective during certain cell cycle phases) and cell-cycle non-specific (effective during all phases of the cell cycle). Based on their specific characteristics and nature of treatment, chemotherapeutic agents can be classified as alkylating agents, anti-metabolites, anthracyclines, antitumor antibiotics, monoclonal antibodies, platinums, or plant alkaloids.

Cancer therapy can be aimed at the cell cycle, which consists of four phases, i.e., the G_1, S, G_2, and M phases. (http://www.mesotheliomaweb.org/categories.htm. Accessed 8-25-09).

Chemotherapy-induced formation of free radicals is well demonstrated most notably with alkylating agents, anthracyclines, epipdophyllotoxins (e.g., etoposide and teniposide), and antitumor antibiotics (mitomycin, bleomycin).

Other agents, **not known to generate free radicals, pose less concern.** These include hormonal therapy, biological agents, antimetabolites, vinca alkaloids, and taxanes.

Antimetabolites

Antimetabolite antineoplastic agents have structures similar to compounds occurring naturally in the body, such as vitamins, amino acids and DNA and RNA precursors. Popular antimetabolite drugs are 5-fluorouracil (5FU), Methotraxate, Thioguanine, Cytarabine, Cladribine, Gemcitabine, and Fludarabine.

Alkylating agents

Having being introduced in the early 1940s, alkylating agents have been one of the most commonly used methods for cancer treatment. Many of these agents are active or dormant nitrogen mustards, which are poisonous agents previously used in military operations. Commonly used alkylating agents are Chlorambucil, Cyclophosphamide, CCNU, Melphalan, Procarbazine, Thiotepa, BCNU and Busulphan and they are effective during all phases of the cell cycle.

Anthracyclines

Anthracycline drugs are daunosamine and tetra-hydronaphthacenedione-based chemotherapeutic agents. Common drugs in this category are daunorubicin, Doxorubicin, Idarubicin, Epirubicin, and Mitoxantrone. Anthracyclines work by generating EMOD-induced apoptosis or by breaking DNA strands and thereby inhibiting DNA synthesis and function.

Anthracyclines (doxorubicin, daunorubicin, epirubicin, and idarubicin) are currently the most effective group of anti-neoplastic drugs used in clinical practice. Of these, doxorubicin (also called adriamycin) is a key chemotherapeutic agent in cancer treatment, although its use is limited as a consequence of the chronic and acute toxicity associated with this drug.

Antitumor antibiotics

Antitumor antibiotics also generate EMODs. The most common antitumor antibiotic is Bleomycin, which is used to treat testicular cancer and Hodgkin's lymphoma.

Bleomycin causes EMOD generation and its effects are blocked by antioxidants (Buettner et al, 1992).

Monoclonal antibodies

One of the newest tumoricidal agents is the monoclonal antibodies, which reportedly works by attaching to certain parts of the tumor specific antigens making them easily recognizable by the body's immune system. They also block the cell receptors to which chemicals called "growth factors" attach promoting growth. Examples are Alemtuzumab (Campath), Bevacizumab (Avastin), Cetuximab (Erbitux), Gemtuzumab (Mylotarg), Ibritumomab (Zevalin), Panitumumab (Vectibix), Rituximab (Rituxan), Tositumomab (Bexxar), and Trastuzumab (Herceptin). Monoclonal antibodies can be combined with other antineoplastic drugs and radioactive particles and deliver them directly to cancer cells.

Platinum derivatives

Platinum-based chemotherapy drugs work by cross-linking DNA subunits. The first generation drug was cisplatin, the second generation drug was carboplatin and the third generation drug was Oxaliplatin.

Plant alkaloids

Plant alkaloid chemotherapy drugs are primarily categorized into four groups: topoisomerase inhibitors, vinca alkaloids, taxanes and epidophyllotoxins. Mesothelioma is treated with the plant alkaloid Vincristine (Oncovin).

Topoisomerase inhibitors

Topoisomerase inhibitors are classified into type I, such as camptothecans (irinotecan and topotecan), which are from the bark and wood of the Chinese tree Camptotheca accuminata. Type II are Amsacrine, etoposide, etoposide phosphate, and teniposide, which are from the roots of May apple plants.

Vinca alkaloids

Vinca alkaloids, from the periwinkle plant, are effective in the M phase of the cell cycle and consist of Vincristine, Vinblastine, Vinorelbine and Vindesine.

Taxanes

Plant alkaloids, the taxanes, also work in the M cell cycle phase and consist of Paclitaxel and docetaxel.

Epipodophyllotoxins

Epipodophyllotoxins are extracted from the May Apple tree and consist of etoposide and Teniposide and are effective in the G1 and S cell cycle phases.

Porphyrin derivatives

Motexafin gadolinium (MGd), an expanded porphyrin, is a tumor-selective redox-mediator that reacts with many intracellular reducing metabolites and induces apoptosis. The mechanism of cytotoxicity was related to induction of apoptosis as demonstrated by alteration in mitochondrial membrane potential and elevated annexin V expression. This was accompanied by depletion of intracellular glutathione and increased EMOD production. Catalase substantially abrogated MGd-induced cell death. (Evens et al, 2005).

Many chemotherapeutic drugs have well-defined mechanisms of actions, including traditional alkylating agents and anthracycline antitumor antibiotics, which generate EMODs. **Depending upon specifics of oxidation/reduction potentials, these EMODs are uniformly subject to transformation to altered compounds by antioxidants through the simple process of electron transfer.**

According to Conklin, when cytochrome c is displaced from the electron transport chain, instead of electrons being transferred to oxygen via cytochrome c oxidase with the formation of water, electrons are diverted from NADH dehydrogenase (Complex I) and reduced coenzyme Q10 to oxygen with the concomitant formation of superoxide radicals. Although superoxide is not highly toxic, mitochondrial superoxide dismutase generates hydrogen peroxide from superoxide and, in the presence of reduced iron that is abundant in mitochondria, highly toxic hydroxyl radicals are formed via Fenton and Haber-Weiss reactions. Thus, all drugs that induce apoptosis by this mechanism generate some degree of oxidative stress, although this does not imply that free radical generation is necessary for a drug to exert its cytotoxic effect on neoplastic cells, because the apoptotic process is initiated by cytochrome c release and superoxide generation occurs secondarily. (Conklin, 2004).

My question at this point is, "If EMODs are so damaging to membranes, how does the mitochondrial membrane survive, especially in the presence of hydroxyl radicals? I do not believe it and there are some who say that the Haber-Weiss reaction does not occur at all under physiological conditions. There is significant data showing the key role of EMODs in antineoplastic activity.

Although approved cytoprotectants (antioxidants) are available, including dexrazoxane for doxorubicin-induced cardiotoxicity, amifostine for cisplatin-induced nephrotoxicity, and mesna for ifosfamide-induced hemorrhagic cystitis, **these agents are not without adverse effects.** To wit, dexrazoxane can reduce the antineoplastic activity of doxorubicin. This most likely results from complex formation and inactivation of doxorubicin, which may also prevent doxorubicin from interfering with CoQ10 biosynthesis and function, thus explaining the cardioprotectant effect of dexrazoxane. **Dexrazoxane is also myelosuppressive and may increase the risk of developing secondary malignancies. Amifostine can induce hypotension, hypocalcemia, and nausea, and administration of mesna is associated with nausea, vomiting, and diarrhea.**

EMOD production by chemotherapeutic agents

EMODs do not activate NF-kB DNA binding

Some studies indicate that EMODs are not involved with certain chemotherapeutic drugs. Investigators have examined the role of EMODs in the pharmacodynamics of chemotherapeutic agents. (Campbell et al, 2006). These investigators found that

EMOD generation is apparently not required for induction of NF-κB DNA binding, implied by the effect of mitoxantrone. Although reactive oxygen species have been

shown to activate NF-κB in a cell context dependent manner, it has been recently shown that many of the compounds used in studies to neutralize free radicals in

themselves could inhibit NF-κB activity. In that regard, N-acetyl-L-cysteine (NAC) and pyrrolidine dithiocarbamate (PDTC), antioxidants commonly used in studies of NF-kB activation, prevented TNF induced NF-kB DNA binding independent of their antioxidant activity (Hayakawa et al, 2003).

NAC was shown to lower the affinity of TNF for its receptor, whilst PDTC inhib-

ited the IkB-ubiquitin ligase activity. In contrast, alternative antioxidants such as epigallocatechingallate (EGCG), the main component of green tea, and trolox, a soluble vitamin E analogue (both strong phenolic radical scavengers) did not affect

TNF induced NF-kB activation. (Hayakawa et al, 2003).

EMODs induce NF-kB DNA-binding

Oxygen free radicals have been shown to induce NF-kB DNA-binding under some circumstances and could potentially represent a key component of the ability of

cytotoxic agents to differentially regulate NF-kB function. (Schreck et al, 1991) (Schoonbroodt et al, 2000) (Brennan, O'Neill, 1995).

Daunorubicin and doxorubicin

Daunorubicin and doxorubicin can undergo redox cycling and produce EMODs, which can have a variety of effects, including damage to cell membranes and DNA-damage. (Gerwirtz, 1999).

Bleomycin and doxorubicin

Bleomycin and doxorubicin are two agents known to generate reactive oxygen species. (Hasinoff, Davey, 1988).

In reactions involving Fe(II) and oxygen, an "activated" bleomycin species is formed that damages DNA through free radical intermediates. (Burger, 1998).

Superoxide and hydrogen peroxide can also react with Fe(II) or Fe(III) bleomycin, respectively, to produce the activated form of the drug. DNA damage from bleomycin and ionizing radiation is similar both in induction and re- pair. (Byfield et al, 1976).

Anthracyclines

NADPH-flavin reductase, cytochrome p450 reductase and mitochondrial NADH reductase can all reduce anthracyclines to a semiquinone radical. (Halliwell, 1989).

This semiquinone radical can donate its free electron to molecular oxygen to generate the superoxide radical ($O_2^{\cdot}$).

Like hydrogen peroxide (H_2O_2), $O_2^{\cdot}$ can generate hydroxyl radicals ($^{\cdot}OH$) upon interaction with metal ions. (Halliwell, 1989).

This results in lipid peroxidation of plasma membranes, leading to a loss of mitochondrial inner membrane potential and consequent cytochrome c release and apoptosis. Reactive oxygen species can also directly damage DNA through generation of strand breaks and oxidized nucleic bases such as guanine to 8-hydroxyguanine, giving rise to G-T transversions.

However, **free radical generation by anthracyclines is thought to be responsible for the cardiotoxicity that limits their therapeutic use.** (Davies, Doroshow, 1986) (Doroshow, Davies, 1986).

CHAPTER FOURTEEN: RADIATION

Radiotherapy produces extensive amounts of EMODs

In tissues exposed to treatment, **radiotherapy produces cytotoxic free radicals and extensive oxidative stress**. (Cook et al, 2004) (Doroshenko et al, 2004).

Ionizing radiation produces a number of reactive oxygen species, including superoxide ion, hydroxyl radical, and hydrogen peroxide; it is currently postulated that the primary therapeutic effects from radiotherapy are mediated through the generation of cytotoxic reactive oxygen species. (Cook et al, 2004) (Lee et al, 2004).

Furthermore, **cancer cells accumulate iron, and radiotherapy elevates intracellular free iron concentrations that can lead to the production of cytotoxic hydroxyl radicals through the Fenton reaction.** (Kwok, Richardson, 2002) (Weijl et al, 2004).

Therefore, **cells exposed to radiotherapy are subjected to heightened oxidative stress.** These cells must either adapt to such conditions or perish. Adaptation often includes induction of biochemical pathways that quench or mediate the destructive effects of reactive intermediates. **In U251 human glioblastoma cells, radiation has been shown to induce the expression of a number of antioxidant enzymes, including superoxide dismutase (twofold) and glutathione peroxidase** (fivefold). (Lee eAntioxidant adaptations noted in U251 human glioblastoma cells are consistent with clinical observations of GBM resistance to radiotherapy. Glioblastoma is one of the most radioresistant tumors. Exposure of cells to ionizing radiation leads to formation of reactive oxygen species (ROS) that are associated with radiation-induced cytotoxicity. ROS scavengers, therefore, are one of the important factors in protecting cells against ROS injury during ionizing radiation exposure. In the present study, they isolated and established a radioresistant variant clone (RRC) from **U251 human glioblastoma cell line** and investigated the potential role of antioxidant enzymes in radioresistance of the glioblastoma cell line. RRC showed a higher radioresistance than the parent cell line as measured by clonogenic survival assay and showed delayed G2/M arrest. Antioxidant enzymes, such as **superoxide dismutase (SOD), catalase, glutathione peroxidase (GPX), glutathione reductase (GR), were activated up to 5-fold in RRC** compared to the parent cells after radiation. **In addition, RRC**

also had cross-resistance to the antitumor agent cisplatin. Therefore, radioresistance and cross-resistance to chemotherapeutic agent in RRC might be due to the highly coordinated activation of antioxidant enzymes rather than a single enzyme alone. (Lee et al, 2004).

Glioblastoma adds another human cancer cell line which is sheltered by antioxidants, in this case, by antioxidant enzymes.

Cancer cells are frequently found in a low-oxygen (hypoxic) environment. **Hypoxic cancer cells are radio-resistant,** which contributes dramatically to the inability of radiotherapy to control neoplastic growth and metastasis. **Methods or therapies that provide increased oxygen to cancer cells help radiation work more effectively by enabling more EMOD or free-radical formation.**

Radiation kills cancer cells by concentrating massive amounts of free radicals directly into tumors.

Ionized radiation releases reactive oxygen species from the water molecule. (Little et al, 1993). Thus, cancer patients who undergo radiation therapy may be exposed to significant quantities of reactive oxygen species.

Radiation therapy produces numerous biological perturbations in cells and treatments are designed to strike a balance between eradicating neoplastic cells and protecting normal cells. Radiotherapy aims to alter cellular homeostasis, modify signal transduction pathways, alter redox states and induce cellular apoptosis.

Clinical radiation therapy utilizes electromagnetic radiation and particulate radiation, mostly electrons and to a lesser extent neutrons and protons, which damages cells by direct ionization of DNA and other cellular targets and by indirect effect **through generation of EMODs.** Exposure to ionizing radiation produces oxygen-derived free radicals including hydroxyl radicals (the most damaging), superoxide anion radicals, hydrogen peroxide and other oxidants. (Borek, 2004).

Even though EMODs are effective in killing tumor cells, they may threaten the integrity and survival of surrounding normal cells, which is dependent upon inherent tissue sensitivity and repair. Intracellular oxygen determines the extent of DNA damage by X-rays and gamma-rays. **To be effective, oxygen must be present during radiation or at least during the lifetime of the free radical (10^{-5} s).**

Without oxygen, the indirect radiation damage can be repaired and thiols, e.g., glutathione, or other antioxidants can compete with this oxidation.

Apoptosis is triggered via a mitochondrial-dependent pathway, with the release of cytochrome C, followed by activation of the caspase cascade, with caspase 3 leading cells to their death. Also, apoptosis can proceed through a mitochondrial-independent pathway, with the ligation of death receptors CD95 (Fas/Apo1/) and the subsequent recruitment of caspases. (Zimmerman et al, 2001).

Therapeutic radiation doses deplete cellular alpha-tocopherol in normal cells, thereby increasing their risk of damage and animal studies show that whole-body exposure to X-ray irradiation or aging decreases tissue concentrations of vitamins C and E. (Umegaku et al, 1995).

A reduction in tissue vitamins E and Se during radiation therapy for breast cancer and a fall in vitamins A, C, E, and Se during breast cancer treatment with EMOD-producing adriamycine **may increase normal tissue sensitivity to radiation damage.** (Borek, 2004).

Antioxidant impact depends on the oxygen partial pressure in a tissue and the reactivity of the antioxidant and beta carotene is an effective chain-breaking antioxidant at low PO$_2$; whereas, at high oxygen pressure it is less efficient and may even act as a prooxidant due to autooxidation. (Young et al, 2001).

A combined treatment with vitamins E and C inhibits apoptosis in human endothelial cells more effectively than each alone, while increasing Bcl-2 and downregulating the pro-apoptotic Bax. (Haendeler et al, 1996).

Adding to the confusion, vitamin E can induce apoptosis in human breast and prostate cancer cells as well as leukemia and glioblastoma cells. (Sigounas et al, 1997) (Borek, Pardo, 2002).

Thus, **EMOD-induced prooxidant apoptosis and the cancer conundrum leave us with unanswered questions regarding their interactions, autooxidation of antioxidants and the prooxidant character of some antioxidants.** (Seifried et al, 2003).

The bottom line is that oxygen and its derivatives are essential for effective radiation therapy and the induction of either apoptosis or necrosis.

EMOD-induced apoptosis (HeLa cell death) with radiation

Oxidative damage is an important mechanism in X-ray-induced cell death. Radiolysis of water molecules is a source of reactive oxygen species (ROS) that contribute to X-ray-induced cell death. In this study, we showed by ROS detection and a cell survival assay that **NADPH oxidase has a very important role in X-ray-induced cell death. Under X-ray irradiation, the upregulation of the expression of NADPH oxidase membrane subunit gp91**[phox] **was dose-dependent.** Meanwhile, the cytoplasmic subunit p47[phox] was translocated to the cell membrane and localized with p22[phox] and gp91[phox] to form reactive NADPH oxidase. Our data suggests, for the first time, that **NADPH oxidase-mediated generation of ROS is an important contributor to X-ray-induced cell death.** This suggests a new target for combined gene transfer and radiotherapy. (Liu et al, 2008). **This study shows that radiation kills cancer cells directly with EMODs and further induces increased levels of EMOD-producing NADPH oxidase.**

No role of nutritional intervention in patients treated with radiotherapy for pelvic malignancy

Up to **12,000 patients** with gynecological, urological and rectal cancer undergo radical pelvic radiotherapy annually in the UK. More than 70% develop acute inflammatory changes causing gastrointestinal symptoms during treatment because healthy bowel tissue is encompassed in the radiation field. In total, 50% go on to develop chronic bowel symptoms, which affect quality of life due to permanent changes in the small and large intestine. Nutritional intervention may influence acute and chronic bowel symptoms but the validity of the advice given to patients is not clear. To assess the incidence and significance of malnutrition and to examine the efficacy of therapeutic nutritional interventions used to manage gastrointestinal side effects in patients undergoing pelvic radiotherapy and those with chronic bowel side effects after treatment, a critical review of relevant original studies on human subjects was carried out using a specific set of mesh terms in MEDLINE and EMBASE databases and the Cochrane Library in September 2003. Full texts of all relevant articles were collected and reference lists were checked. Sources of grey literature including conference abstracts and web-based information were also reviewed. **A total of 36 papers published in peer-reviewed journals between 1966 and 2003 were identified. In all, 14 randomized controlled trials, 12 prospective cohorts, four retrospective, two qualitative, one validation, one pilot study and two case reports were obtained.** These included 2,646 patients. Eight articles including three conference abstracts and web-based information were found. None of the studies was definitive because of weakness in methodology. No studies could be combined because the interventions and the end points were different. **There is no evidence base for the use of nutritional interventions to prevent or manage bowel symptoms attributable to radiotherapy.** Low-fat diets, probiotic supplementation and elemental diet merit further investigation. (McGough et al, 2004). **This seems to be in contrast to the conclusions of Block and Conklin.**

Radiation and apoptosis

Apoptosis is activated as a result of radiation-induced cellular signaling and structural changes in normal and tumor cells. A few older animal studies showed vitamin C can be used with radiotherapy. (Seifter et al, 1984) (Taper et al, 1996).

Limited old animal data on vitamin E suggests that typical therapeutic doses (<1,200 IU) enhance the effect of radiation therapy while extremely high doses (35,000IU) may have the opposite effect. (Kagreud, Peterson, 1981).

Vitamin A (cis-retinoic acid) and radiotherapy improved the tumor response rate in a clinical trial of locally advanced cervical cancer compared to historical controls. (Park et al, 1998).

A randomized human trial of 50 patients evaluated the effect of combined Vitamin C 5gms/day and radiotherapy in different tumor types and noted **more complete responses to radiation in the vitamin C group.** (Hanck, 1988). **These inconsistencies makes interpretation of the data even more difficult.**

Radiotherapy coadministered with melatonin 20 mg./day in 30 patients with glioblastoma demonstrated improved survival at one year compared to radiation therapy alone. Fewer radiation- induced side effects were observed in the melatonin treated group. (Lissoni et al, 1996).

Patients randomized to receive intravenous glutathione (1200 mg.) administered just prior to adjuvant pelvic radiotherapy for endometrial cancer showed a significant reduction in radiation induced diarrhea compared to controls receiving radiation only. (De Maria et al, 1992).

Patients are increasingly self-prescribing antioxidant therapy during chemotherapy and radiation therapy as a result of market forces and aggressive advertising by antioxidant manufacturers.

In the above older data, only a limited number of human trials of antioxidant supplementation had been completed in patients with breast and lung cancer. These trials had demonstrated an increase in survival but were seriously limited by their small sample sizes, limited duration, and comparisons based on historical controls.

Based on the older studies, patients should **avoid combining antioxidant therapy only with those chemotherapeutic agents known to induce formation of free radicals, and with radiation therapy**.

Alkylating agents, antitumor antibiotics, and *topisomerase II inhibitors* depend on the generation of free radicals for their therapeutic action.

Ionizing radiation generates free radicals that damage DNA. Therefore, concurrent administration of antioxidants would theoretically, not be advisable for:

Alkylating Agents: Busulfan, Carmustine, Lomustine, Chlorambucil, Cyclophosphamide, Cisplatin, Carboplatin, Ifosamide, Mechlorethamine, Melphalan, Thiotepa, Dacarbazine, Procarbazine

Antitumor Antibiotics: Bleomycin, Dactinomycin, Daunorubicin, Doxorubicin, Idarubicin, Mitomycin, Mitoxantrone, Plicamycin.

Topoisomerase II inhibitor: Etoposide, Teniposide

RADIOTHERAPY- ANTIOXIDANT INTERACTIONS:
a biased review

Carmia Borek, Ph.D., Professor of Community Health, and Director, Nutrition and Infectious Diseases, Tufts University School of Medicine, Boston, MA, reviewed background material on antioxidants and radiation therapy. **Approximately 60% of cancer patients in the United States receive radiotherapy,** mostly ionizing radiation (IR) or to a lesser extent particle beam radiation (PR). Radiotherapy is a local treatment confined to the area of affected cells and activates a variety of genes, including NfkB, thereby activating cytokines and causing inflammation. **An important goal of radiotherapy is to administer enough radiation to kill tumor cells without killing adjacent normal cells.** DNA is the primary target of radiotherapy; damage to DNA occurs through a direct effect but mostly (two-thirds of damage) through **an indirect effect, by free radicals [superoxide, hydroxyl radical (the most toxic), and nitric oxide metabolites].** Cells are most sensitive to radiation damage in the G1-mol/L phase of the cell cycle; **oxygen**

248

concentration and cyclins will modify radiation response. Irradiation of nondividing or slow-dividing cells causes apoptotic death.

Antioxidants, including vitamins, help normal cells to withstand oxidative stress and *may* modify tumor-cell response to radiation. Depending on the tissue and the presence and level of free radicals, specific vitamins may be of greater benefit. To illustrate, beta-carotene is an effective antioxidant at low levels of pO_2, and vitamin E is more effective at high levels of pO_2. Radiation reduces tissue antioxidant levels; in animals, radiation exposure reduces vitamin E levels in cells. In other studies, bone marrow vitamin C and E levels are reduced, and in breast cancer studies, vitamin A, C, and E and selenium levels fall during cancer radiotherapy. **Whether supplementing antioxidants during radiotherapy is beneficial to cancer patients or has an adverse effect is not known.**

Studies of antioxidants in radiation therapy provide interesting insights into the amount of protection that is possible with supplementation. **Selenium increases the number of antioxidant enzymes in normal cells but not in cancer cells.** A study using ultraviolet light as the source of radiation on human cell lines indicates that functional *p53* increases, causing increased DNA repair in these cells.

Vitamin E protects cells from radiation-induced chromosome damage, reduces side effects of radiotherapy, reduces the expression of *ras* oncogenes, prevents apoptosis in normal cells by increasing *bcl2* and decreasing *bax*, and induces apoptosis in cancer cells. In the brain, vitamin E plays an important role in protecting neurons and acetylcholine receptors from free radical damage and prevents apoptosis in neural cells. In glioblastoma, vitamin E may help increase apoptosis and activates capsase-3 enzyme activity.

Cancer is generally an age-related disease, and plasma antioxidant levels decrease with age; it is important to take this into consideration during radiotherapy. Recent human experiments show that plasma proteins containing thiols are radioprotective and there is an inverse relation between plasma radioprotective ability and age.

Phytochemicals found in fruits and vegetables include many with antioxidant potential (e.g., flavonoids and carotenoids) that also have an important role in reducing oxidative stress. For example, S-allyl cysteine is a water-soluble compound in garlic that increases glutathione in cells and stimulates apoptosis in prostate cancer cells. A trial in England is investigating a compound in grape-seed extract that may protect against fibrosis after radiation treatment for breast cancer. Tea compounds are also a rich area of investigation in the search for agents to increase apoptosis in cancer cells.

It is important to remember that radiation does cause cancer and that vitamin E and selenium protect against radiation-induced malignancy in vitro. This may be the direction of future research because radiotherapy will remain a part of cancer therapy. The use of antioxidant combinations can help decrease damage expected from radiotherapy, especially high-dose radiotherapy (Borek, 2004).

Borek neglects to mention that many of the above antioxidants also have prooxidant activity.

Redox-Sensitive Signaling Factors and Antioxidants: How Tumor Cells Respond to Ionizing Radiation

David Gius, Center for Cancer Research, NCI

David Gius, M.D., Ph.D., Chief, Molecular Radiation Oncology Branch, Center for Cancer Research, NCI, NIH, Rockville, MD, discussed the molecular aspects of redox signaling and the role of antioxidants in this process regarding radiation exposure. There is a paradigm that ionizing agents induce the expression of prosurvival genes and that activation of these genes can alter phenotypes in cells. A model utilizing AP-1 DNA-binding transcriptional complex, containing a protein from the *fos* family and a protein from the *jun* family, was used to illustrate this paradigm. Various outside factors that produce oxidative stress, such as ionizing radiation, activate this complex. Hydroxyl radicals produced from water by ionizing radiation probably act as a signal that the cell has been initiated by oxidative stress.

Ionizing radiation (IR) causes the formation of reactive oxygen intermediates that are thought to initiate several redox-sensitive signaling cascades in response to the damaging and cytotoxic effects of IR. Because IR appears to activate redox-sensitive signaling factors, it is logical to hypothesize that critical cysteine residues contained in thioredoxin and thioredoxin reductase (TRX/TR) might mediate these signaling pathways.

Antioxidants and oxidative stress activate proteins such as thioredoxin and thioredoxin reductase Ref-1 through modification of sulfur atoms on cysteines, primary targets for redox reactions. The critical redox-sensitive signaling proteins and their cysteines transport a signal from the cytoplasm to the nucleus to turn on the transcription factor. For example, thioredoxin interacts in the nucleus with a second signaling protein, Ref-1 (i.e., an endonuclease), a protein that has a 5'-critical cysteine that is necessary for its signaling activity. Investigations confirm this observation.

Hydrogen peroxide stimulates many cytoplasmic signaling factors (e.g., *erk* families, *p38, ras,* and *raf*). Hence, it seems logical to determine whether activation of these factors by hydrogen peroxide and ionizing radiation is important in the response to the damaging effects of oxidative stress.

Based on these results, it is appealing to hypothesize that TR is a signaling factor in a cascade that begins with IR-induced free radicals in the cytoplasm, then activates transcription factors in the nucleus, which, in turn, regulate downstream genes that protect the cell from the oxidative stress induced by free radicals. In this model, subtle changes in cellular redox potential induced by a stressing agent could alter the flow of electrons through the cysteine residues of TR and TRX, causing profound changes in protein activity. These critical cysteines would appear to act as redox-sensitive "sulfhydryl switches" that reversibly modulate protein activity and allow signal transduction cascades to redirect metabolism in response to radiation-induced stress using redox-sensitive transcription factors.

To summarize the model, hydrogen peroxide and ionizing radiation produce free radicals; the NADP level is altered in cytoplasm and mitochondria (not proven); thioredoxin reductase is activated and passes the signal on to thioredoxin, which is transported into the nucleus; thioredoxin forms a physical interaction with REF1; REF1 passes the signal to the AP-1 transcriptional complex, which is composed of *fos* and *jun*, each of which have critical cysteine in the DNA-binding domain; and DNA-binding activity increases. (Nelson, 2004).

Suggested antioxidant radiotherapy safety measures

Those reviewing some of the older studies suggest the following safety measures:

- Avoid high doses of vitamin C with methotrexate and DTIC
- Avoid vitamin A, vitamin C, selenium, and N-acetyl cysteine, with doxorubicin
- Avoid beta carotene with 5-FU
- Avoid N-acetylcysteine with cisplatin
- Avoid citrus bioflavinoid supplements with tamoxifen

Some suggest that for chemotherapeutic agents which induce free radical production, **the introduction of antioxidants could be timed so as to avoid a critical period defined by the pharmacodynamic properties of the chemotherapeutic agent involved.** Still, I believe that even this should be approached with great caution.

CHAPTER FIFTEEN:

Photodynamic therapy

Photodynamic therapy (PDT)

Photodynamic therapy (PDT) holds considerable promise in treating cancer but current terminology leads to confusion.

First, we need a definition of terms:

Phototherapy - light, UV, etc., is shown on to the skin, such as treating hyperbilirubinemia in babies.

Photochemotherapy - uses a photosensitizer like, psoralin

Photodynamic therapy - uses a photosensitizer given to the patient to produce
$^1O_2^*$.

Photo-oxidative therapy - also referred to as photo irradiative therapy, uses UV
light shown on blood which is returned to the body.

Bio-oxidative therapy - aerobic exercise.

Autohemotherapy - ozone.

Photodynamic effect - a photon is absorbed by a photosensitizer and raises it to its lowest triplet excited state, it diffused until it collides with O_2 and raises it to its lowest singlet state.

The basic elements of PDT are as simple as 1-2-3: Photosensitizer + Visible light + Oxygen = Tissue Response. The unique property of photosensitizers to selectively accumulate in malignant and dysplastic tissues is exploited in the treatment of malignancies. PDT can selectively destroy tumors with this simple concept.

In biological systems, singlet oxygen has a short lifetime of <0.04 ms and has also been shown to have a short radius of action of <0.02 mm. (Moan, J. and Berg, K. The photodegradation of porphyrins in cells can be used to estimate the lifetime of singlet oxygen. Photochem Photobiol 1991; 53: 549-553). Cytosolic delivery of macromolecules is called photochemical internalization and this technique allows $^1O_2^*$ to oxidize biomolecules in the membranes of endosomes and lysosomes, resulting in the subsequent release of these contents into the cytosol. (Selbo et al, 2002).

Compared to surgery and conventional thermal Yag and argon laser treatment, there is much less damage and disruption of the underlying and adjacent normal tissue structures with photodynamic therapy, since **there is essentially no thermal damage to the tissues**. Superficial treatments do not require sterile theatre conditions and can be delivered in an outpatient setting. There is little post-treatment discomfort and **the only significant side effect is residual photosensitivity (protection from direct sunlight is necessary for a period of time).**

Photodynamic therapy (PDT) is a novel therapeutic method for the treatment of malignant tumors, which utilizes EMOD generation and in particular singlet oxygen ($^1O_2^*$). By combining PDT with hyperoxygenation, any underlying hypoxic condition is improved and the cell killing rate at various time points after PDT is dramatically enhanced. (Al-Waili et al, 2006) (Tomiselli et al, 2001).

When generated under carefully controlled conditions using exogenous sensitizers and light in the visible range (400 -700 nm), $^1O_2^*$ **can be exploited for therapeutic purposes, as for example, in antineoplastic photodynamic therapy (PDT).**

Singlet oxygen molecules exist ~3-4 msec in aqueous solution; which corresponds to a mean diffusion distance of 90-100 nm.. O_2^- effectively quenches $^1O_2^*$. In a cell with quenchers abounding, $^1O_2$ lifetime is <50 nsec with a diffusion distance <10 nm from its point of origin, which is less than 0.1% of the radius of an average eukaryotic cell.

Remember, that **all antibodies go through a singlet oxygen and ozone step.** Antibodies can generate hydrogen peroxide (H_2O_2) from singlet molecular oxygen ($^1O_2^*$). This process is **catalytic**, and we identify the electron source for a **quasi-unlimited generation of H_2O_2. Antibodies produce up to 500 mole equivalents of H_2O_2 from $^1O_2^*$, without a reduction in rate. This work shows the enormous potential for H_2O_2 production by antibodies.** (Wentworth et al, 2001) (Wentworth et al, 2002).

Ultraviolet blood irradiation is also called: photoluminescence, photopheresis, photo-oxidation, hemo-irradiation or even photodynamic therapy. It reportedly stimulates immunity and kills bacteria. **UV irradiation of blood is FDA approved to treat cutaneous T cell lymphoma.**

Apoptosis and PDT

In 1991, investigators described an apoptotic response to PDT. (Agarwal et al, 1991).

However, **malignant cell types often exhibit an impaired ability to undergo apoptosis.** PDT-mediated oxidative stress induces a transient increase in the downstream early response genes c-fos, c-jun, c-myc, and egr-1. (Luna et al, 1994). The in vivo tumoricidal reaction after PDT is accompanied by a complex immune response.

Vascular shutdown is clearly an important aspect of PDT. (Henderson, Dougherty, 1992).

Availability of ground state oxygen within the tumor can dramatically influence and limit direct tumor cell kill. (Zilberstein et al, 1997).

Oxidizing species, especially singlet oxygen, produced by photosensitization or derived from cytotoxic agents, can **activate apoptotic pathways.** (Kochevar et al, 2000).

Photodynamic therapy-mediated tumor cell death also requires the presence of oxygen and **cells are not killed under anoxic conditions**. The critical threshold below which progressively reduced cell death was observed varied from 15 to 35 mmHg, probably **because of the reduced production of singlet oxygen ($^1O_2*$)** species and different sensitivities to the treatment in different cell lines. (Henderson, Fingar, 1987) (Chapman et al, 1991). This means that because of the utilization of oxygen by PDT, it is a self-limiting process. In contrast, the **Howes Singlet Oxygen Cancer Therapy System** brings its own oxygen supply with it and is, therefore, not self-limiting.

The probability of cell inactivation per quantum of absorbed light is widely different among PDT sensitizers. (Berg et al, 1992). Thus, **the PDT system is much more difficult to predict and quantitate than the Howes Singlet Oxygen Delivery System.**

PDT is a highly effective means of generating tumor-sensitized immune cells that can be recovered from lymphoid sites distant to the treated tumor at protracted time intervals after PDT, which asserts their immune memory character. (Korebelic, Dougherty, 1999) (Korbelik, 1996).

CHAPTER SIXTEEN:

Hyperbaric oxygen therapy (HBO)

Hyperbaric oxygen therapy using pressures at or less than 2.5 ATA do not significantly increase ROS in the presence of normal anti-oxidant defenses.

Hyperbaric oxygen increases the oxygen in tumor tissue, as well as EMOD levels, and appears to enhance the efficiency of PDT. (Tomaselli et al, Lasers Surg Med. 2001) (Maier et al, 2000).

Hyperoxygenation appears to provide effective ways for improving PDT efficiency by oxygenating both preexisting and treatment-induced cell hypoxia. (Chen et al, 2002).

Results with hyperbaric oxygen is similar to that obtained by the Baylor investigators using intra-arterial and intra-venous H_2O_2.

PDT/HBO increases EMODs and tumoricidal activity on malignant bronchial stenosis

Photodynamic tumor therapy (PDT) is based upon a photochemical reaction that is limited by the availability of molecular oxygen in the target tissue. The use of hyperbaric oxygenation (HBO) increases the amount of oxygen available for the process may thereby enhance the efficacy of PDT. They proved in a prospective, non-randomized clinical pilot study the acute effects **on malignant bronchial stenosis** and the technical feasibility of combined PDT/HBO. **Forty patients** (29 males, 11 females, mean age: 64.3 years; range 39-82 years) with inoperable, advanced malignant bronchial tumor stenosis were studied prospectively. Photosensitization was carried out using a hematoporphyrin-derivative 2 mg/kg bw 48 h prior to PDT. The light dose was calculated as 300 J/cm fiber tip. The assessment of outcome 1 and 4 weeks after PDT/HBO was done by endoscopy, chest X-ray, spirometry, laboratory parameters, subjective report of dyspnea and Karnofsky performance status. At 1 and 4 weeks after the treatment the patients felt a significant improvement of dyspnea and hemoptysis alongside with an objective subsiding of poststenotic pneumonia, though spirometric parameters revealed no significant difference. A significant reduction of tumor stenosis ($P<0.05$) and an improvement of the Karnofsky performance status ($P<0.05$) were documented 1 and 4 weeks after PDT/HBO. **No therapy related complications were observed.** CONCLUSION: Although the small number of patients does not allow to draw definitive conclusions, the results suggest that **combined PDT/HBO represents a new, safe and technically feasible approach.** It enables efficient and rapid reduction of the endoluminal tumor load and helps conditioning the patient for further treatment procedures. (Tomiselli et al, 2001).

PDT/HBO increases EMODs and esophageal tumoricidal activity

The photochemical reaction of photodynamic therapy **(PDT) depends on the presence of molecular oxygen. Due to anoxic regions in tumor tissue and vascular shutdown during PDT the efficiency is limited.** Therefore, the use of hyperbaric oxygen which increases the oxygen in tumor tissue, as well as the amount of singlet oxygen, may enhance the efficiency of PDT. According to this prospective non-randomized study, combined PDT/HBO represents a new approach in the treatment of esophageal and cardia cancer which appears to have enhanced the efficiency of PDT. (Maier et al, 2000). **My singlet oxygen delivery system circumvents the problems associated with both PDT/HBO.**

PDT/HBO increases EMODs and lung tumoricidal activity

Photodynamic tumor therapy (PDT) is based upon a photochemical reaction that is limited by the availability of molecular oxygen in the target tissue. The use of hyperbaric oxygenation (HBO) increases the amount of oxygen available for the process may thereby enhance the efficacy of PDT. Although the number of patients (30) was small it does not allow to draw definitive conclusions to be drawn, the results suggests that combined PDT/HBO represents a new, safe, and technically feasible approach. It enables efficient and rapid reduction of the endoluminal tumor load and helps conditioning the patient for further treatment procedures. (Tomaselli et al, Lasers Surg Med. 2001).

PDT tumoricidal activity improved by HBO in C3H mice with transplanted mammary carcinoma

Photodynamic therapy (PDT) requires molecular oxygen during light irradiation to generate reactive oxygen species. Tumor hypoxia, either preexisting or induced by PDT, can severely hamper the effectiveness of PDT. Lowering the light irradiation dose rate or fractionating a light dose may improve cell kill of PDT-induced hypoxic cells but will have no effect on preexisting hypoxic cells. In this study hyperoxygenation technique was used during PDT to overcome hypoxia. **C3H mice with transplanted mammary carcinoma tumors** were injected with 12.5 mg/kg Photofrin and irradiated with 630 nm laser light 24 h later. Tumor oxygenation was manipulated by subjecting the animals to 3 atp (atmospheric pressure) hyperbaric oxygen or normobaric oxygen during PDT light irradiation. The results show a significant improvement in tumor response when PDT was delivered during hyperoxygenation. With hyperoxygenation up to 80% of treated tumors showed no regrowth after 60 days. In comparison, when animals breathed room air, only 20% of treated tumors did not regrow. To explore the effect of hyperoxygenation on tumor oxygenation, tumor partial oxygen pressure was measured with microelectrodes positioned in preexisting hypoxic regions before and during the PDT. The results show that hyperoxygenation may oxygenate preexisting hypoxic cells and compensate for oxygen depletion induced by PDT light irradiation. In conclusion, hyperoxygenation may provide effective ways to improve PDT efficiency by oxygenating both preexisting and treatment-induced cell hypoxia. (Chen et al, 2002). **The foregoing papers illustrate the principle taught in my previous books which demonstrate the tumoricidal activity of EMODs, especially singlet oxygen.**

PDT, iron and HBO act synergistically to kill human leukemic cells

Photodynamic therapy (PDT) is a new therapeutic approach for the treatment of malignant tumors. Hyperbaric oxygen (HBO(2)) shows beneficial effects in various modalities of cancer interventions. **Tumor cells tend to accumulate large amount of iron.** There is interaction between tissue content of oxygen, iron, free radical production and tissue damage. **Accumulation of intracellular iron is necessary for the production of oxygen radicals. HBO(2) increases tissue oxygen and hydrogen peroxide production in the cells. Malignant cells require iron**, and exhibit more transferrin receptors. The photodynamic sensitization of **human leukemic cells** is achieved with accumulation of porphyrins stimulated by 5-aminolaevulinic acid (ALA) plus hemin. Further, **a significant improvement in tumor response is obtained when PDT is delivered during hyperoxygenation. When PDT is combined with hyperoxygenation, the hypoxic condition is improved and the cell killing rate at various time points after PDT is significantly enhanced.** Photosensitization with use of porphyrins is used with HBO(2) and PDT for treatment of certain tumors. PDT with ALA is used for treatment of actinic keratosis (AK). The combination of iron administration (by injection or oral route), hemin, or transferrin, as a source for iron, HBO(2) as a source of oxygen under pressure and PDT as a source of generating free-radical tissue damage may be useful in the treatment of tumors. The possibility of combining HBO(2), iron, light and local photosensitizers to overcome skin tumors deserve extensive laboratory and clinical research work. Conclusively, **iron, HBO(2), and PDT may have synergistic effect to** hamper tumor cells (**Phototherapy and malignancy: Possible enhance-ment by iron administration and hyperbaric oxygen.** Al-Waili, NS and Butler, GJ. Med Hypotheses, 2006;67(5):1148-58). **I believe** that this conforms my belief that a combinatorial approach to increase EMOD levels is effective in killing cancer. It may be possible to increase iron and vitamin C intake to a level needed to oxidatively kill cancer and still be safe.

The outcome of 5-ALA-mediated photodynamic treatment in mela-noma cells is influenced by vitamin C and heme oxygenase-1. (Grimm et al, 2011)

Photodynamic therapy (PDT) is an important clinical approach for cancer treatment. It involves the administration of a photosensitizer, followed by its activation with light and induction of cell death. **The underlying mechanism is an increased production of reactive oxygen species (ROS) leading to oxidative stress, which is followed by cell death. However, effectiveness of PDT is limited due to an initiation of endogenous rescue response systems like heme oxygenase-1 (HO-1) in tumor cells.** In recent years, **consuming of antioxidant supplements has become widespread,** but the effect of exogenously applied antioxidants on cancer therapy outcome remains unclear. Thus, this study was aimed to investigate if exogenous antioxidants might decrease ROS-induced cytotoxicity in photodynamic treatment. **Lycopene, b-carotene, vitamin C, N-acetylcysteine, trolox, and N-tert-butyl-a-phenylnitrone in different doses were administered to human melanoma cells prior exposure to photodynamic treatment. Supplementation with vitamin C resulted in a significant decrease of the cell death rate,** whereas **the other tested antioxidants had no effect on cell viability and oxidative stress markers. The simultaneous application of vitamin C with the HO-1 activity inhibitor zinc protoporphyrine IX (ZnPPIX) caused a considerable decrease of photodynamic treatment-induced cytotoxicity compared to ZnPPIX alone.** It can be summarized that exogenously applied antioxidants do not have a leading role in the protective response against photodynamic treatment. (Grimm et al, 2011).

The Howes Singlet Oxygen ($^1O_2^*$) Cancer Therapy System

Howes proposed a singlet oxygen generating system composed of physiological agents for the eradication of cancer, which did not have the limitations of conventional photodynamic therapy or chemotherapeutic systems. In a pilot study at Tuft's Medical School, athymic mice, which had received human squamous carcinoma, experienced a 22.7% tumor disappearance rate in the "high dose group" following injection with the singlet oxygen producing system. (Howes, 2005).

Even more encouraging results were seen, with an initial 80% disappearance rate, when basal cell skin cancers were similarly injected with this singlet oxygen delivery system. (Howes, Farber, 2005).

PDT generates similar products, in particular $^1O_2^*$, with similar chemical reactivity as the **Howes Singlet Oxygen Delivery system.**

Commonality Between PDT and the Howes Singlet Oxygen Therapy system

Pioneering work by Howes and Steele on microsomal lipid peroxidation. (Howes, Steele, 1971) **and aryl-hydroxylations** (Howes, Steele, 1972) demonstrated evidence for the generation and participation of electronic excitation states, namely singlet oxygen.

This was the first demonstration of a functional generation of an electronic excitation state, exclusive of vision, in mammalian systems. Their proposal, that singlet oxygen is the identity of the long sought out "active oxygen" acting on the cytochrome P 450 microsomal mixed function oxidases, has recently been supported by the work of Yasui et al (Yasui et al, 2002).

While studying widely divergent biological electronic excitation generating systems, such as the microsomal mixed function oxidases, the neutrophil respiratory burst (Howes et al, 1976) and proline hydroxylation for collagen biosynthesis, one of our investigators (Howes) believed that these oxidative systems shared a point of convergence, expressed in the Howes Excytomer Pathway, involving superoxide anion and electronically excited singlet oxygen (Howes et al, 1977).

Furthermore, **Howes saw an additional commonality with generation of singlet oxygen produced by the steady-state physiological oxidative reagents containing an organic peroxide and the salt of hypohalous acid.** (Howes, Steele, 1976).

Subsequently, Howes reasoned that the peroxide/hypochlorite oxidative system may represent an ideal method of singlet oxygen delivery for effectively treating premalignant and malignant lesions, while simultaneously eliminating many of the drawbacks associated, not only with PDT, but with all other conventional methods of cancer therapy. The peroxide/hypochlorite oxidative system has been shown to generate singlet oxygen exclusively, as opposed to hydroperoxide/hypochlorite systems which have been shown to produce peroxyl and alkoxyl radicals. (Noguchi et al, 2002).

**The living/breathing cell holds within it
the answers to every query
the physician can ever perceive or fathom.
He struggles to tease out its secret cures,
whilst the scientist suffers to know "why?"**
R. M. Howes, M.D., Ph.D.
9/7/09

SECTION FIVE:

EMOD induced apoptosis, continued

CHAPTER SEVENTEEN:

EMOD-inducing apoptotic agents

PCI-24781 (histone deacetylase (HDAC) inhib)

Investigators examined the cytotoxicity and mechanisms of cell death of the broad-spectrum histone deacetylase (HDAC) inhibitor PCI-24781, alone and combined with bortezomib in **Hodgkin lymphoma and non-Hodgkin lymphoma cell lines** and primary lymphoproliferative (CLL/SLL) cells. **PCI-24781 resulted in increased EMODs** and NF-κB inhibition, leading to caspase-dependent apoptosis. They showed that bortezomib is synergistic with PCI-24781. This combination or PCI-24781 alone has potential therapeutic value in lymphoma. (Bhalla et al, 2009).

Chaetocin

Investigators found that Chaetocin, a thiodioxopiperazine natural product previously unreported to have anticancer effects, was found to have potent antimyeloma activity in IL-6–dependent and –independent myeloma cell lines in freshly collected sorted and unsorted patient CD138⁺ **myeloma cells and in vivo.** Chaetocin displays superior ex vivo antimyeloma activity and selectivity than doxorubicin and dexamethasone, and dexamethasone- or doxorubicin-resistant myeloma cell lines are largely non–cross-resistant to chaetocin. Mechanistically, chaetocin is dramatically accumulated in cancer cells via a process **inhibited by glutathione** and requiring intact/unreduced disulfides for uptake. **Its anticancer activity appears mediated primarily through the imposition of oxidative stress and consequent apoptosis induction**. The selective antimyeloma effects of chaetocin appear not to reflect heightened sensitivity of myeloma cells to the cytotoxic effects of imposed oxidative stress. (Isham et al, 2007).

Elesclomol (formerly STA-4783) triggers oxidative apoptosis

Elesclomol (formerly STA-4783) is a novel small molecule undergoing clinical evaluation in a pivotal phase III **melanoma trial** (SYMMETRY). In a phase II randomized, double-blinded, controlled, multi-center trial in 81 patients with stage IV metastatic melanoma, treatment with elesclomol plus paclitaxel showed a statistically significant doubling of progression-free survival time compared with treatment with paclitaxel alone. Although elesclomol displays significant therapeutic activity in the clinic, the mechanism underlying its anticancer activity has not been defined previously. Here, we show that elesclomol induces apoptosis in cancer cells through the induction of oxidative stress. **Treatment of cancer cells in vitro with elesclomol resulted in the rapid generation of reactive oxygen species (ROS) and the induction of a transcriptional gene profile characteristic of an oxidative stress response.** Inhibition of oxidative stress by the antioxidant N-acetylcysteine blocked the induction of gene transcription by elesclomol. In addition, **N-acetylcysteine blocked drug-induced apoptosis, indicating that ROS generation is the primary mechanism responsible for the proapoptotic activity of elesclomol.** Excessive ROS production and elevated levels of oxidative stress are critical biochemical alterations that contribute to cancer cell growth. Thus, **the induction of oxidative stress by elesclomol exploits this unique characteristic of cancer cells by increasing ROS levels beyond a threshold that triggers cell death.** (Kirshner et al, 2008).

Glioma pathogenesis-related protein 1 (GLIPR1), a p53 target gene

Glioma pathogenesis-related protein 1 (GLIPR1), a novel p53 target gene, is down-regulated by methylation in prostate cancer and has p53-dependent and -independent proapoptotic properties in tumorous cells. Investigators reported that the expression of GLIPR1 is significantly reduced in **human prostate tumor** tissues compared with adjacent normal prostate tissues and in multiple human cancer cell lines and that overexpression of GLIPR1 in cancer cells leads to suppression of colony growth and induction of apoptosis. Mechanistic analysis indicated that GLIPR1 up-regulation **increases EMOD production leading to apoptosis** through activation of the c-Jun–NH$_2$ kinase (JNK) signaling cascade. These results identify GLIPR1 as a proapoptotic tumor suppressor acting through the ROS-JNK pathway and support the therapeutic potential for this protein. (Li et al, 2008).

Imexon

Investigators studied the identity biomarkers that may be predictive for the clinical activity of the redox-active antitumor agent imexon. Both cDNA microarray and quantitative real-time PCR showed the up-regulation of many antioxidant genes, including thioredoxin reductase-1, glutaredoxin-2, and peroxiredoxin-3 in PBMCs collected from patients treated with imexon. The antitumor agent imexon activates antioxidant gene expression, which is **evidence for an oxidative stress response.** Together, these results show that a predominant biological effect of imexon is **a change in redox state** that can be detected in surrogate normal tissues as increased redox-sensitive transcription factor binding and increased antioxidant gene expression. (Baker et al, 2007).

Zinc

Zinc is becoming increasingly important in regulating cancer cell growth and proliferation. Investigators showed that the anticancer agent motexafin gadolinium (MGd) disrupted zinc metabolism in **A549 lung cancer cells**, leading, in the presence of exogenous zinc, to cell death. They reported the effect of MGd and exogenous zinc on intracellular levels of free zinc, oxidative stress, proliferation, and cell death in exponential phase human B-cell lymphoma and other hematologic cell lines. They found that **increased levels of oxidative stress and intracellular free zinc precede and correlate with cell cycle arrest and apoptosis**. (Lecane et al, 2005).

Doxorubicin, arsenic-induced apoptosis and 2-Methoxyestradiol induced apoptosis

Antineoplastic therapy can be based on the cell cycle, which is broken up into four phases, i.e., the G_1, S, G_2, and M phases or it can be based on the involvement of electronically modified oxygen derivatives (EMODs), which have formerly been called oxygen free radicals or reactive oxygen species. These **EMOD reactants can induce apoptosis** and appear to be essential as activators for removing or killing cells that have accumulated mutations. (Tsang et al, 2003) (Liu et al, 2003) (Djavaheri-Mergny et al, 2003).

Apoptosis (cellular suicide) has been shown to be one of the most important means of eliminating precancerous and cancerous cells from the body. (Howes, Philica. Feb 26, 2007).

Cancer therapy seeks to utilize the sensitivity of transformed cells towards apoptotic signals, which allows the execution of apoptotic cell death. (Nicholson, 297–301. 1996) (Nicholson, 810-816. 1996).

Ideal treatment should aim to selectively kill the cancer cells, without harming normal cells. Elegant regulation of EMOD levels may be a means to this exalted goal.

Contrary to the free radical theory, EMODs have been found to play a crucial role in intracellular apoptotic execution (cellular suicide). (Fluery et al, 2002) (Clement et al, 1998) (Hirpara et al, 2001) (Simizu et al, 1998) (Mansat-De Mas et al, 1999).

Tamoxifen, doxorubicin, mitomycin C, etoposide and cisplatin

Many chemotherapeutic drugs, such as tamoxifen, doxorubicin, mitomycin C, etoposide and cisplatin are superoxide (EMOD) generating agents and induce oxidative stress and apoptosis. (Ferlini et al, 1999) (Yokomizo et al, 1995).

Likewise, radiotherapy and photodynamic therapy generate EMODs within treated carcinoma cells, which appear essential for induction of apoptosis of the neoplastic cells.

EMOD induced cell death in B16F10 melanoma cells treated with TNP-470

TNP-470 is an acknowledged anti-angiogenic factor, and was studied clinically as an anti-cancer drug. Investigators previously reported on an additional property of this molecule: the intracellular generation of reactive oxygen species in B16F10 melanoma cells. They showed that **a massive generation of EMODs (ROS) occurred in the first few hours after treatment with TNP-470 and that this event was critical to subsequent cell death.** In this study, they analyzed the process of cell death and noticed an atypical pattern of death markers. Some of these, such as DNA fragmentation or condensation of chromatin, were characteristic for programmed cell death, while others (the lack of phosphatidylserine flip-flop but permeability to propidium iodide, the maintenance of adhesion to the substratum, no change in mitochondrial transmembrane potential, no effect of the panspecific caspase inhibitor) rather suggested a necrotic outcome. They concluded that TNP-470 induced at least some pathways of programmed cell death. However, increasing damage to critical cell functions appears to cause a rapid switch into the necrotic mode. **Their data is similar to that in other reports describing the action of ROS-generating agents.** They hypothesize that **this rapid programmed cell death/necrosis switch is a common scenario following free radical stress.** (Okroj et al, 2006).

EMOD action of the fumagillin analog, TNP-470, in the B16F10 murine melanoma

TNP-470, a semisynthetic derivative of fumagillin, is an acknowledged angiogenesis inhibitor, presently undergoing clinical trials. **It exerts an anti-proliferative effect directed against endothelial cells.** This effect is known to be based on cell cycle inhibition effected by the p53/p21 pathway. They observed short-term toxicity of TNP-470 in the **B16F10 murine melanoma cell line** in vitro and investigated the mechanism of action. Cell death occurred as soon as 2 h after the addition of TNP-470, without typical apoptotic features. The toxic effect could be modulated and it depended on the type of culture medium or supplementation with anti-oxidants. **Addition of N-acetylcysteine protected B16F10 cells from TNP-470-induced death and inhibited an increase in the generation of reactive oxygen species (ROS),** which are detected by the 2',7'-dichlorodi-hydrofluorescein diacetate probe. They conclude that **TNP-470 can induce intracellular generation of ROS, which act toxically inside B16F10 cells.** The possibility of its modulation gives a prospect for controlling the action of this potential drug and probably its derivatives. (Okroj et al, 2005). **As I had predicted, the action of TNP-470 is via EMOD production.**

SECTION SIX:

More antioxidant debate

CHAPTER EIGHTEEN:

Pros and cons of antioxidants

Effects of Oncological Treatment and Mechanisms of Action of Antioxidants

The principal therapeutic effect of radiation occurs indirectly via the ionization of water molecules in the cytoplasm to reactive oxygen species, for example, super-oxide and hydroxyl radicals. These free radicals react with nuclear DNA, thereby creating structural bonds that are potentially fatal to cells. Some of this radiation damage can be repaired, leaving a cell that remains viable and that can proliferate. **It takes only a millisecond for the free radical–DNA reaction to occur, and a normal cell that is not killed outright can repair the damage in as few as 6 hours.** (Hall, 2000).

Antioxidants are compounds that can counteract free radicals and prevent them from causing tissue and organ damage. (Ratnam et al, 2006).

They function through a variety of mechanisms: as preventative agents that suppress the formation of free radicals, as radical scavenging agents that inhibit chain initiation and/or propagation, as repair and de novo enzymes that repair and reconstitute cell membranes, and as adaptation agents that generate appropriate antioxidant enzymes and transfer them to the necessary site of action. (Papas et al, 1999).

Antioxidants—whether produced endogenously (e.g., alpha-lipoic acid, ubiquinone) or consumed in the diet (e.g., alpha-tocopherol, ascorbic acid)—must be present in the cell during the free radical–DNA reaction, and at a sufficient concentration, to be effective in blocking free radical–mediated DNA damage. **Although antioxidants, by definition, scavenge free radicals, it is important to recognize that most also act via other mechanisms to affect cell proliferation, apoptosis, angiogenesis, and other processes relevant to tumor growth and metastasis.**

Although antioxidants may play a role in the primary prevention of cancer in part by reducing the oxidative modification of DNA, the same action might be expected to be counterproductive against radiation therapy and chemotherapeutic agents that **act solely via the production of reactive oxygen species and induction of apoptosis** (Ratnam et al, 2006).

These agents include the **anthracyclines (e.g., doxorubicin), platinum-containing complexes (e.g., cisplatin, carboplatin), alkylating agents (e.g., cyclophosphamide, ifosfamide), and cytotoxic antibiotics (e.g., bleomycin, mitomycin-C).**

Dietary antioxidants comprise a variety of chemical classes, **including carotenoids, polyphenols, tocols, and triterpenes,** and they display an array of biologic activities. Thus, it is not possible to make broad generalizations about whether or how they might interact with oncological treatments. Nonetheless, **these nutrients are defined by their shared capacity for quenching reactive oxygen and nitrogen species** even though their in vivo potency and selectivity can vary substantially by class, bioavailability, dose, and duration, as well as by route of administration. (Ratnam et al, 2006).

For example, the most readily bioavailable form of **the antioxidant lycopene is in cooked rather than raw foods, and ascorbic acid acts as an antioxidant when taken orally but as a prooxidant when administered intravenously at high doses.** (Ratnam et al, 2006) (Padayatty et al, 2004).

Individual variations (e.g., polymorphisms) in the expression of antioxidant enzymes such as superoxide dismutase and catalase further complicate potential interactions between oncological treatments and the antioxidant defense network. For example, some polymorphisms in the gene encoding glutathione-S-transferase, an antioxidant enzyme, can decrease the antioxidant activity of the enzyme.

Laboratory evidence indicates that the effect of dietary antioxidants on tumors is dose dependent. **In the absence of radiotherapy or chemotherapy, high doses of dietary antioxidants often inhibit the growth of cancer cells without affecting the growth of normal cells.** (Salganik, 2001) (Prasad et al, 1999) (Prasad et al, 2001).

However, data from some studies indicate that **antioxidant supplementation at doses that are intermediate to dietary intakes (relatively low doses) and high supplemental doses may reduce the efficacy of x-irradiation against cancer cells.** (Sakamoto, Sakka, 1973) (Witenberg et al, 1999) or stimulate tumor cell growth (Prasad, Kumar, 1996).

Interpretation of these experimental data is difficult because the doses that inhibit tumor cell growth vary between species and tumor types and the distribution of antioxidants varies between tumor cells and nor-

mal cells. (Prasad, Kumar, 1996) (Hanck, 1988) (Liede et la, 1998) (Agus et al, 1999) (Piyathilake et al, 2000) (Picardo et al, 1996) (Langemann et al, 1989).

They attempted to identify all published randomized clinical trials that have investigated the possible radio-modifying effects (ie, increasing or decreasing radio-sensitivity) of concurrent administration of supplemental antioxidants on normal tissues and tumors.

Bairati et al. (Bairati et al, 2005 Apr 6) reported that among 540 head and neck cancer patients who were randomly assigned to receive either alpha-tocopherol with or without beta-carotene vs placebo concurrent with their radiation therapy, **those who received both antioxidants had a statistically significant 38% reduction in severe, acute side effects.** However, **this benefit appeared to be offset by reductions of 29% and 56% in the local tumor control rates for alpha-tocopherol and alpha-tocopherol plus beta-carotene, respectively.** It is interesting to note **that in a recently reported subgroup analysis of these patients,** (Meyer et al, 2008), **the interactions between antioxidant supplementation and cigarette smoking during radiation therapy were associated with an increase in both disease and cancer-specific mortality.** There was no increase in either of these outcome measures for the nonsmokers.

The most concerning data are presented in a subsequent publication by Bairati et al. (Bairati et al, 2006) on the same cohort of patients. In this article, **they demonstrate that the patients who received antioxidants had statistically significant poorer overall survival. Some believe that this study is the most important randomized clinical trial, to date, on the use of a supplemental antioxidant and radiation therapy.**

Several other studies have provided evidence that antioxidants can decrease the effectiveness of radiation therapy. For example, Ferreira et al. randomly assigned 54 head and neck cancer patients who were undergoing radiation therapy to receive an oil-based oral rinse that contained either vitamin E or placebo before and after each daily dose of radiation. **Although the vitamin E supplementation was associated with a 36% reduction in symptomatic mucositis, the authors also reported a decrease in 2-year overall survival** (32% with supplemental vitamin E vs 63% with placebo; $P = .13$). This concerning decrease in overall survival, albeit **not statistically significant**, may have been confounded by the greater percentage of patients with stage 3 and 4 tumors found in the vitamin E group. (Ferreira et al, 2004).

In another study, **Lesperance et al.** investigated a historical cohort of 90 patients with nonmetastatic breast cancer who received conventional treatment (e.g., surgery, chemotherapy, radiation therapy, and hormonal therapy) either alone or in combination with high doses of beta-carotene, vitamin C, niacin, selenium, coenzyme Q10, and/or zinc. (Lesperance et al, 2002). **Breast cancer–specific survival (ie, patients censored only at death from breast cancer) and disease-free survival were shorter in the nutrient-supplemented group than in the nonsupplemented group, but the differences were not statistically significant** (hazard ratio of breast cancer death = 1.75, 95% CI = 0.83 to 2.69, and hazard ratio of relapse = 1.55, 95% CI = 0.94 to 2.54, respectively). Despite the substantial limitations of these studies, **it is troubling that both reported results suggesting poorer survival with concurrent administration of antioxidants and cytotoxic therapy**, even though these results are at odds with other studies.

For example, **two randomized trials—Misirlioglu et al**. (Misirlioglu et al, 2006), **testing pentoxifylline and alpha-tocopherol in patients with non–small cell lung cancer, and Lissoni et al**. (Lissoni et al, 1996), **testing melatonin in patients with brain glioblastomas—found that radiotherapy combined with alpha-tocopherol or melatonin supplementation increased survival.**

However, **this suggestion of radiosensitization of tumors was not confirmed by Berk et al. in a randomized trial of radiation therapy and high-dose melatonin in brain metastases.** (Berk et al, 2007).

Despite concerns about current recommendations supporting the use of antioxidant supplementation during oncological treatments, some antioxidants, such as **amifostine (WR-2721), a thiol-containing antioxidant that has been approved by the Food and Drug Administration to increase the radioresistance of salivary gland tissues**, show promise as cotherapies. Although some preclinical studies have shown that amifostine increases the radioresistance of tumors, **neither the randomized clinical trials nor the meta-analyses of this agent have provided conclusive evidence of increased radioresistance of tumors.**

Mell et al. stated that their "...results suggest that any effect of amifostine (an antioxidant which has been pulled from clinical use) on reducing overall response [to radiation therapy], if it exists, is no larger than a 3% relative risk reduction. (Mell et al, 2007).

They identified **16 randomized clinical trials that studied the concurrent use of antioxidant supplements and chemotherapy;** 6 of those trials included a placebo control. Although no decrements in tumor response rates or survival rates were observed in the studies that reported response data, none of those studies were powered to evaluate these endpoints. For example, Pathak et al. (Pathak et al, 2005) examined whether the concurrent administration of a high-dose antioxidant mixture containing vitamins C and E and beta-carotene with paclitaxel and cisplatin improved tumor response and survival in 136 patients with advanced non–small cell lung cancer and observed no survival or tumor response benefits with the antioxidants. However, **the authors' conclusion that the antioxidant supplementation was safe is not warranted because the study was not sufficiently powered to evaluate a reduction in survival or tumor response.**

In a systematic review of the randomized trials of antioxidants and chemotherapy, Ladas et al. found such a wide range of cancer diagnoses, chemotherapy regimens, and antioxidant supplementation that **they could not draw definitive conclusions about the safety and efficacy of the antioxidant interventions.** (Ladas et al, 2004).

FREE RADICALS: THE PROS AND CONS OF ANTIOXIDANTS

Summary Report February 13, 2004 (Final). NIH Campus Bethesda, MD June 26-27, 2003.

Some of the following material was excerpted, abstracted or modified from: **FREE RADICALS: THE PROS AND CONS OF ANTIOXIDANTS. Division of Cancer Prevention National Cancer Institute. Division of Cancer Treatment and Diagnosis, National Cancer Institute. National Cancer Institute. National Center for Complementary and Alternative Medicine National Institutes of Health. Office of Dietary Supplements National Institutes of Health.**

Note: This version can be found at http://www.nutrition.org, References to the published, final version of this manuscript should include the following citation: J. Nutr. 134:3143S-3163S, 2004.

Mechanisms for determining when an antioxidant becomes a pro-oxidant are largely unknown and this will need to be established before recommending nutritional or nutritional/pharmacologic interventions. Doses are important and the underlying oxidant properties of the tissue being looked at are extremely critical.

Antioxidants Suppress Apoptosis

Steven Zeisel, University of North Carolina–Chapel Hill

Steven Zeisel, M.D., Ph.D., Professor and Chairman, Department of Nutrition, Associate Dean, Research School of Public Health, University of North Carolina–Chapel Hill, discussed antioxidants and the mechanisms for suppressing apoptosis (cell suicide) and apoptotic signaling. There is a growing body of evidence that there are signaling systems that physiologically use ROS as intermediate signals. **ROS not only regulate the signaling for apoptosis, but are capable of activating apoptotic pathways upstream and many of the drugs and treatments that we use to kill cancer cells (chemotherapy and radiation) work by generating ROS to activate apoptotic pathways and kill cells. These pathways involve activation of a caspase upstream**, a mitochondrial depolarization that generates ROS, which can then activate the caspase, as well as activation of downstream signals that end in final common pathways for cell suicide.

Choline deficiency involves an apoptotic pathway that uses ROS as an intermediary message and a nuclear factor kappa-B (NFkB) signal downstream. If there is little antioxidant content in liver cells that are also choline deficient, apoptosis is induced. **If an antioxidant is added, such as N-acetylcysteine, apoptosis is inhibited by blocking the ROS signal. N-acetylcysteine also blocks transforming growth factor beta-1 (TGF-beta-1) induced apoptosis, which also uses a ROS to produce an intermediary signal from the mitochondria during the signaling cascade for apoptosis.**

Studies using a mouse model with a mutated retinoblastoma (Rb) protein show that mice fed a diet low in vitamin E and other antioxidants had higher rates of apoptosis and reduced tumor volume. Other researchers have reported that **antioxidants such as vitamin E and N–acetylcysteine delay and inhibit apoptosis in a number of models, including pancreatic cells and PC-12 cells. There is some data in the literature suggesting that when we want to kill cells with chemotherapy or radiation, the mechanism we are using is the generation of excess levels of EMODs (ROS) that then activate cell death. If we gave antioxidants during these treatments, we would reduce the amount of cell death produced.**

Studies have investigated the effects of antioxidant supplementation on cancer therapy. Studies on cisplatin indicate that it kills breast cancer cells by apoptosis and necrosis, and that the addition of vitamin E blocks much of the apoptotic process. **High-dose vitamin E reduces the efficacy of cisplatin**, although the normal cells involved would be protected by vitamin E. Lymphoma cells treated with 5 Gy of radiation die or stop dividing, but **if N-acetylcysteine is added to the media, the lymphoma cells keep growing. Vitamin E succinate also protects cells against the effects of radiation in vitro.**

There has been no conclusive evidence to show which antioxidant doses or mixtures protect cells against DNA damage and lipid and protein oxidation but do not interfere with apoptosis signaling pathways. There may be a threshold beyond which DNA is protected against oxidants because the ROS oxidants produced are being quenched and there may be a higher dose needed to suppress signaling. **Oversupplementation may actually produce an environment that is beneficial to the tumor and allow it to survive.**

I firmly believe that antioxidants can also produce deficiencies of EMODs and allow for the manifestation of cancer in otherwise normal patients. Thus, to a significant degree, antioxidants block prooxidant prevention and control of cancer.

Before recommending that individuals take antioxidants for chemoprevention, a better understanding of free radical-mediated damage must be considered.

Zeisel's approach - antioxidants suppress apoptosis

The production of **excess levels of EMODs is important for activation of internal cell programs for cell suicide (apoptosis)** that are important protection mechanisms that kill cancer cells (Weijl, et al, 1997) (Kuipers, Lafleur, 1998).

Also, **this mechanism is critical for effective cancer chemotherapy and radiation treatment** (Kuipers, Lafleur, 1998) (Blumenthal et al, 2000).

Thus, before cancer patients supplement their diets with antioxidants, suppression of apoptosis and an EMOD insufficiency by antioxidants needs to be considered as having a negative effect on cancer therapy.

Apoptosis is triggered when internal monitors recognize neoplasia, damage or malfunction and initiate signaling cascades that eventually activate caspases and endonucleases that kill the cell (Kokileva, 1994) (Zhivotovsky et al, 1994) (Wyllie, 1987) (Arends et al, 1990).

An important functions of apoptosis is the elimination of preneoplastic and neoplastic cells. (Lowe et al, 1993) (Thompson, 1995) (Tomlison, Bodmer, 1995).

In most forms of cell suicide, the signaling cascade utilizes reactive oxygen species (EMODs) as essential intermediate messenger molecules. (Albright et al, 2003) (Vrablic et al, 2001) (Slater et al, 1995) (Johnson et al, 1996) (Sugiyama et al, 1996).

This is the reason that **antioxidants are capable of inhibiting apoptosis.** Antioxidants such as **alpha-tocopherol, which partition into the lipid compartment of cells, or N-acetylcysteine, a free radical scavenger that partitions into the aqueous phase of the cytosol, can delay or inhibit apoptosis.** (Hawkins et al, 1998) (Takahashi et al, 1998).

Thus, **it is logical and prudent to suggest that removal of antioxidants from the diet might enhance apoptosis, and thereby inhibit tumor growth**.

Recently, colleagues extended this observation to another cancer type, breast cancer, by showing that **dietary depletion of vitamin E and vitamin A inhibits mammary tumor growth and metastasis in transgenic mice.** (Albright et al, 2004). Thus, **the presence of the antioxidants, vitamin E and A, were sheltering the breast tumor cells.**

Using a transgenic mouse model of mammary tumorigenesis with defined rates of tumor growth and lung-targeted metastasis, they determined that dietary antioxidant depletion inhibited tumor growth and diminished metastasis. Compared with control **mice** fed a standard diet, **mice fed an antioxidant-depleted diet exhibited tumor-targeted generation of reactive oxygen species; the number of apoptotic cells in tumors increased 5-fold, and the percentage of tumor cells undergoing mitosis decreased by half.** The mice fed the antioxidant-depleted diet had more small primary tumors and fewer large primary tumors than did controls, and they also had <30% of the number of lung metastatic tumor foci compared with mice fed the control diet.

Cells contain endogenous antioxidant enzymes (e.g., catalase, superoxide dismutase, and glutathione peroxidase), and **many, but not all, human cancer cell types have decreased antioxidant enzyme levels compared to their normal tissue counterparts** (Coursin et al, 1996) (Oberley et al, 1996) (Oberley, Oberley, 1997).

The concentrations of free oxygen radicals are reportedly higher in malignant cells than in normal cells. (Sztarovski et al, 1991) (Toyokune et al, 1995).

Thus, cancer cells should be more sensitive to generated EMODs, and **this may be a useful selective difference that can be exploited when attempting to kill cancer cells but spare normal cells.** Even a moderate increase in the accumulation of oxygen radicals in malignant cells of animals fed an antioxidant-poor diet could increase EMODs to the critical level required for progression of apoptosis. (Slater et al, 1995) (Johnson et al, 1996) (Sugiyama et al, 1996).

Conversely, **even modest quenching or reduction of EMODs by dietary antioxidants could block initiation or completion of apoptosis.**

Antioxidants, by preventing oxidant-mediated damage to diverse targets (DNA, RNA, proteins, and lipids), may logically play a protective role in healthy individuals; however, by inhibiting apoptosis, **these same antioxidants may exert a cancer-promoting effect in cancer patients and in individuals with pre-cancerous DNA changes**.

Inhibition of apoptosis by antioxidants may explain why, in several studies in heavy smokers, **vitamin E and beta-carotene enhanced carcinogenesis in the lung.** (DeLuca et al, 1996) (Heinonen et al, 1998) (where, presumably, smoking had not caused precancerous lesions that predated antioxidant treatment).

Even though some speculate that early administration of antioxidants may help prevent the initiation and progression of cancer by quenching the action of potentially mutagenic reactive free radicals, **administration of antioxidants subsequent to a mutagenic event may effectively intercept free radicals (EMODs) that are critical in promoting apoptosis.** This imbalance may allow the rate of proliferation in tumors to exceed the capacity for apoptosis. It seems reasonable to suggest that **the potential risks and benefits of high-dose antioxidants in cancer patients should be approached with significant caution and indiscriminate use of antioxidant dietary supplements should be avoided.** (Zeisel, 2004).

During a 2004 conference, Zeisel said, "Studies have investigated the effects of antioxidant supplementation on cancer therapy. Studies on cisplatin indicate that it kills breast cancer cells by apoptosis and necrosis, and that the addition of vitamin E blocks much of the apoptotic process. High-dose vitamin E reduces the efficacy of cisplatin, although the normal cells involved would be protected by vitamin E. Lymphoma cells treated with 5 Gy of radiation die or stop dividing, but if N-acetylcysteine is added to the media, the lymphoma cells keep growing. Vitamin E succinate also protects cells against the effects of radiation in vitro.

There is no conclusive evidence to show which antioxidant doses or mixtures protect cells against DNA damage and lipid and protein oxidation but do not interfere with apoptosis signaling pathways. **Oversupplementation (with antioxidants) may actually produce an environment that is beneficial to the tumor and allow it to survive**."

However, Kedar N. Prasad, Ph.D., Professor, Department of Radiology, University of Colorado Health Sciences Center, Denver, presented his views on the use of high-dose multiple antioxidants as an adjunct to radiotherapy and chemotherapy. The use of antioxidants in cancer therapy is driven by two opposing hypotheses. One hypothesis states that the use of dietary multiple antioxidants and micronutrients improves the efficacy of treatment; the opposing hypothesis states that the use of antioxidants and micronutrients protects cancer cells against free radical damage. These opposing hypotheses have grown out of generalized experimental data.

Prasad feels that antioxidant dose levels and combinations need to be investigated.

Do antioxidants reduce EMOD levels in cancer patients?

Investigators assessed the blood levels of reactive oxygen species as a marker of free radicals producing oxidative stress and the most relevant of the physiological body enzymes counteracting reactive oxygen species, namely glutathione peroxidase and superoxide dismutase. They carried out an **open non-randomized study on 28 advanced stage cancer patients** (stage III, 10.7%, and stage IV, 89.3%) with tumors at different (8) sites: all were hospitalized in the Medical Oncology Dept, University of Cagliari Interventions. The patients were divided into 5 groups and a different antioxidant treatment was administered to each group. **The selected antioxidants were: alpha lipoic acid 200 mg/day orally, N-acetylcysteine 1800 mg/day i.v. or carboxycysteine-lysine salt 2.7 g/day orally, amifostine 375 mg/day i.v., reduced glutathione 600 mg/day i.v., vitamin A 30000 IU/day orally plus vitamin E 70 g/day orally plus Vitamin C 500 mg/day orally.** The antioxidant treatment was administered for 10 consecutive days. *Results.* Their results show that **all but one of the antioxidants tested were effective in reducing reactive oxygen species levels** and 2 of them (cysteine-containing compounds and amifostine) had the additional effect of increasing glutathione peroxidase activity. Comprehensively, **the "antioxidant treatment" was found to have an effect both on reactive oxygen species**

levels and glutathione peroxidase activity. The antioxidant treatment also reduced serum levels of IL-6 and TNF. Patients in both ECOG PS 0-1 and ECOG PS 2-3 responded to antioxidant treatment. (Mantovani et al, 2002). **Although this was a small study, it showed that antioxidants definitely reduce EMOD levels in cancer patients.**

Antioxidant vitamins can pose a significant potential danger to cancer patients both on and off of chemotherapy, radiation therapy and photodynamic therapy. While the intention of taking an antioxidant supplement would seem like a good idea, **voluminous research has shown that taking certain antioxidants with certain cancers actually block cancer cell kill and promote tumor spread.**

Is there a need for cancer patients to avoid antioxidant supplements?

Please refer to: SUMMARY: Points *against* the use of antioxidants with chemo or radiation therapy

The Royal College of Radiologists advise patients to avoid antioxidant supplements, especially in high doses, during their conventional cancer therapy.

According to Breastcancer.org, **this can alter the cancer treatment process and seriously compromise prognosis and survival.** Taking any medication or antioxidant supplement can pose considerable health risks when undergoing cancer treatment. Thus, it may be prudent not take any unnecessary risks. (http://www.livestrong.com/article/318898-vitamins-cancer-chemotherapy/#ixzz1AZiaGLw0. accessed 1-9-11).

Antioxidant vitamins A, E, C, plus glutathione, and selenium are extremely dangerous to take with chemotherapy. According to Bastyr Center for Natural Health, these antioxidants reduce the desirable toxicity of chemotherapy, a necessary effect for killing cancer cells and shrinking tumors in the cancer patient. (D'Andrea, 2005). (http://bastyrcenter.org/content/view/902/. accessed 1-9-11).

These antioxidants actually protect the cancer cells by presenting a buffer between the healthy cells and the cancer-fighting oxygen free radicals (EMODS) in chemotherapy. **The vitamins work against both the patient's immune system and the chemotherapy actually providing an excellent environment for the cancer cells to flourish and grow.** (Parker-Pope, 2005).

Even cancer patients that are also deficient in nutrients are generally advised against taking antioxidant vitamins or mineral supplements on or off of chemotherapy treatments. **Multivitamin supplements for example, were shown to feed cancerous tumors.** Breastcancer.org suggests that the only vitamin that has not been linked to cancer spread is vitamin D. I believe that vitamin D is safe because it efficiently generates EMODs.

All other vitamins have shown considerable elevation of risk among patients with prostate and breast cancers with advanced metastases and premature death. Even multivitamins, which also contain antioxidants, are not recommended for cancer patients. (http://www.breastcancer.org/ symptoms/types/recur_metast/ask_expert/conf_2007_10/question_24.jsp. accessed 1-9-11).

There may be some vitamins or complementary treatments allowed during cancer treatments, yet antioxidants A, E, and C may need to be stopped. Not only can these antioxidant vitamins and supplements interrupt the activity of the chemotherapy and radiation, but the disease could ultimately get much worse because of them and lead to premature death.

To repeat, **the following was taken from the website for the American Cancer Society:** http://www.**cancer.org**/Treatment/TreatmentsandSideEffects/ TreatmentTypes/Chemotherapy/ChemotherapyPrinciplesAnIn-depthDiscussiono ftheTechniquesanditsRoleinTreatment/chemotherapy-principles-selecting-chemo-drugs-to-use?ssDomainNum=5c38e88&docSelected=chemotherapy-principles-add-res&print=true. Last medical review and update 9/28/10. Accessed 1-9-11.

*Because most people think of vitamins as a safe way to improve health, it is not surprising that many people with cancer take high doses of one or more vitamins. But **few realize that some vitamins might make their chemotherapy less effective.***

Certain vitamins, such as A, E, and C act as antioxidants. This means that they can prevent formation of ions (free radicals) that damage DNA. This damage is thought to have an important role in causing cancer. There is some evidence that getting enough of these vitamins (through a balanced diet and, perhaps, by taking vitamin supplements) may help reduce the risk of developing some types of cancer.

*On the other hand, some chemotherapy drugs (as well as radiation treatments) work by producing these same types of ions. These ions severely damage the DNA of cancer cells so the cells are unable to grow and reproduce. **Some scientists believe that taking high doses of antioxidants during treatment may make chemotherapy or*** *radiation less effective. Few studies have been done to thoroughly test this theory. Until we know more about the effects of vitamins on chemotherapy drugs, many oncologists recommend the following during chemotherapy:*

- *If your doctor has not prescribed vitamins for a specific reason, it is best not to take any.*

- *A simple multivitamin is probably OK for people who want to take a vitamin supplement, but always check with your doctor first.*

- ***It is safest to avoid taking high doses of antioxidant vitamins during cancer treatment.** Ask your doctors if and when it might be safe to start such vitamins after treatment is finished.*

- *If you are concerned about nutrition, you can usually get plenty of vitamins by eating a well-balanced diet.*

The American Cancer Society experts believe that antioxidant vitamins and supplement shouldn't be used during cancer treatment. A 2005 report in the medical journal *CA* cites several studies that show the use of vitamins by cancer patients doesn't help and may even cause harm.

According to the Linus Pauling Institute website, "When *Cancer and Vitamin C* was first published in 1979, Drs. Cameron and Pauling noted that little information was available on the interaction between vitamin C and chemotherapeutic drugs. **They cautioned that patients undergoing aggressive chemotherapy expected to be curative should refrain from taking large doses of vitamin C at the same time in case the vitamin interfered with the drug action.** Dr. Chan Park has found that the growth of leukemic cells from some leukemia patients put into culture was enhanced by vitamin C. The growth of cells taken from other leukemia patients was either inhibited or unaffected by vitamin C." (http://lpi.oregonstate.edu/s-s00/vitaminc.html. accessed 1-9-11).

In vitro evidence does suggest that **cancer cells take in more vitamin C than do normal neighboring cells; cancer cells also resist oxidative injury more successfully after treatment with vitamin C.** (D'Andrea, 2005).

Also, there is general agreement that **endogenous antioxidants such as glutathione and antioxidant enzyme-elevating agents may protect cancer cells against cytotoxic therapy.** (Pradad, 2004).

"Can vitamin and herbal supplements reduce the adverse effects of cancer treatment, decrease the risk of cancer recurrence or improve a patient's chances of survival? **We don't really know.** Research into these matters has been minimal," said senior author Cornelia (Neli) Ulrich, Ph.D., an associate member of the Hutchinson Center's Public Health Sciences Division. "While supplement use may be beneficial for some patients, such as those who cannot eat a balanced diet, **research suggests that certain supplements may actually interfere with treatment or even accelerate cancer growth**," she said in an article published Feb. 1, 2008 in the *Journal of Clinical Oncology*.

The researchers also found that many people initiate the use of vitamins and supplements after cancer diagnosis; between 14 percent and 32 percent start taking them after learning they have cancer. **"Some vitamins, such as folic acid, may be involved in cancer progression while others, such as St. John's wort, can interfere with chemotherapy.**

Antioxidants could be beneficial in people with innate or acquired high baseline levels of reactive oxygen species but be harmful in people with lower innate levels. (Salganik, 2001).

Meta-analyses of randomized clinical trials have not shown that antioxidant supplements reduce cancer incidence. (Bjelakovic et al. 2004) (Bjelakovic et al, Lancet 2004) (Caraballoso et al, 2003) (Bjelakovic et al, 2006).

2-methoxyoestradiol and polyunsaturated fatty acids (PUFAs) inhibit SODs and cause an increase of $O_2^{\cdot-}$ in tumor cells leading to their death. In addition, PUFAs (especially gamma-linolenic acid), 2-methoxyoestradiol and thalidomide may possess anti-angiogenic activity. **This suggests that free radicals can suppress angiogenesis.** Limited clinical studies done with gamma-linolenic acid showed that it can regress human brain gliomas without any significant side-effects. Thus, PUFAs, thalidomide and 2-methoxyoestradiol or their derivatives may offer a new radical approach to the treatment of cancer. (Das, 2002). **I believe that this is in conformity with my UTOPIA theory and of the fact that high levels of EMODs are needed to protect us from neoplasia.**

Antioxidant use or avoidance with Cancer Therapy

Despite nearly two decades of research investigating the use of dietary antioxidant supplementation during conventional chemotherapy and radiation therapy, controversy remains about the efficacy and safety of this complementary treatment. **Several randomized clinical trials have demonstrated that the**

concurrent administration of antioxidants with chemotherapy or radiation therapy reduces treatment-related side effects. Some data indicate that antioxidants may protect tumor cells as well as healthy cells from oxidative damage generated by radiation therapy and some chemotherapeutic agents. However, other data suggest that antioxidants can protect normal tissues from chemotherapy- or radiation-induced damage without decreasing tumor control. We review some of the data regarding the putative benefits and potential risks of antioxidant supplementation concurrent with cytotoxic therapy. **On the basis of our review of the published randomized clinical trials, we conclude that the use of supplemental antioxidants during chemotherapy and radiation therapy should be discouraged because of the possibility of tumor protection and reduced survival.**

In the absence of good evidence of benefit, it is contrary to the principle of **primum non nocere** to advise patients to continue a potentially harmful intervention.

In this report published in 2008, researchers cautioned that cancer patients should avoid use of antioxidant supplements during radiation and <u>chemotherapy</u>. According to the report's authors, **antioxidant supplements may reduce the anticancer effects of therapy** (Lawenda et al, 2008).

Several clinical studies have reported modest decreases in treatment-related side effects when supplemental antioxidants—either dietary or pharmaceutical—are administered concurrently with cytotoxic regimens. (Sieja, 2000) (Pace et al, 2003) (Conklin, 2005) (Branda et al, 2004) (Bairati et al, J Clin Oncol. 2005) (Ferreira et al, 2004).

However, **concern has been expressed that the action of supplemental antioxidants might not be restricted to reducing the oxidative damage to normal tissues generated by radiation therapy and certain chemotherapeutic agents.** (D'Andrea, 2005) (Seifried et al, 2003).

Theoretically, **antioxidants can exert their effects on all tissues to some degree, thereby protecting tumor cells as well as healthy ones. Experimental and clinical studies** (Bairati et al, J Clin Oncol. 2005) (Ferreira et al, 2004) (Fantappie et al, 2004) (Sakamoto, Sakka, 1973) (Mothersill et al, 1986) (Wiernik et al, 1992) (Lesperance et al, 2002) (Lawenda et al, 2007) (Salganik, 2001) **lend support to this hypothesis, with some clinical data also suggesting that cancer patients who use antioxidant supplements during radiation or chemotherapy have worse survival than those who do not**

(Bairati et al, J Clin Oncol. 2005) (Ferreira et al, 2004) (Lesperance et al, 2002) (Bairati et al, 2006).

Data is presented on the use of supplemental antioxidants during chemotherapy or radiation therapy and highlights the reasons why this combined treatment approach should be avoided until it is shown to be safe.

Antioxidant depletion reduces brain tumor size and metastatic lesions

In 2000, Salganik observed a reduction in **brain tumor size in the TgT (121) transgenic mouse model,** which spontaneously develops brain cancer, when these mice were fed diets depleted of antioxidants; there was enhanced apoptosis within tumors and showed that **dietary antioxidant depletion enhances tumor EMODs (reactive oxygen species, ROS) and apoptosis, resulting in a reduction in brain tumor size** in the TgT_{121} transgenic mouse model, a non-metastatic tumor model. (Salganik et al, 2000).

As stated before, in 2004, Salganik showed that in a transgenic mouse model of mammary tumorigenesis with defined rates of tumor growth and lung-targeted metastasis, we determined the ability of dietary antioxidant depletion to inhibit tumor growth and metastasis. Compared with control mice fed a standard diet, **antioxidant-depleted mice exhibited tumor-targeted generation of ROS manifested by increased levels of oxidatively modified DNA/RNA (8- hydroxy-2'-deoxyguanine, 8-hydroxyguanine) and lipid peroxidation (4-hydroxy-2-nonenal) in primary and metastatic tumor foci.** In addition to increased tumor-targeted ROS, the number of apoptotic cells was increased approximately 500% and terminal dUTP nucleotide DNA end-labeling–positive cells 200% in mice fed the antioxidant-depleted diet, whereas the percentage of tumor cells undergoing mitosis was >50% lower than in controls. The proportional distribution of small (<1.5 cm) and large (≥1.5 cm) primary mammary tumors differed. **The mice fed the antioxidant-depleted diet had more small primary tumors and fewer large primary tumors.** Importantly, **they also had fewer lung metastatic tumor foci compared with mice fed the control diet.** These findings may be important in understanding the role of dietary antioxidant vitamins in tumor growth and metastasis (Albright et al, 2004).

Antioxidant Supplements and Increased Risk of Death

In 2004, investigators studied **14 randomized trials with 170,525 participants** to establish whether antioxidant supplements reduce the incidence of gastrointestinal cancer and mortality. **In seven high-quality trials (n=131 727), the fixed-effect model showed that antioxidant significantly increased mortality. b-carotene and vitamin A (1 29, 1 14–1 45) and b-carotene and vitamin E (1 10, 1 01–1 20) significantly increased mortality, whereas b-carotene alone only tended to increase mortality. They could not find evidence that antioxidant supplements can prevent gastrointestinal cancers on the contrary, they seem to increase overall mortality.** (Bjelakovic et al, Lancet 2004).

Taking antioxidant supplements containing beta-carotene, vitamin E, and vitamin A may be linked to an increased risk of death, according to a 2007 review and meta-analysis of 68 trials including a total of 232,606 participants. Although no increased mortality risk was associated with vitamin C supplementation, researchers didn't find any evidence that vitamin C supplements increased longevity either. Selenium supplementation, meanwhile, appeared to reduce the risk of death. (Bjelakovic et al, 2007).

To illustrate the complex relationship of dose, agent, and microenvironment, consider the following **two large randomized studies** that have assessed the efficacy of ß-carotene as a preventative agent in patients at high risk of malignancy. The Alpha-Tocopherol, Beta-Carotene cancer prevention trial randomly assigned 29,133 male smokers to supplementation with a-tocopherol, ß-carotene, both, or placebo, and **unexpectedly found an increased risk of lung cancer in participants who received ß-carotene supplementation.** Supplementation with a-tocopherol alone in this study appeared to have no adverse effect on lung cancer incidence. (The ATBC Cancer Prevention Study Group, 1994).

In addition, *the beta-Carotene and Retinol Efficacy trial randomly assigned 18,314 men and women at high risk of developing lung cancer to the combination of daily ß-carotene and retinyl palmitate (vitamin A) or placebo. This large study was stopped early because of evidence of a significant increase in the risk of lung cancer and lung cancer mortality in the treatment group* compared with the placebo group. (Omenn et al, 1996).

It is hypothesized that the increased incidence of lung cancers seen in both of these large, randomized studies is **at least partially due to the pro-oxidant nature of ß-carotene** when used at high doses or in oxygen-rich environments, such as the lung. (Palazzo et al, 2003). (RMH Note: Some investigators can not bring themselves to admit that antioxidants can have any harmful effects at all. In their minds, only prooxidants can cause harm.)

Beta-carotene is an antioxidant at low oxygen concentrations; however, it acts as a pro-oxidant at high oxygen concentrations. (Palazzo et al, 2003).

How do the preclinical findings that antioxidants improve the efficacy of radiotherapy translate into clinical outcomes? Numerous clinical studies investigating the effects of antioxidants in combination with radiotherapy or after radiotherapy have now been completed, with **various degrees of success**. In the adjuvant setting, antioxidants have been used to manage a wide range of radiation-induced normal tissue toxicities with varying success. Clinical studies of antioxidants delivered concurrent with radiotherapy have also been completed with the hopes of reducing normal tissue toxicity in a variety of settings, including **head and neck cancers** (Ferreira et al, 2004) (Mills, 1988), **bladder cancers** (Sanchiz et al, 1996), **and in the prevention of alopecia and radiation dermatitis during brain radiotherapy** (Metz et al, 2004) (Halperin et al, 1993).

Although promising efficacy in the prevention of normal tissue toxicity has been reported with antioxidant supplementation, **it is important to consider the effects of this treatment on the ability to achieve the primary goal of radiotherapy: the local cure of the tumor**. In the 2005 issue of the *Journal of Clinical Oncology*, Bairati et al reported the results of a **randomized trial evaluating alpha-tocopherol and beta-carotene supplementation during and after radiotherapy for head and neck cancer**. (Bairati et al, J Clin Oncol. 2005).

This double-blind, placebo-controlled, randomized study was initiated to determine the effect of antioxidant supplementation on the development of second cancers and to determine if concurrent administration of these agents with radiotherapy reduces normal tissue toxicity. A total of **540 patients** were included in this trial and observed for evidence of acute toxicity. Adherence to the assigned treatment was assessed with pill counting and assays of plasma a-tocopherol and ß-carotene levels. ß-carotene supplementation was discontinued after the results of the Alpha-Tocopherol, Beta-Carotene trial and ß-Carotene and Retinol Efficacy trial became available. To assess the effects of supplementation on normal tissue toxicity, acute toxicity and quality of life were measured in each study participant during, at the completion of, and 1 month after radiotherapy. **With regard to outcomes, supplementation with alpha-tocopherol and ß-carotene appeared to reduce the toxicity encountered by study participants significantly.**

Of significant concern is the finding of an increased risk of local recurrence in the supplemented group, suggesting decreased efficacy of radiotherapy with supplementation.

A smaller **randomized trial** evaluating daily mouth rinsing with **alpha-tocopherol solution during radiotherapy to prevent mucositis in head and neck cancer** patients has been published recently. (Ferreira et al, 2004).

This study included **54 patients with oral cavity and oropharynx cancers** and found a significant improvement in symptomatic mucositis. The rates of local recurrence are not discussed in the report of this trial; however, **a trend toward a decrease in survival in the experimental arm is reported at a median follow-up of 12 months. The authors attribute this trend toward decreased survival in patients receiving alpha-tocopherol mouth rinse to the higher number of patients with advanced disease in that arm.**

Where do these findings leave us? With the results of Bairati et al, it appears that supplementation with beta-carotene is not justified for reduction in mucositis **given the concerns for a decrease in the efficacy of radiotherapy for head and neck cancers in addition to the concerns of increasing the risk of lung cancers in a group of patients who are already at an elevated risk.** Similarly, the results of Bairati et al with alpha-tocopherol in combination with the results observed by Ferreira et al suggest that additional randomized trials using antioxidants for normal tissue cytoprotection in patients with head and neck cancers are not warranted. Furthermore, the issue of patient self-supplementation with antioxidants during radiotherapy must also be addressed in more detail given the results of this study. **Without any definitive data on this issue, a reasonable approach would be to avoid unnecessary supplementation during and after radiotherapy.**

Bairati et al are to be commended for their work in attempting to increase the therapeutic ratio of radiation therapy for head and neck cancers. However, what should be apparent from these data is the difficulty in determining from preclinical data **which agents will be protectors of normal tissue without providing protection to tumor tissue in clinical trials.** These issues are of primary concern for future trials designed to test a potential radiation protector. Perhaps future investigations of antioxidant supplementation and radioprotectors to prevent normal tissue toxicity should be performed initially in patients with diseases with high rates of salvage. In these participants, the **possible unintentional tumor protection** and resultant recurrence may not lead to significant decrements in survival if effective salvage therapy was available.

This **raises significant concerns about the possible inadvertent simultane-ous protection of tumor tissues.**

Cyanidin-3-rutinoside, a Natural Polyphenol Antioxidant, Selectively Kills Leukemic Cells by Induction of Oxidative Stress

Prevention of malignant transformation: Anthocyanins prevent cellular malignant transformation. Moreover, anthocyanins have been probed to induce apoptosis in some malignant cells. This characteristic is extremely important since, as was shown above, anthocyanins are protective for normal cells. A recent publication from Feng et al (Feng 2007) brings light over this apparent contradiction and re-inforces the selectivity of anthocyanins anti-tumorous activity. Feng found that **Cyanidin-3-rutenoside selectively kills leukemic cells (HL-60 cells) by induction of oxidative stress. Anthocyanins induce peroxide accumula-tion and apoptosis in HL-60 cells.** In addition, cyanidin-3-rutinoside treatment resulted in reactive oxygen species (ROS)-dependent activation of p38 MAPK and c-jun NH2-terminal kinase (JNK), which contributed to cell death by activating the mitochondrial pathway mediated by Bim. Notably, cyanidin-3-rutinoside treatment did not lead to increased ROS accumulation in normal human peripheral blood mononuclear cells and had no cytotoxic effects on these cells (Feng 2007).

Molecular mechanisms behind the chemoprotective effects of anthocyanins can be inferred from all the biological effects already mentioned. Hou et al (Hou et al, 2004) proposed similar mechanisms including modulation of MAPK pathway, AP-1 factor, NF-kB pathway, Cyclooxigenase-2 gene and JNK-mediated caspase activation. Though more information is available every day; the current information should be enough to support the use of anthocyanines. (Feng et al, 2007). **I believe that this is just one more example of so-called antioxidants causing can-cer cell death but they are doing it prooxidatively, because it increases peroxide accumulation.**

Delphinidin 3-sambubioside, a Hibiscus anthocyanin, induces apoptosis in human leukemia cells through reactive oxygen species-mediated mitochondrial pathway

Delphinidin 3-sambubioside (Dp3-Sam), a Hibiscus anthocyanin, was iso-lated from the dried calices of Hibiscus sabdariffa L. **Dp3-Sam could induce a dose-dependent apoptosis in human leukemia cells (HL-60)** as character-ized by cell morphology, DNA fragmentation, activation of caspase-3, -8, and -9, and inactivation of poly(ADP)ribose polymerase (PARP). Molecular data showed that

Dp3-Sam induced Bid truncation, mitochondrial membrane potential (DeltaPsi(m)) loss, and cytochrome c release from mitochondria to cytosol. Moreover, **Dp3-Sam caused a time- and dose-dependent elevation of intracellular reactive oxygen species (ROS) level in HL-60 cells, and antioxidants such as N-acetyl-L-cysteine (NAC) and catalase could effectively block Dp3-Sam-induced ROS generation, caspase-3 activity, and DNA fragmentation.** These data indicate that Dp3-Sam might induce apoptosis in HL-60 cells through a ROS-mediated mitochondrial dysfunction pathway. These findings enhance our understanding for anticancer function of Hibiscus anthocyanins in herbal medicine (Hou et al, 2005). **I believe that this confirms the prooxidant activity of anthocyanins and the fact that it can be blocked by NAC. HL-60 cells are human promyelocytic leukemia cells.**

Anthocyanin induces apoptosis in human leukemia cells via EMODs

Anthocyanins block colon cancer cells

Department of Nutrition and Food Science, University of Maryland, College Park, MD.

Anthocyanin-rich extracts, potent antioxidants and **commercially available food coloring agents,** have been reported to inhibit growth of various cancer cell lines. We investigated the effect of semipurified anthocyanin-rich extract from fruits of Aronia meloncarpa, on **normal colon and colon cancer cell lines.** A 24-h exposure to 50 mg monomeric anthocyanin/ml of Aronia extract resulted in **60% growth inhibition of human HT-29 colon cancer cells.** The treated cells showed a blockage at G1/G0 and G2/M phases of the cell cycle. The cell cycle arrest coincided with an increased expression of the p21WAF1 and p27KIP1 genes and decreased expression of cyclin A and B genes. Prolonged exposure to the extract resulted in no further change in the cell number, indicating a cytostatic inhibition of cell growth. NCM460 normal colon cells demonstrated <10% growth inhibition at the highest concentration of 50 mg/ml extract. **A 35% decrease in the cyclooxygenase-2 gene expression was observed within 24 h of exposure of HT-29 cells** but did not translate into decreased protein levels or protein activity. These results support the need for further research to identify the specific component(s) in this extract that suppress cancer cell growth and the genes affected by these natural compounds. (Malik et al, 2003).

Anthocyanins prevent cellular malignant transformation

Prevention of malignant transformation: Anthocyanins prevent cellular malignant transformation. Moreover, anthocyanins have been probed to induce apoptosis in some malignant cells. This characteristic is extremely important since, as was shown above, anthocyanins are protective for normal cells. A recent publication from Feng et al (Feng 2007) brings light over this apparent contradiction and reinforces the selectivity of anthocyanins anti-tumorous activity. **Feng found that Cyanidin-3-rutenoside selectively kills leukemic cells (HL-60 cells) by induction of oxidative stress. Anthocyanins induce peroxide accumulation and apoptosis in HL-60 cells.** In addition, cyanidin-3-rutinoside treatment resulted in reactive oxygen species (ROS)-dependent activation of p38 MAPK and c-jun NH2-terminal kinase (JNK), which contributed to cell death by activating the mitochondrial pathway mediated by Bim. Notably, cyanidin-3-rutinoside treatment did not lead to increased ROS accumulation in normal human peripheral blood mononuclear cells and had no cytotoxic effects on these cells (Feng et al, 2007). Molecular mechanisms behind the chemoprotective effects of anthocyanins can be inferred from all the biological effects already mentioned. Hou et al (Hou et al, 2004) proposed similar mechanisms including modulation of MAPK pathway, AP-1 factor, NF-kB pathway, Cyclooxygenase-2 gene and JNK-mediated caspase activation. Though more information is available every day; the current information should be enough to support the use of anthocyanines.

(Feng et al, 2007).

A polyphenol antioxidant (anthocyanin) kills by increasing EMODs

Anthocyanins are a group of naturally occurring phenolic compounds widely available in fruits and vegetables in human diets. **They have broad biological activities including anti-mutagenesis and anticarcinogenesis, which are generally attributed to their antioxidant activities.** We studied the effects and the mechanisms of the most common type of anthocyanins, cyanidin-3-rutinoside, in several leukemia and lymphoma cell lines. We found that cyanidin-3-rutinoside extracted and purified from the black raspberry cultivar Jewel **induced apoptosis in HL-60 cells in a dose- and time-dependent manner. Paradoxically, this compound induced the accumulation of peroxides, which are involved in the induction of apoptosis in HL-60 cells**. In addition, cyanidin-3-rutinoside treatment resulted in reactive oxygen species (ROS)-dependent activation of p38 MAPK and JNK, which contributed to cell death by activating the mitochondrial pathway mediated by Bim. Down-regulation of Bim or overexpression of Bcl-2 or Bcl-x$_L$

considerably blocked apoptosis. Notably, **cyanidin-3-rutinoside treatment did not lead to increased ROS accumulation in normal human peripheral blood mononuclear cells and had no cytotoxic effects on these cells.** These results indicate that cyanidin-3-rutinoside has the potential to be used in leukemia therapy with the advantages of being widely available and selective against tumors. (Feng et al, 2007). **This is the pattern which I see over and over again. EMODs kill cancer cells selectively and do not harm normal cells.**

Thioredoxin blocks EMOD-induced apoptosis for human neuroblastoma

Human neuroblastoma cells, SH-SY5Y, contain relatively low levels of thioredoxin (Trx); thus, they serve favorably as a model for studying oxidative stress-induced apoptosis. Interestingly, **thioredoxin is upregulated by cGMP/protein kinase G in human neuroblastoma cells, protecting cells from oxidative stress–induced apoptosis** (Andoh et al, 2003).

Vitamin E blocks cinnamaldehyde induced apoptosis in human hepatoma cells

Cinnamaldehyde has been shown to be effective in inducing cell apoptosis in a number of human cancer cells. The aim of the present study was to investigate the effect of vitamin E on the apoptotic signalling mechanism induced by cinnamaldehyde in **human hepatoma PLC/PRF/5 cells.**

Using the XTT assay, cinnamaldehyde exhibited a powerful antiproliferative effect on PLC/PRF/5 cells. Apoptosis was elicited when cells were treated with 1 μmol/L cinnamaldehyde, as characterized by the appearance of phosphatidylserine on the outer surface of the plasma membrane.

The apoptotic effect induced by cinnamaldehyde could be further supported by the release of cytochrome c, Smac/Diablo and Omi/HtrA2 from mitochondria to the cytosol and activation of caspase 3. Cinnamaldehyde also upregulated the expression of pro-apoptotic protein (Bax) and down-regulated the levels of anti-apoptotic proteins, such as Bcl-2 and the inhibitor of apoptosis protein family (X-linked inhibitor of apoptosis protein (XIAP), cellular inhibitor of apoptosis protein (cIAP)-1 and cIAP-2).

Cinnamaldehyde induces the generation of EMODs (reactive oxygen species, ROS) in cells. Following the pre-incubation of PLC/PRF/5 cells with antioxidants, it was found that 100 μmol/L **vitamin E significantly diminished the**

effect of cinnamaldehyde-induced apoptosis, whereas a lesser effect was seen with on 100 μmol/L N-acetyl-l-cysteine. Vitamin E effectively blocked the release of cytochrome *c*, Smac/Diablo and Omi/HtrA2 from mitochondria to the cytosol in cells treated with cinnamaldehyde. Vitamin E also markedly suppressed caspase 3 activation. The expression of apoptotic inhibitors (XIAP, cIAP-1, cIAP-2) and anti-apoptotic (Bcl-2) and pro-apoptotic (Bax) proteins was affected by vitamin E pretreatment.

Taken together, the results suggest that cinnamaldehyde triggers apoptosis possibly through the mitochondrial pathway. **Pretreatment with vitamin E markedly prevented cinnamaldehyde-mediated apoptosis,** which was associated with the modulation of XIAP, cIAP-1, cIAP-2, Bcl-2 and Bax protein activity. (Wu et al, 2004).

Cinnamaldehyde (cinnamic aldehyde) is the main component in cassia oil as well as cinnamon bark oil and is used in flavoring compounds to impart a cinnamon flavor. Considerable safety data exist from the food and flavoring industry which utilizes food grade cinnamaldehyde in non-alcoholic beverages, ice cream, candy, baked goods, chewing gum, condiments and meats at levels ranging from 9 ppm to 4900 ppm. Cinnamaldehyde is Generally Recognized As Safe (GRAS) by the Flavoring Extract Manufacturers' Association and is approved for food use (21 CFR 182.60) by the Food and Drug Administration (FDA). Cinnamon oil, which contains 70% to 90% cinnamaldehyde, is also classified as GRAS, and, like cinnamaldehyde, is used in the food and flavoring industry. (Wu et al, 2004).

Data consistently shows that EMODs kill human cancer cells and this effect is blocked by antioxidants.

Antioxidants mimic the ability of chorionic gonadotropin to suppress apoptosis

Dharmarahan et al. have recently reported that members of the bcl-2 gene family are expressed and estradiol regulated in **rabbit luteal cells during corpus luteum (CL)** regression, and that **estradiol and hCG are effective inhibitors of apoptosis** in the rabbit CL in vivo and in vitro. As **Bcl-2 and related proteins are known to regulate levels of reactive oxygen species** or their intermediates in cells as one possible mechanism to control apoptosis, the present studies were designed to examine if oxidative stress plays a role in luteal cell apoptosis during CL regression in the rabbit. In the first set of experiments, healthy CL obtained from day 11 pseudopregnant rabbits were incubated in serum-free medium for 2 h in the absence or presence of superoxide dismutase (SOD; 1.5-150

U/ml), ascorbic acid (1-100 mM), N-acetyl-L-cysteine (25 and 50 mM), or catalase (10-1000 U/ml). Cells within CL incubated in medium alone exhibited extensive apoptosis (examined by analysis of extracted DNA using 3'-end labeling), and **this onset of apoptosis was blocked in a dose-dependent fashion by treatment with SOD, ascorbic acid, N-acetyl-L-cysteine, or catalase**. In the second set of experiments, expression of bax and bcl-x in CL after in vitro treatment without and with 100 U/ml SOD was examined. Although **SOD treatment did not alter the levels of bcl-x messenger RNA (mRNA) over the 2-h incubation period**, this antioxidant enzyme significantly reduced the levels of bax mRNA in incubated CL. In the final set of experiments, they observed that expression of mitochondrial- or manganese-containing SOD was significantly increased by treatment of isolated CL with 1 microg/ml hCG in vitro, whereas bax mRNA levels were significantly reduced under the same culture conditions. Collectively, these data indicate that the gonadotropin-mediated inhibition of apoptosis in rabbit luteal cells involves enhanced expression of the oxidative stress response gene, manganese-containing SOD, whose protein product may then function to protect luteal cells directly from the damaging effect of reactive oxygen species and/or indirectly by acutely down-regulating expression of Bax, a prooxidant member of the Bcl-2 protein family. (Dharmarahan et al, 1999).

NAC blocks tumoricidal activity of adaphostin and EMOD apoptosis

B-cell chronic lymphocytic leukemia (CLL) is characterized by accumulation of clonal lymphocytes resistant to apoptosis. **The antioxidant N-acetylcysteine blocked both adaphostin-induced ROS generation and apoptosis. Adaphostin induces apoptosis selectively in CLL B-cells through a mechanism that involves EMOD (ROS) generation**, but also demonstrate its ability to augment the effects of fludarabine. (Shanafelt et al, 2005).

Enter adaphostin, also originally thought to be an agent that would work primarily by inhibiting the substrate of the Bcr/abl kinase. However, this agent is also known to cause an elevation of reactive oxygen species **(ROS), and can induce DNA single-strand breaks and DNA damage responses.** (Kay, 2006). Consistent with this Bcr/abl-independent mechanism, adaphostin has been found to result in the induction of **apoptosis and/or killing of chronic lymphocytic leukemia (CLL) lymphocytes and acute myeloid leukemia (AML) blasts. (Chandra et al, 2003)** (Shanafelt et al, 2005).

In those studies, the antioxidant **N-acetylcysteine (NAC) was shown to protect leukemic cells from the lethal impact of adaphostin** providing **further**

evidence for the importance of EMODs (ROS). Chandra and colleague's report now extends the spectrum of adaphostin killing of **leukemic cells to IM-resistant leukemic lymphoid and myeloid cells.** In Chandra et al's work, **both NAC and Trolox (water-soluble vitamin E) protects these cells from apoptosis** or other functional damage and provides further evidence for the importance of ROS in adaphostin cytotoxicity. Their report also shows that adaphostin can induce down-regulation of both wild-type (WT) and mutant Bcr/abl protein but independent of ROS generation. Does this mean that the former activity can still contribute to IM-resistant cell killing? We agree with the investigators that their findings strongly encourage further studies of unique agents that work by the up-regulation of ROS. Encouragingly, **earlier studies by this group have shown relative selectivity of this drug for leukemic and not normal cells.** (Shanafelt et al, 2005) (Mow et al, 2002). **Again I believe that this illustrates the ability of antioxidants to block apoptosis and promote cancer.**

Alpha lipoic acid prooxidant apoptosis is blocked by antioxidants

The **antioxidant alpha-lipoic acid (ALA)** has been shown to affect a variety of biological processes associated with oxidative stress including cancer. We determined in **HT-29 human colon cancer cells** whether ALA is able to affect apoptosis, as an important parameter disregulated in tumor development. Exposure of cells to ALA or its reduced form dihydrolipoic acid (DHLA) for 24 h dose dependently increased caspase-3-like activity and was associated with DNA-fragmentation. DHLA but not ALA was able to scavenge cytosolic O_2^- in HT-29 cells whereas **both compounds increased O_2^--generation inside mitochondria.** Increased mitochondrial O_2^--production was preceded by an increased influx of lactate or pyruvate into mitochondria and resulted in the down-regulation of the anti-apoptotic protein bcl-X_L. **Mitochondrial O_2^--generation and apoptosis induced by ALA and DHLA could be prevented by the O_2^--scavenger benzoquinone.** Moreover, when the lactate/pyruvate transporter was inhibited by 5-nitro-2-(3-phenylpropylamino) benzoate, ALA- and DHLA-induced mitochondrial ROS-production and apoptosis were blocked. In contrast to HT-29 cells, **no apoptosis was observed in non-transformed human colonocytes in response to ALA or DHLA addition.** In conclusion, our study provides evidence that **ALA and DHLA can effectively induce apoptosis in human colon cancer cells by a prooxidant mechanism that is initiated by an increased uptake of oxidizable substrates into mitochondria.** (Wenzel et al, 2005).

Again, this shows death to cancer cells and no harm to normal cells via EMOD induced apoptosis.

Bortezomib EMOD induced cancer apoptosis blocked by antioxidant Tiron

Bortezomib, a proteasome inhibitor, shows substantial anti-tumor activity in a variety of tumor cell lines, is in phase I, II, and III clinical trials and has recently been approved for the treatment of patients with multiple myeloma. The sequence of events leading to apoptosis following proteasome inhibition by bortezomib is unclear. **Bortezomib effects on components of the mitochondrial apoptotic pathway were examined: generation of reactive oxygen species (ROS), alteration in the mitochondrial membrane potential (Δc_m), and release of cytochrome c from mitochondria.** With **human H460 lung cancer cells**, bortezomib exposure at 0.1 µM showed induction of apoptotic cell death starting at 24 h, with increasing effects after 48-72 h of treatment. **After 3-6 h, an elevation in EMOD (ROS) generation,** an increase in (Δc_m) and the release of cytochrome c into the cytosol, were observed in a time-dependent manner. Co-incubation with rotenone and antimycin A, inhibitors of mitochondrial electron transport chain complexes I and III, or with cyclosporine A, an inhibitor of mitochondrial permeability transition pore, resulted in inhibition of bortezomib-induced ROS generation, increase in (Δc_m) and cytochrome c release.

Tiron, an antioxidant agent, blocked the bortezomib-induced EMOD (ROS) production, (Δc_m), and cytochrome c release. Tiron treatment also protected against the bortezomib-induced PARP protein cleavage and cell death. Benzyloxycarbonyl-VAD-fluoromethyl ketone, an inhibitor of pan-caspase, did not alter the bortezomib-induced ROS generation and increase in (Δc_m) although it prevented bortezomib-induced poly(ADP-ribose) polymerase cleavage and apoptotic death. In PC-3 prostate carcinoma cells (with overexpression of Bcl-2), a reduction of bortezomib-induced ROS generation, (Δc_m) was correlated with cellular resistance to bortezomib and the attenuation of drug-induced apoptosis. The transient transfection of wild type p53 in p53 null H358 cells caused stimulation of the bortezomib-induced apoptosis but failed to enhance ROS generation and (Δc_m). Thus, EMOD (**ROS**) generation plays a critical role in the initiation of the bortezomib-induced apoptotic cascade by mediation of the disruption of (Δc_m) and the release of cytochrome c from mitochondria. (Ling et al, 2003). **I believe that this again demonstrates the danger of antioxidants in blocking apoptosis, which controls human cancer.**

Antioxidants and vitamin C block endometrial carcinoma cells apoptosis

Investigators recently demonstrated that proteasome inhibitors can be effective in inducing apoptotic cell death in endometrial carcinoma cell lines and primary culture explants. **Increasing evidence suggests that reactive oxygen species are responsible for proteasome inhibitor-induced cell killing. Antioxidants can thus block apoptosis (cell death) triggered by proteasome inhibition.** Here, we have evaluated the effects of different antioxidants (edaravone and tiron) on **endometrial carcinoma cells** treated with aldehyde proteasome inhibitors (MG-132 or ALLN), the boronic acid-based proteasome inhibitor (bortezomib) and the epoxyketone, epoxomicin. We show that **tiron specifically inhibited the cytotoxic effects of bortezomib,** whereas edaravone inhibited cell death caused by aldehyde-based proteasome inhibitors. We have, however, found that edaravone completely inhibited accumulation of ubiquitin and proteasome activity decrease caused by MG-132 or ALLN, but not by bortezomib. Conversely, tiron inhibited the ubiquitin accumulation and proteasome activity decrease caused by bortezomib. These results suggest that edaravone and tiron rescue cells of proteasome inhibitors from cell death, by inhibiting blockade of proteasome caused by MG-132 and ALLN or bortezomib, respectively. We also tested other antioxidants, and we found **that vitamin C inhibited bortezomib-induced cell death.** Similar to tiron, vitamin C inhibited cell death by blocking the ability of bortezomib to inhibit the proteasome. Until now, all the antioxidants that blocked proteasome inhibitor-induced cell death also blocked the proteasome inhibitor mechanism of action. (Llobet et al, 2008).

In conclusion, our studies provide evidence that **ascorbic acid by its antioxidative capacity reduces drastically the production of EMODs in mitochondria that are required for the execution of drug-induced apoptosis. The data consequently raises the question of whether a high intake of ascorbic acid during chemotherapy of tumors is beneficial.**

Quercetin

Quercetin blocks EMOD induced apoptosis

The **antioxidant**, rather than prooxidant, activities of quercetin on normal cells:
- quercetin protects mouse thymocytes from glucose oxidase-mediated apoptosis. (Lee J, et al, 2003). **This indicates that the FRS drink advertised and promoted by Lance Armstrong is capable of blocking the oxidative killing of cancer cells.**

Quercetin can act as a prooxidant

The effects of **carnosine, rutin and quercetin on oxidative processes and metmyoglobin (MetMb)-reducing activity** in a beef model system were investigated. Ground beef was mixed with antioxidant solution at two concentrations. Storage period and antioxidant treatment negatively affected colour, colour stability and thiobarbituric acid-reactive substances values. Carnosine, rutin and to lesser extent quercetin accelerated discolouration, accumulation of MetMb and lipid peroxidation in the meat. The results suggest that **these antioxidants acted as a pro-oxidants under the specified experimental conditions.** The pro-oxidant activities were in the following order: carnosine>rutin>quercetin. The MetMb-reducing activity was not correlated with storage time, color parameters, MetMb (%) or lipid oxidation. The MetMb-reducing activity was significantly reduced by 1 mM carnosine. However, there was no association between MetMb-reducing activity and colour stability during post-mortem storage. (Bekhit et al, 2004).

This is just another example of the confusion in redox studies. Antioxidants can have significant prooxidant activity and I believe that the prooxidant activity is responsible for tumoricidal effects attributible to them. Thus, there are many studies reporting antioxidant induced apoptosis, which is a misinterpretation of the data, when it is actually the prooxidant properties that lead to apoptotic cancer cell death.

Antioxidant and prooxidant effects of quercetin on GPDH

Anti- and prooxidant properties of quercetin under different conditions were investigated using glyceraldehyde-3-phosphate dehydrogenase, a glycolytic enzyme containing essential cysteine residues. **Quercetin was shown to produce hydrogen peroxide** in aqueous solutions at pH 7.5, this resulting in the oxidation of the cysteine residues of the enzyme. Quercetin significantly increased oxidation of GAPDH observed in the presence of ferrous ions, particularly when FeSO(4) was added to the solution containing GAPDH and quercetin. The results suggest **the formation of hydroxyl radical in the case of the addition of FeSO(4) to a quercetin solution.** At the same time, quercetin protects GAPDH from oxidation in the presence of ascorbate and Fe(3+). In the absence of metals, quercetin protects SH-groups of GAPDH from oxidation by the superoxide anion generated by the system containing xanthine/xanthine oxidase. (Food and chemical toxicology, 2007).

Acai is an anthocyanin antioxidant may interfere with chemo

Researchers at Texas A&M University confirm that acai contains **anthocyanins, the antioxidant found in grapes, cranberries and other purple and red-purple fruits.** Research has shown that the antioxidant occurs in levels roughly the same as in grapes and in a form that is usable by the human body. But it does not show that acai's <u>antioxidants</u> are any better than those found in less expensive and more widely available fruits such as blueberries and raspberries.

Beware of Marketing Claims

Researchers at the University of Florida exploring the other possible uses of acai note that acai has antineoplastic (anticancer) effects in the laboratory when placed with certain types of leukemia cells. However, **they do not know whether acai or its extracts will work in treating human subjects with leukemia.**

Some companies have claimed that acai berries can cure cancer. **The U.S. Food and Drug Administration (FDA) has found no evidence that acai can reduce or eliminate cancer cells.** In fact, the **Memorial Sloan-Kettering Cancer Center issued a statement that acai may lessen the positive effect of chemotherapy by interfering with the drugs used to eradicate the cancer.** Do not use any acai products if you are undergoing chemotherapy without first consulting with your doctor.

Many Internet websites boast of acai's effectiveness as a weight-loss agent, usually paired with a colon cleansing product. Some weight loss is often seen; however, determining whether the weight loss is due to the acai or is the result of the laxative effects of the colon cleansing is difficult. To date, no research has substantiated the effectiveness of acai as a weight-loss product.

While acai may be a beneficial addition to a daily diet, **it has not been proven to cure anything,** and it should not replace a well-balanced, healthy diet.

Side Effects, Adverse Reactions

Many marketing websites claim that acai has no side effects. Any substance can have side effects, adverse reactions or adverse interactions with other substances. **AARP's Drug Directory recommends using acai with caution if you are taking antineoplastic medications, antioxidants or anti-inflammatory drugs or herbs.** Acai may increase the actions of these medications/herbs to unsafe levels. Problems with hypertension may occur or increase, and fluid retention and swelling may be seen. Acai may cause gastrointestinal ulcers or bleeding. Allergic reactions may occur if an individual is allergic to pollens or any of acai's by-products, such as palm hearts.

CHAPTER NINETEEN:

Opponents to antioxidant avoidance in cancer patients

Some of the following was excerpted from: J. Nutr. Nov. 1, 2004. Vol. 134. No. 11, pp. 3143S-3163S.

Chemotherapy and Antioxidants: An Overview (by an antioxidant fan)

Conklin

Kenneth A. Conklin, M.D., Ph.D., Clinical Professor, Jonsson Comprehensive Cancer Center, David Geffen School of Medicine, University of California—Los Angeles, discussed the controversy surrounding the use of antioxidants during chemotherapy. Approximately 300 to 400 preclinical studies have been published on this topic, and **most show that antioxidants do not interfere with the mechanism of action of therapeutic agents.** However, **too few clinical studies have been done to draw any definitive conclusions.**

Antioxidants (e.g., vitamins C and E) act as reducing agents to neutralize free radicals. **If a therapeutic agent works by releasing free radicals, it is possible that antioxidants may interfere with its action. Some antioxidants are also strong nucleophiles (e.g., GSH, *N*-acetyl cysteine, and a-lipoic acid), and they may interfere with the anticancer effects of platinum coordination complexes (e.g., cisplatin and carboplatin) and alkylating agents.**

Doxorubicin (Adriamycin), a very versatile antineoplastic agent, is an anthracycline that is reduced to a semiquinone that can **generate superoxide radicals.** Anthracyclines are important in the study of antioxidant effects because they form large amounts of free radicals and induce oxidative stress. Regarding the mechanism of action of anthracyclines, the most compelling evidence shows that at clinically relevant concentrations they intercalate with double-stranded DNA and inhibit the function of topoisomerase II. Free radicals produced by doxorubicin may play a role in cancer therapy, but **preclinical studies suggest that antioxidants do not interfere with the anticancer actions of the drug.**

The side effect of greatest concern when doxorubicin is administered is cardiac toxicity. In heart cells, doxorubicin forms a deoxyaglycone that can replace coenzyme Q10 (CoQ10) in the electron transport chain and act as an electron acceptor. This disrupts the energetics of cardiac mitochondria, leading to reduced generation of ATP, and accounts for the commonly seen side effects of acute cardiac toxicity (arrhythmias and reduced ejection fraction). The effect of doxorubicin on cardiac mitochondria is uniquely different from its effect on mitochondria of other cells. This is most likely due to the unique structure of cardiac mitochondria, which contain an NADH dehydrogenase on the outer surface of the inner membrane; this organization is not found in noncardiac mitochondria.

Animal studies show that doxorubicin generates EMODs (ROS) in cardiac mitochondria for at least 1 wk after the drug is administered. This causes the formation of mitochondrial DNA-adducts that can suppress gene expression and reduce synthesis of critical components of the mitochondrial electron transport systems. This may irreversibly damage cardiac mitochondria and be responsible for the development of chronic cardiac toxicity (congestive heart failure that is not responsive to digitalis).

The platinum coordination complexes also generate free radicals that can damage the kidney. Animal model studies with antioxidants (reducing agents) show that they do not reduce the toxicity of platinum drugs such as cisplatin. However, **several studies suggest that the nucleophilic antioxidant GSH, administered intravenously, ameliorates renal toxicity without interfering with the antineoplastic action of the drug.** (Conklin, 2004).

I believe that Conklin ignores substantial in vitro and in vivo work, plain and simple.

Some argue that, although many chemotherapy drugs do induce the formation of free radicals, their anticancer effects do not, in general, seem to depend on the formation of these free radicals. Consequently, antioxidant supplementation may in some circumstances help prevent free-radical-induced side effects without inhibiting the positive effects of the chemotherapy. I thoroughly discussed this in my review article entitled, Cancer therapy, and countered this view. (Howes R : Cancer Therapy, 2010).

Weijl

However, this is consistent with the findings of **Weijl et al., who found that antioxidants such as vitamin C, vitamin E, coenzyme Q10, glutathione, and selenium can reduce the toxicity of free radicals.** (Weijl, et al, 1997).

In studies in humans with cancer, coenzyme Q10 prevented the heart damage that often occurs with the cancer drug adriamycin without inhibiting its anticancer effect. (Cortes EP, Gupta M, Chou C et al. Adriamycin cardiotoxicity: early detection by systolic time interval and possible prevention by coenzyme Q10. *Cancer Treat Rev* 1978;62:887-91). (Judy et al, 1984).

Please keep in mind that the literature shows that CoQ10 can serve as a prooxidant and generate EMODs.

Sieja

In another study of women with ovarian cancer, supplementation with selenium along with chemotherapy (cisplatin plus cyclophosphamide) prevented the loss of appetite, hair loss, vomiting, and decline in white blood cell counts that occurred when the chemotherapy was given by itself. (Seija et al, 2004). Similarly, selenium can serve as a prooxidant and generate EMODs.

Prasad

Defenders of high doses of dietary antioxidants in cancer patients cite pilot data in humans that show that **high-dose multiple dietary antioxidants given adjunctively with radiation or chemotherapy actually enhance the effect of conventional cancer treatments, although the mechanism remains unknown**. (Pradad, 2004).

If this is true, I believe that it is due to a prooxidant effect of the high doses used. It is know that both vitamin C and beta carotene can have prooxidant activity in high doses.

Based on these and other data, researchers have proposed nutritional protocols for both the active treatment phase and follow-up maintenance, consisting of varying doses of vitamins A, B, C, D, E, beta-carotene, and certain minerals, administered orally, twice daily. **This contrasts with other research indicating that patients receiving megadoses of vitamin and mineral combinations fared worse in terms of survival**. (Lesperance et al, 2002). Cited in: (D'Andrea, 2005).

Moss

Should patients undergoing chemotherapy and radiotherapy be prescribed antioxidants? (Moss, 2006).

In September 2005, *CA: A Cancer Journal for Clinicians* published a warning by Gabriella D'Andrea, MD, (D'Andrea, 2005) against the concurrent use of antioxidants with radiotherapy and chemotherapy. However, several deficiencies of the *CA* article soon became apparent, not least the selective omission of prominent studies that contradicted the author's conclusions. While acknowledging that only large-scale, randomized trials could provide a valid basis for therapeutic recommendations, the author sometimes relied on laboratory rather than clinical data to support her claim that harm resulted from the concurrent use of antioxidants and chemotherapy. She also sometimes **extrapolated from chemoprevention** studies rather than those on the concurrent use of antioxidants per se. The article **overstated** the degree to which the laboratory data diverged in regard to the safety and efficacy of antioxidant therapy: in fact, the preponderance of data suggests a synergistic or at least harmless effect with most high-dose dietary antioxidants and chemotherapy. The practical recommendations made in the article to avoid the general class of antioxidants during chemotherapy **are inconsistent**, in that if antioxidants were truly a threat to the efficacy of standard therapy, **antioxidant-rich foods, especially fruits and vegetables, ought also be proscribed during treatment**. Yet no such recommendation is made. Furthermore, the **wide-scale use by both medical and radiation oncologists of synthetic antioxidants (e.g., amifostine) to control the adverse effects of cytotoxic treatments is similarly overlooked**. In sum, this *CA* article is **incomplete**: there is far more information available regarding antioxidant supplements as an appropriate adjunctive cancer therapy than is acknowledged. Patients would be well advised to seek the opinion of physicians who are adequately trained and experienced in the intersection of 2 complex fields, that is, chemotherapeutics and nutritional oncology. Physicians whose goal is comprehensive cancer therapy should refer their patients to qualified integrative practitioners who have such training and expertise to guide patients. **A blanket rejection of the concurrent use of antioxidants with chemotherapy is not justified by the preponderance of evidence at this time and serves neither the scientific community nor cancer patients.**

Simone

Antioxidants and other nutrients do not interfere with radiation or chemotherapy

Some in the oncology community contend that patients undergoing chemotherapy and/or radiation therapy should not use food supplement antioxidants and other nutrients. Oncologists at an influential oncology institution contended that **antioxidants interfere with radiation and some chemotherapies because those modalities kill by generating free radicals that are neutralized by**

antioxidants, and that folic acid interferes with methotrexate. This is despite the common use of amifostine and dexrazoxane, 2 prescription antioxidants, during chemotherapy and/or radiation therapy. DESIGN: To assess all evidence concerning antioxidant and other nutrients used concomitantly with chemotherapy and/or radiation therapy. The MEDLINE and CANCERLIT databases were searched from 1965 to November 2003 using the words vitamins, antioxidants, chemotherapy, and radiation therapy. Bibliographies of articles were searched. All studies reporting concomitant nutrient use with chemotherapy and/or radiation therapy (280 peer-reviewed articles including 62 in vitro and 218 in vivo) were indiscriminately included. RESULTS: Fifty human clinical randomized or observational trials have been conducted, involving **8,521 patients using beta-carotene; vitamins A, C, and E; selenium; cysteine; B vitamins; vitamin D3; vitamin K3; and glutathione as single agents or in combination.** CONCLUSIONS: **Since the 1970s, 280 peer-reviewed in vitro and in vivo studies, including 50 human studies involving 8,521 patients, 5,081 of whom were given nutrients, have consistently shown that they do not interfere with therapeutic modalities for cancer.**

Furthermore, non-prescription antioxidants and other nutrients enhance the killing of therapeutic modalities for cancer, decrease their side effects, and protect normal tissue. **In 15 human studies, 3,738 patients who took non-prescription antioxidants and other nutrients actually had increased survival.** (Simone et al, 2007).

Some **found it surprising that a recent review** (Simone, Simone, Simone, 2007) (Simone et al, 2007) **definitively concludes that antioxidants (and other supplemental nutrients), when given concurrently with chemotherapy and/or radiation therapy, 1) do not interfere with chemotherapy and/or radiation therapy, 2) enhance the cytotoxic effects of chemotherapy and radiation therapy, 3) protect normal tissues, and 4) increase patient survival.**

In the concluding sentence of this review, **the authors recommend that "Antioxidant and other nutrient food supplements are safe and can help to enhance cancer patient care"** (Simone et al, 2007).

Others caution antioxidant use in cancer patients.

Such a recommendation merits close examination of the evidence because it is at odds with other authoritative reviews on this topic

(D'Andrea, 2005) (Ladas et al, 2004) (Block et al, 2007) (Dennert, Horneber, 2006) (Sagar, 2005).

Of the 52 clinical studies Simone et al. reviewed, **36 were observational**, a study design that is limited by selection bias and unknown confounders. Of the 16 randomized controlled trials they reviewed, **10 included fewer than 50 patients, a sample size too small to inspire confidence** in findings of equivalent survival. Indeed, if antioxidant supplements interfered completely with an agent associated with an absolute increase in survival of 5%, a suitably powered trial would require approximately 2000 patients. The six remaining reports reviewed by Simone et al were randomized trials with at least 50 patients, and, of these, **only one** (Cascinu et al, 1995) **tested an antioxidant**. In this trial (n = 50), **glutathione improved response rates and decreased neurotoxicity in advanced gastric cancer patients who received cisplatin**. This is an interesting result, but it must be confirmed in a larger study.

A challenge to these considerations is the absence of any consistent pattern of serum status of vitamins C and E, beta-carotene, or selenium in cancer patients receiving chemotherapy. (Ladas et al, 2004).

It is noteworthy that although the initiation of anticancer therapies may lower plasma antioxidant concentrations by altering dietary intakes, **an increase in plasma antioxidant levels has been associated with a reduction in the cancer burden.** (Jonas et al, 2000).

Block

Impact of antioxidant supplementation on chemotherapeutic efficacy: a systematic review of the evidence from randomized controlled trials

Much debate has arisen about whether antioxidant supplementation alters the efficacy of cancer chemotherapy. Some have argued that antioxidants scavenge the reactive oxygen species integral to the activity of certain chemotherapy drugs, thereby diminishing treatment efficacy. Others suggest antioxidants may mitigate toxicity and thus allow for uninterrupted treatment schedules and a reduced need for lowering chemotherapy doses. The objective of this study was to systematically review the literature in order to compile results from randomized trials that evaluate concurrent use of antioxidants with chemotherapy.

DESIGN: MEDLINE, Cochrane, CinAhl, AMED, AltHealthWatch and EMBASE databases were searched. Only **randomized, controlled clinical trials** that reported survival and/or tumor response were included in the final tally. The literature searches were performed in duplicate following a standardized protocol. No meta-analysis was performed due to heterogeneity of tumor types and treatment protocols used in trials that met the inclusion criteria.

RESULTS: Of 845 articles considered, 19 trials met the inclusion criteria. Antioxidants evaluated were: glutathione (7), melatonin (4), vitamin A (2), an antioxidant mixture (2), vitamin C (1), N-acetylcysteine (1), vitamin E (1) and ellagic acid (1). Subjects of most studies had advanced or relapsed disease.

CONCLUSION: None of the trials reported evidence of significant decreases in efficacy from antioxidant supplementation during chemotherapy. Many of the studies indicated that antioxidant supplementation resulted in either increased survival times, increased tumor responses, or both, as well as fewer toxicities than controls; however, **lack of adequate statistical power was a consistent limitation.** Large, well-designed studies of antioxidant supplementation concurrent with chemotherapy are warranted. (Block et al, 2007).

Low doses of individual antioxidants may stimulate cancer cell proliferation

On the other end of the spectrum, **low doses of individual antioxidants may stimulate cancer cell proliferation in certain instances.** (Pradad, 2004) (Lawenda et al, 2008).

Kedar N. Prasad, PhD, at the Center for Vitamin and Cancer Research at the University of Colorado Health Sciences Center stated that **"It is likely that recommendation of low doses of multiple vitamins containing low doses of micronutrients including antioxidants after therapy may increase the risk of recurrence of the primary tumor among those who are in remission.**

On the other hand, **more than 60% of cancer patients use vitamins, and the majority combines them with standard therapy, mostly without the knowledge of their oncologists.** This practice may also be harmful because **a multiple-vitamin preparation may contain antioxidants such as glutathione-elevating agents, including alpha-lipoic acid and N-acetylcysteine (NAC), and antioxidant enzyme-elevating agents such as excess of**

selenium, which is a cofactor for glutathione peroxidase, or dietary antioxidants such as vitamin E or vitamin C, which, at low doses, may protect cancer cells against free radical damage produced by chemotherapeutic agents or x-irradiation. Neither oncologists nor patients are aware
of these potential dangers of taking antioxidants without any scientific rationale."
(Pradad, 2004).

Moss says antioxidants do not interfere with radiation therapy

Ralph Moss says that until recently, research attention has focused primarily on the interaction of antioxidants with chemotherapy; relatively
little attention has been paid to the interaction of antioxidants with radiotherapy. He reviewed the clinical literature that has addressed whether antioxidants do in fact interfere with radiation therapy. Studies have
variously investigated the use of alpha-tocopherol for the amelioration
of radiation-induced mucositis; pentoxifylline and vitamin E to correct
the adverse effects of radiotherapy; melatonin alongside radiotherapy
in the treatment of brain cancer; retinol palmitate as a treatment for
radiation-induced proctopathy; a combination of antioxidants (and other
naturopathic treatments) and external beam radiation therapy as definitive treatment for prostate cancer; and the use of synthetic antioxidants,
amifostine, dexrazoxane, and mesna as radioprotectants.

With few exceptions, most of the studies draw positive conclusions
about the interaction of antioxidants and radiotherapy. Although further
studies are needed, the preponderance of evidence supports a provi-
sional conclusion that dietary antioxidants do not conflict with the use
of radiotherapy in the treatment of a wide variety of cancers and may
significantly mitigate the adverse effects of that treatment. (Moss, Sept
2007).

However, a 2010 study shows that significant reduction in plasma levels
of selenium is recorded in 209 breast cancer patients undergoing radiotherapy. Multivariate analysis showed statiscally significant difference
in the plasma selenium concentration before and after radiotherapy for
age, BMI, smoking, alcoholism, chemotherapy, and clincial stage. (Franka
et al, 2010).

I believe that this shows that selenium levels are affected by a wide
range of factors, especially the effect of radiation. It is not known if this
has a positive or a negative outcome for the patients.

Moss points out that oncologists have no objection to using **xenobiotic antioxidants** during chemotherapy. This includes **Amifostine** which decreases the toxicity of radiation but **is too toxic on its own and is not used**; **Mesna,** a drug used around the world to protect against the toxic side effects of ifosfamide which damages the urinary system; and **Cardiozane**, which counters Adriamycin's toxicity. There are over 500 papers showing the safety of the latter drug. In one clinical trial using a drug similar to Adriamycin, one-quarter of the patients suffered damage to their hearts. When given Cardiozane concurrently only 7% did. Thus, **it appears that only orthomolecular or natural antioxidants are potentially dangerous. Synthetic antioxidants protect against the toxic effect of drugs but do not increase their therapeutic value**.

Are vitamin supplements beneficial in patients with breast cancer?

One of the most controversial recommendations to support chemotherapy and radiation therapy is the recommendation to use antioxidant nutrients during the active phase of the treatment. I also have concern with using excessive antioxidant nutrients before and after the completion of a course of chemotherapy or radiation treatment, especially in patients with premalignant conditions or proven cancer.

The concern of many oncologists is that antioxidant nutrients will interfere with the effectiveness of conventional therapies. However, some do not believe that this concern is justified. (Prasad et al, 1999) (Lamson, Brignall, 1999).

Prasad feels that "based on results of our studies and others, we have proposed a hypothesis that **supplementation with high doses of multiple antioxidant vitamins, together with diet modification and lifestyle changes may improve the efficacy of standard and experimental cancer therapies by reducing their toxicity on normal cells and by enhancing their growth-inhibitory effects on cancer cells**."

The conclusion in a study in patients with small-cell lung cancer using combination chemotherapy of cyclophosphamide, Adriamycin (doxorubicin), and vincristine with radiation and a combination of antioxidants, vitamins, trace elements, and fatty acids was that the nutritional support significantly prolonged the survival time of patients. (Jaakkola et al, 1992).

A new cohort study by Nechuta et al is fresh off the press and it is likely to stimulate considerable discussion. Thus, I have included it, along with my analysis of it.

Prof Randolph M. Howes MD, PhD

Vitamin supplement use during breast cancer treatment and survival: a prospective cohort study.

Antioxidants may protect normal cells from the oxidative damage that occurs during radiotherapy and certain chemotherapy regimens, however, the same mechanism could protect tumor cells and potentially reduce effectiveness of cancer treatments. Investigators evaluated the association of vitamin supplement use in the first six-months after breast cancer diagnosis and during cancer treatment with total mortality and recurrence. **METHODS:** They conducted a population-based **prospective cohort study of 4,877 women** aged 20-75 years diagnosed with invasive breast cancer in Shanghai, China between March 2002 and April 2006. Women were interviewed approximately six-months after diagnosis and followed-up by in-person interviews and record linkage with the vital statistics registry. **RESULTS:** During a mean follow-up of 4.1 years, 444 deaths and 532 recurrences occurred. Vitamin use shortly after breast cancer diagnosis was associated with reduced mortality and recurrence risk, adjusted for multiple lifestyle factors, sociodemographics, and known clinical prognostic factors. **Women who used antioxidants (vitamin E, vitamin C, multivitamins) had 18% reduced mortality risk and 22% reduced recurrence risk. The inverse association was found regardless of whether vitamin use was concurrent or non-concurrent with chemotherapy**, but was only present among patients who did not receive radiotherapy. **CONCLUSIONS:** Vitamin supplement use in the first six months after breast cancer diagnosis may be associated with reduced risk of mortality and recurrence. Impact: Our results do not support the current recommendation that breast cancer patients should avoid use of vitamin supplements. (Nechuta et al, 2010).

My analysis of the Nechuta study:

- patients who used antioxidants (vitamin E, vitamin C, multivitamins) had an 18% reduction in their mortality risk
- the risk for recurrence was decreased by 22%. This association was observed whether vitamin use was concurrent or non-concurrent with chemotherapy
- this benefit was only seen in patients who did not receive radiotherapy
- complete information was not available for dosages taken. How can one evaluate the effects of the vitamins if one does not know "what kind and how much" they were taking?
- 2 studies that examined the use of multivitamins and breast cancer risk came to very different conclusions: One study found that their use de-

creased the risk for breast cancer, and the other study showed that vitamin supplementation actually increased the risk for breast cancer

- this study is not a randomized trial
- this study was conducted in a population of women in Shanghai, China, so there may be issues such as diet, culture, genetics, and so forth that could affect outcome
- the risks have always been theoretical
- this study does not settle the question of complete safety
- results from this single observational study are not adequate to change the guidelines of vitamin use during cancer treatment
-women who did undergo radiotherapy showed slightly worse outcomes, but the results were not statistically significant
- patients treated with radiotherapy and who used antioxidant vitamins also had non-significant increased risk for mortality and recurrence

CHAPTER TWENTY:

Additional points *for* the use of antioxidants with chemo or radiation therapy

1) **Critics tend to ignore the fact that the majority of these sorts of studies show predominantly beneficial effects.** (not supported by the literature)

Vitamin E at commonly used dosages does not interfere with radiation therapy or chemotherapy and actually appears to enhance the success of these treatment. (Kagreud, Peterson, 1981) (Perez Ripoll et al, 1986).

A higher usual dietary beta carotene intake can reduce the occurrence of severe adverse effects of radiation therapy and decrease local cancer recurrence." (Meyer et al, 2007).

2) **The selective omission of prominent studies that contradicted the author's conclusions.**

In September 2005, CA: A Cancer Journal for Clinicians published a warning by Gabriella D'Andrea, MD, against the concurrent use of antioxidants with radiotherapy and chemotherapy and critics resorted to the above criticism.

3) Authors sometimes **extrapolate from chemoprevention studies rather than those on the concurrent use of antioxidants per se.**

4) **If antioxidants were truly a threat to the efficacy of standard therapy, antioxidant-rich foods, especially fruits and vegetables, ought also be proscribed during treatment.** Yet, no such recommendation is made.

5) **The wide-scale use by both medical and radiation oncologists of synthetic antioxidants (e.g., amifostine) to control the adverse effects of cytotoxic treatments is similarly overlooked.** (not supported by the literature)

6) **A blanket rejection of the concurrent use of antioxidants with chemotherapy is not justified by the preponderance of evidence at this time and serves neither the scientific community nor cancer patients.** (Moss, 2006). (not supported by the literature)

7) **Hyperbolic warnings against antioxidant use for cancer patients.** (not supported by the literature)

8) **Over-hyped negative conclusions.** (not supported by the literature)

9) **Sensational-but-flawed nutrient studies.** (not supported by the literature)

10) **Most such warnings are overblown.** (not supported by the literature)

Additional points *against* the use of antioxidants with chemo or radiation therapy

1) **Vitamin E reduces effectiveness of radiation therapy**

When vitamin E is given to mice at dosages not likely to be achieved with normal supplementation in humans (e.g., dosage greater than 35,000 IU) it can **reduce the effectiveness of radiation therapy.** (Sakamoto, Sakka, 1973).

2) **NAC (N-acetylcysteine - a derivative of the naturally occurring amino acid cysteine) has not been shown to significantly effect treatment outcome and carries with it some risk of inhibiting chemotherapy agents** (e.g., cisplatin). (Olson et al, 1983) (Roller, Weller, 1998).

3) **Selenium supplements are frequently used by cancer patients. Selenium is an essential trace element and is involved in antioxidant protection and redox-regulation in humans.**

Several adverse effects of radiotherapy and chemotherapy in cancer patients as well as cellular processes that maintain chronic lymphoedema have been linked to oxidative cell damage in the human body. Selenium has recently been investigated as a remedy against chemotherapy and radiotherapy-associated side effects as well as its effects on lymphedema. SELECTION CRITERIA: **Randomized-controlled trials of selenium mono-supplements in cancer patients undergoing tumor specific therapy such as chemotherapy, radiotherapy or surgery.** MAIN RESULTS: Two trials have been included, a **randomized controlled trial** with **60 participants** at the beginning of the study investigating secondary lymphedema and an ongoing trial with preliminary results of **63 participants** investigating radiotherapy induced diarrhea as a secondary outcome. Both trials had drawbacks with regard to study quality and reporting. The trial on secondary lymphedema reported a decreased number of recurrent erysipela infections in the selenium supplementation group compared to placebo. However, results must be interpreted with caution and cannot be generalized to other populations. The ongoing trial on radiotherapy associated diarrhea preliminarily reported a lower incidence of diarrhea in patients receiving selenium supplementation concomitant to pelvic radiation, however, no data were presented. **No randomized controlled trials were found studying the effect of selenium supplementation on other therapy-associated toxicities or quality of life or performance status in cancer patients.** AUTHORS' CONCLUSIONS: **There is insufficient evidence at present that selenium supplementation alleviates the side effects of tumor specific chemotherapy or radiotherapy treatments. Or, that it improves the after effects of surgery, or improves quality of life in cancer patients or reduces secondary lymphedema.** To date research findings do not provide a basis for any recommendation in favor or against selenium supplementation in cancer patients. Potential hazards of supplementing a trace mineral should be kept in mind (Selenium for alleviating the side effects of chemotherapy, radiotherapy and surgery in cancer patients. (Dennert, Horneber, 2006).

4) A conclusion followed by a clarification:

A paper on the interaction of antioxidants and radiation therapy was published in the International Journal of Cancer. In April 2005, Isabelle Bairati, MD, PhD, and colleagues at the Hotel-Dieu de Quebec Research Centre and the Universite Laval completed a ten-year study on the interaction of dietary antioxidants and radiation therapy. This was hailed as the first placebo-controlled, double-blind, randomized trial assessing the effect of supplementation with antioxidant vitamins during radiation therapy. The study concluded that supplements of synthetic beta-carotene (30 mg per day) or alpha tocopherol (400 IU per day) had a harmful effect on cancer patients. The authors claimed that the cancer recurrence rate was 40% higher among patients who had been randomly assigned to the supplementation arm of the trial. **They therefore called on patients and physicians to exert caution in using antioxidants until new evidence could be provided by future trials.**

Next came the clarification.

In April 2008, Dr. Bairati published a modification of their previous conclusions. Further analysis revealed that the danger of synthetic antioxidants was limited to one particular sub-population: cigarette smokers--specifically, those who continued to smoke during radiation treatment. The authors analyzed the outcome in 540 patients who had been given radiation for head and neck cancers. During the follow-up period, 119 patients had a recurrence of their disease, and 179 died. Smokers were the group with the worst prognosis. However, smoking in the period leading up to or following radiation therapy did not modify the effects of the two supplements. It was only smoking during the course of radiation therapy that led to a statistically significant increase in the risk of a recurrence. It was a large enough increase to skew the statistics for the group as a whole, and Bairati and her colleagues now say, "Particular attention should be devoted to prevent patients from both smoking and taking antioxidant supplements during radiation therapy."

5) Investigators compared plasma levels of antioxidants and oxidative stress biomarkers in **head and neck squamous cell carcinoma (HNSCC)** patients with healthy controls. **Seventy-eight HNSCC patients and 100 healthy controls** were included in this study. **High relative increase in plasma levels of d-ROMs and high relative decrease in FRAP during radiotherapy are also positively associated with survival.** (Sakhi et al, 2009). **I believe that this important study shows that increased plasma EMODs and lowered plasma antioxidants are associated with increased survival in HNSCC.**

6) Antineoplastic agents are prime suspects for the toxic side-effects of acute or chronic chemotherapy. The present study was undertaken to test whether vitamins C and E (VCE) supplementation protect against some of the harmful effects of In a commonly used anticancer drugs in breast-cancer patients. **Conclusion:** the presence of breast-cancer and chemotherapy. **DNA damage was also reduced by VCE.** The results suggest that VCE should be useful in protecting against chemotherapy-related side-effects and a randomized control trial to evaluate the effectiveness of VCE in breast-cancer patients using clinical outcomes would be appropriate. (Suhail et al, 2011). **I believe that this shows that antioxidant supplementation restores harmful levels of antioxidants and this is verified by the reduced levels of DNA damage. In short, they are counteracting EMOD effects and apoptosis.**

7) **Vitamin K3 (VK3) is a well-known anticancer agent**, but its mechanism remains elusive. In the present study, VK3 was found to simultaneously induce cell death, reactive oxygen species (ROS) generation, including superoxide anion (O_2.-) and hydrogen peroxide (H_2O_2) generation, and histone hyperacetylation in human leukemia HL-60 cells in a concentration- and time-dependent manner. **Catalase (CAT), an antioxidant enzyme that specifically scavenges H_2O_2, could significantly diminish both histone acetylation increase and cell death caused by VK3,** whereas superoxide dismutase (SOD), an enzyme that specifically eliminates O_2.-, showed no effect on both of these, leading to the conclusion that H_2O_2 generation, but not O_2.- generation, contributes to VK3-induced histone hyperacetylation and cell death. This conclusion was confirmed by the finding that enhancement of VK3-induced H_2O_2 generation by vitamin C (VC) could significantly

promote both the histone hyperacetylation and cell death. Collectively, **these results demonstrate a novel mechanism for the anticancer activity of VK3, i.e., VK3 induced tumor cell death through H_2O_2 generation, which then further induced histone hyperacetylation**. (Lin et al, 2005).

8) Tumor-targeted induction of oxystress for cancer therapy

Reactive oxygen species (ROS), such as superoxide anion radicals ($O_2.-$) and hydrogen peroxide (H_2O_2) are potentially harmful by-products of normal cellular metabolism that directly affect cellular functions. ROS is generated by all aerobic organisms and it seems to be **indispensable for signal transduction pathways that regulate cell growth and reduction-oxidation (redox) status**. In fact, **many antitumor agents, such as vinblastine, cisplatin, mitomycin C, doxorubicin, camptothecin, inostamycin, neocarzinostatin and many others exhibit antitumor activity via ROS-dependent activation of apoptotic cell death, suggesting potential use of ROS as an antitumor principle. Thus, a unique anticancer strategy named "oxidation therapy" has been developed by inducing cytotoxic oxystress for cancer treatment. This goal could be achieved mainly by two methods, namely, (i) inducing the generation of ROS directly to solid tumors and (ii) inhibiting the antioxidative enzyme (defense) system of tumor cells.** Since 1950s, many strategies have been employed based on the first method, namely, administration of ROS per se (e.g. H_2O_2) or ROS generating enzyme to tumor bearing animals. However, no successful and practical results were obtained probably because of the lack of tumor selective ROS delivery and hence resulting in subsequent induction of severe side effects. To overcome these obstacles, we developed polyethylene glycol (PEG) conjugated $O_2.-$ or H_2O_2-generating enzymes, xanthine oxidase (XO) and D-amino acid oxidase (DAO) (PEG-DAO) respectively. More recently, a pegylated (PEG) zinc protoporphyrin (PEG-ZnPP) and a highly water soluble micellar formulation of ZnPP based on amphiphilic styrene maleic acid (SMA) copolymer, SMA-ZnPP, are prepared, which are potent inhibitors of heme oxygenase-1 (HO-1). **HO-1 is a major antioxidative enzyme of tumors, that is different in mechanism of catalase or superoxide dismutase (SOD).** Consequently, both PEG-enzymes and PEG-ZnPP exhibited superior in vivo pharmacokinetics than their parental molecules, particularly in tumor delivery by taking advantage of the EPR effect of macromolecular nature, and thus showed remarkable antitumor effects suggesting the potentials of this anticancer therapeutic for clinical application. Furthermore, **it has been well known that many antioxidative enzymes such as catalase, SOD are down-regulated in most solid tumors in vivo.** On the contrary, **HO-1 is highly upregulated and it plays a very important role of antioxidation, because HO-1 generates biliverdin, which being converted to**

bilirubin exhibits a very potent antioxidative effect, and hence antiapoptosis in tumors. Thus this oxidation therapy, by inhibiting this HO-1 dependent antioxidant (bilirubin) formation by ZnPP, and by enhancing ROS generation, is expected to offer a powerful therapeutic modality for future anticancer therapy. (Fang et al, 2007).

9) Oxystress inducing antitumor therapeutics via tumor-targeted delivery of PEG-conjugated D-amino acid oxidase

Investigators developed a H_2O_2 generating enzyme, polyethylene glycol conjugated D-amino acid oxidase (PEG-DAO), which exhibited potent antitumor activity by generating toxic reactive oxygen species, namely oxidation therapy, subsequently **showed remarkable antitumor effect on murine Sarcoma 180 solid tumor,** by taking advantage of the enhanced permeability and retention effect. Along this line, they reported the preparation of PEG-DAO by use of recombinant DAO and its antitumor activity by using various tumor cell lines and tumor models. Recombinant DAO (rDAO) was obtained from E. coli BL21 (DE3) carrying the porcine DAO expression vector with high yield (20 mg/l) and high enzyme activity (5.3 U/mg). Pegylated rDAO (PEG-rDAO) showed high stability against sonication, repeated freezing/thawing, lyophilization and exhibited superior in vivo pharmacokinetics. PEG-rDAO had a molecular size of 65 kDa and existed as nanoparticles in aqueous solution with mean particle diameter of 119 nm. In vitro experiments showed strong cytotoxicity of PEG-rDAO against various tumor cells, whereas less cytotoxicity was found against various normal cells. In vivo antitumor treatment was carried out **using 2 mice tumor models, namely colon 38 tumor and Meth A tumor model.** PEG-rDAO was administered i.v. and after an adequate lag time, D-proline (the substrate of DAO) was injected i.p. to the tumor-bearing mice. Consequently, preferential generation of H_2O_2 **in the tumor was successfully achieved,** which **resulted in remarkable suppression of tumor growth without any visible side effects.** These findings suggest a potential of PEG-rDAO as a novel anticancer strategy toward clinical development. (Fang et al, 2008).

SECTION SEVEN:

General discussion

CHAPTER TWENTY ONE:

Generalities

Physicians who wish to approach the issue with the most conservative viewpoint should caution patients about extreme antioxidant therapies, with multiple high dose supplemental or synthetic antioxidants. However, while it can be reasonable for physicians to offer cautions about use of herbs, vitamins, and antioxidants, they must also be careful not to warn people away from potentially usefully adjunct therapies, although I have yet to see clear verification of this.

At the earliest indication that a specific therapy may be harmful, the physician is obligated to assess the evidence about whether the putative benefit outweighs the potential harm. It is contrary to the principle of "primum non nocere (First, do no harm.) to advise patients to continue a potentially harmful intervention. Safety remains the top priority.

Lest we forget, oxygen and prooxidant EMODs play a central protective role against pathogens, as well as a crucial role in cancer therapy.

With radiation, **the primary damage to the tumor comes from generation of a huge number of free radicals that interact with cellular components and disrupt them, thereby killing the tumor.**

The very large amount of antioxidant research conducted over the past decade clearly shows that these substances have limited impact for several diseases and they harbor the potential to do harm. The potential to treat diseases have not been very successful and the prevention of diseases has had minimal or negligible effects.

Polymorphonuclear cells require oxygen to kill organisms by producing prooxidant superoxide, hydrogen peroxide, singlet oxygen and other products via the respiratory burst. (Barbior, 1974).

The PMN is protected by detoxifying free radicals with superoxide dismutase, catalase and glutathione. **It has been shown in numerous studies that the degree of polymorphonuclear cell function in killing of bacteria is directly dependent on oxygen tension.** (DeChatelet, 1975), (Hohn, 1997).

Oxygen enhanced environments have been shown to be bactericidal for most clostridia species and inhibit alpha toxin release. Hyperbaric oxygen has been shown to be a beneficial adjunct to therapy in Bacteroides fragilis, Fusobacterium infections and nonclostridial anaerobic infections. (Schreiner, 1974).

Measuring Cancer Therapy Success With Oxygen

In August of 2008, scientists at The Ohio State University (OSU) identified a way to predict very early in the treatment process the outcome of radiation and chemotherapy for cervical cancer patients -- based on oxygen levels within the tumor.

According to Jian Z. Wang, Assistant Professor at OSU and the Director of the Radiation Response Modeling Program at the OSU James Cancer Hospital and Solove Research Institute, the oxygenation of a tumor is critical for the success of cancer treatment because the amount of oxygen in a cell is directly correlated with the ability of that cell to repair radiation damage. Under hypoxic conditions, the lethal biological changes in tumor cells produced by radiation can be repaired and tumor recurrence is probable. However, adequate oxygen can react to produce EMODs, which causes that damage to be "permanent and irreparable." Wang stated that, "Inevitably, those well-oxygenated tumor cells die, tumors are less likely to return, and patient survival rates rise."

In their study of 88 women with cervical cancer, Dr. Wang and his colleagues measured the level of hemoglobin, and the blood supply to the tumor with MRI scans. Cancer recurrence rates were tracked for up to 9 years. Measurements of tumor oxygenation just 2 weeks into treatment provided the best predictor of tumor control and disease-free survival. The research was described in the talk, "When Does the Oxygen Level Matter Most During Radiation Therapy of Cervical Cancer?" presented July 31, 2008 at the 50th annual meeting of the American Association of Physicists in Medicine.

Why Some Prostate Cancer Returns

In May of 2009, men with a low oxygen supply to their tumor had a higher chance of the prostate cancer returning, as found by increasing prostate-specific antigen (PSA) levels following treatment, according to Benjamin Movsas, M.D., senior study author and chair of the Department of Radiation Oncology at Henry Ford Hospital. Moreover, recent studies suggested the same finding also appears to apply to patients treated with surgery. Their studies showed that oxygen levels to the tumor were significantly related to the patient's outcome. Movsas stated that "A tumor's oxygen supply can significantly predict outcome following treatment, independent of tumor stage or Gleason score (a classification of the grade of prostate cancer). (Movsas. 2009).

Solid Tumor Cells Not Killed By Radiation And Chemotherapy Become Stronger

In June of 2008,because of the way solid tumors adapt the body's machinery to bring themselves more oxygen, chemotherapy and radiation may actually make these tumors stronger. According to Mark W. Dewhirst, D.V.M., Ph.D., professor of radiation oncology at Duke University Medical Center. "Unless the treatment is very effective in killing many if not most tumor cells, you are shooting yourself in the foot."

Radiation and chemotherapy do kill most solid tumor cells, surviving cells have an increase in a regulatory factor called HIF1 (hypoxia-inducible factor 1), which cells use to get the oxygen they need by increasing blood vessel growth into the tumor. Solid tumors generally have low supplies of oxygen, Dewhirst explained and HIF1 helps them get the oxygen they need and that blocking HIF1 would provide a clear mechanism for killing solid-tumor cells, particularly cells that are proving resistant to radiation or chemotherapy treatments.

Oxygen levels naturally cycle up and down in individual blood vessels as well as large tumor regions and this instability in the tumor's oxygen levels can increase HIF-1 production and cause radiation therapy to fail, Dewhirst said.

"It is my opinion that the whole tumor grows more aggressively because of this pulsation of oxygen at low levels," Dewhirst said. The Duke team argues that blocking HIF1 is the consistent answer to tumor growth problems, which interferes with the tumor's ability to undergo glycolysis (energy production) in low-oxygen conditions, which blocks tumor growth.

Study Of Hypoxia And New Gene Reveals Early-stage Action Of P53 Tumor Suppressor Gene

In January of 2004, it was known that the p53 tumor suppressor gene was important for killing cells as they proliferate under low-oxygen conditions inside tumors. As tumors grow they outstrip their oxygen supply. If a cell has a normal p53 gene, the p53 protein will eliminate cancerous cells, keeping tumor growth at bay. Under conditions of stress to the cell, such as radiation or chemotherapy and hypoxia, p53 normally eliminates tumors.

Hypoxia induces p53 to mutate, such that the less oxygen, the more mutations in the p53 gene, so cancer cells are not killed and instead, they proliferate. A team led by Wafik El-Deiry, MD, PhD, Associate Professor, Departments of Medicine, Genetics, and Pharmacology with the Abramson Cancer Center of the University of Pennsylvania, discovered a gene related to p53 called Bnip3L that can also cause cell death and is turned on by p53 and a second transcription factor called hypoxia inducible factor (HIF). The team silenced Bnip3L in cells with normal p53 and exposed cells to low oxygen conditions and the tumors with silenced Bnip3L grew more aggressively in low oxygen conditions than cells and tumors with intact Bnip3L. El-Deiry and Peiwen Fei, MD, PhD report their findings in the December issue of Cancer Cell. They think one of the ways that p53 suppresses tumors at their earliest stages is by turning on Bnip3L, and that's new. Understanding how cells die after they are starved for oxygen is important for fighting cancer as well as other diseases.

In short, consideration of oxygen levels in cancer chemotherapy is crucial for successful eradication of neoplasia.

CHAPTER TWENTY TWO:

Ozone therapy

My coverage of ozone will be only marginal. There is significant data available to demonstrate the beneficial effect of ozone in treating many disease maladies.

http://en.wikipedia.org/wiki/Ozone_therapy#cite_note-77

Countries that allow ozone therapy

Ozone therapy is a well established alternative and complementary therapy in most mainland European countries where health authorities have tolerated its practice. The European Cooperation of Medical Ozone Societies, founded in 1972 publishes guidelines on medical indications and contraindications of ozone and hosts training seminars. In the early 1980's a German survey and investigation into ozone therapy by the University Klinikum in Giessen and the Institute for Medical Statistics, published in the Empirical Medical Acts revealed over 5 million ozone treatments had been delivered to some 350,000 patients, by more than 1000 therapists, of this number about half were medical doctors. Although ozone is used in a complementary capacity by a significant number of doctors in Italy, Switzerland, Austria and Germany it has still not gained popular support with main stream industry policy makers in those countries, it is not covered by health insurance, nor is it part of the curriculum at most esteemed medical schools. Proposals to include ozone therapy in German health insurance schemes invoked hostile objections from pharmaceutical researchers who question its evidence base. In general Countries with more socialist style health systems seem to have had less difficulty in accepted ozone as a medicine. No prohibition of ozone therapy is evident in Bulgaria, Cuba, Czech Republic, France, Germany, Greece, Israel, Italy, Japan, Malaysia, Mexico, Poland, Romania, Russia, Switzerland, Turkey, United Arab Emirates and Ukraine. In the USA, recently passed Alternative Therapy Legislation has made ozone therapy an option for patients in some states. In Alaska, Arizona, Colorado, Georgia, Minnesota, New York, New Jersey, North Carolina, Ohio, Oklahoma, Oregon, South Carolina, and Washington Physicians can legally use ozone treatments in their practice without fear of prosecution.

The American Cancer Foundation has always strongly advised cancer patients against resorting to ozone therapy. In its last reviews of Ozone therapy in 1993/94 it insisted although ozone has been subject to legitimate research there is no evidence that ozone is effective for the treatment of cancer in humans and could possibly have harmful effects. This remains the American Cancer Foundation's policy to date. (CA Cancer J Clin, 1993) (CA Cancer J Clin, 1994).

Other industry opinion leaders in the UK and Australia as recently as 2001 also suggest that knowledge regarding the potential benefit and harm of ozone in cancer patients is insufficient. Therefore such therapy can't be recommended as an alternative form of treatment for cancer patients. (Ernst, 2001).

With regards to the small amount of research of ozone in the treatment of cancer that has been done. In 1980 laboratory studies by main stream cancer researchers at Washington University discovered ozone inhibited growth of lung, breast and uterine cancer cells in a dose dependent manner while healthy tissues were not damaged by ozone. (Sweet et al, 1980).

Dr. Boguslaw Lipinski, Boston Cardiovascular Health Center and the Tufts University School of Medicine, offered support for the use of ozone in treating cancer in the following statement: "Preliminary clinical studies indicate that oxidative therapy might produce desirable results in cancer treatment....Exposure of patient's blood in vitro to ozone and subsequent injection is a medical procedure used for successful treatment of cancer in one Swiss clinic [Roka clinic] since 1960...Although these preliminary findings do not constitute proof in themselves, they may certainly encourage clinical researchers and practitioners to try this unorthodox but apparently promising modality."

Although these very encouraging preliminary findings have long been argued justified funding for further research it should not be assumed that ozone would be similarly effective in vivo and could cure cancer.

In 1990 pre-clinical French studies reported ozone enhanced the treatment of chemo resistant tumors and seemed to act adjunctively to chemotherapy in tumors derived from the colon and breast. (Zanker, Kroczek, 1990).

Although the Warburg hypothesis is not considered the cause of cancer, tumor hypoxia or oxygen deficiency is still implicated by modern cancer researchers in the growth of tumors and is a known adverse factor in the effectiveness of conventional radiation and chemotherapy. (Gray et al, 1953) (Dunn, 1997).

Recent research by radiation and oncology researchers has shown ozone therapy can improve oxygenation in hypoxic tumors. (Clavo et al, 2004) (Bocci et al, 2005).

In 2004 Oxford University reported of a Spanish cancer research institutes human trial of ozone therapy. Involving 19 patients with incurable head and neck tumors receiving radiotherapy and tegafur, plus either chemotherapy (12 patients) or ozone therapy (7 patients). Those receiving ozone intravenously during radiotherapy where on average 10 years older and their tumors significantly more abundant and progressed than the chemotherapy group. But on average the ozone group survived slightly longer than those receiving chemotherapy. They conclude these results warrant further researcher of ozone as a treatment for cancer. (Clavo, Ruiz et al, 2004).

There are reports that ozone maybe useful in treating the debilitating side effects of orthodox cancer treatment. Radiation-induced injuries has been successfully treated with ozone application. (Clavo et al, 2005).

Recent Cuban experiments on rats have shown that ozone treatment can alleviate the adverse effects of <u>Cisplatin</u> a popular modern anticancer drug, that has been well documented to induce extreme toxicity and acute damage in the kidneys of animals and humans. (Borrego et al, 2004) (Gonzalez et al, 2004) (Borrego et al, 2006).

Human trials at the Department of Oncology, Nizhni Novgorod State Medical in Russia also report benefits of complimentary ozone treatment and with regards to drug complications. (Potanin et al, 2000) (Grechkanev et al, 2002).

Female researchers at the same institute also report "We have followed up on 52 women with breast cancer, 32 patients along with cytostatic therapy have undergone a course of ozone therapy. 20 women were on only conventional polychemotherapy. The groups were compatible according to age, stage of the disease and accompanying pathology. Involvement of ozone therapy diminished the incidence and degree of cytostatics toxical side effects, improve their life quality and immunological parameters and significally increase the activity of antioxidant defence system". (Kontorschikova et al, 2001).

Also, please refer to the comprehensie book by Bocci: Oxygen-ozone therapy: a critical evaluation. Velio Bocci. Kluwer Academic Publishers. 2002. However, I do not know of any RCTs which utilize ozone cancer therapy. Thus, its use is still considered speculative and theoretical. Yet, it has received good clinical evaluations by physicians using it.

Exercise

I have shown where cancer cells like low levels of oxygen (hypoxia) and have shown the benefits of hyperbaric oxygen. **Even more impressive is the effect of excess oxygen consumption associated with exercise.** Exercise alone is one of the greatest deterrents of cancers of all types.

Exercise increases oxygen consumption by 10-15 fold, which results in marked increase in EMOD production. I believe that this is the mechanism whereby oxygen works it magic in association with exercise.

A March 1, 2011 report by the BBC Health News said, **"People who take regular exercise were 16% less likely to develop bowel polyps and 30% less likely to develop large or advanced polyps."**

Polyps - also known as adenomas - are growths in the bowel and while they are not cancerous in themselves they can develop into cancer over a long period of time. Cancer Research UK says most bowel cancers develop from a polyp and about 1 in 4 of us have one or more by the age of 50, while about half of us have them by the time we are 70. But only a small fraction of polyps develop into cancer and it takes years for that to happen.

Exercise link

Professor Kathleen Wolin, one of the lead authors of the research, says the evidence now shows a clear link between exercise and a reduced risk of bowel cancer but it is not yet clear exactly why that link exists. **I believe that link is a direct one with EMOD generation and EMOD induced apoptosis.** Still, most authors are unaware of the pivotal role of oxygen in controlling cancer prevention and cure.

"There are a number of likely pathways but we don't know exactly. So for example exercise reduces inflammation in the bowel, which has been linked to bowel cancer.

"But exercise also reduces insulin levels and improves the body's response to hyperinsulinaemia (excess levels of insulin circulating in the blood), which again increases polyp risk.

"It also enhances the immune system (which functions oxidatively) and because people who exercise often do so outside, they get vitamin D (a prooxidant), which is also important for bowel cancer.

"The reality is that exercise is acting through more than one mechanism. The upside is there are so many benefits all over the body, it is hard to pinpoint." **Such is the beauty of oxygen.**

Sara Hiom, director of health information at Cancer Research UK, says the evidence shows that keeping active could help prevent thousands of cases of cancer every year.

"We'd recommend doing at least half an hour's moderate exercise a day - such as brisk walking or anything that leaves you slightly out of breath. Getting enough physical activity will also help you keep a healthy weight, which is one of the most important ways of reducing the risk of cancer."

Mark Flannagan, Chief Executive of Beating Bowel Cancer, backed the study and said it was clear that lifestyle was an important factor in protecting yourself from cancer.

"Although the majority of polyps are not cancerous, it is thought that almost all bowel cancers develop from polyps. Therefore we recommend taking 30 minutes of physical activity each day, along with a healthy diet and lifestyle, to reduce your risk of developing bowel cancer."

Deborah Alsina, Chief Executive of Bowel Cancer UK, said the report was good news.

"Evidence also shows that the combination of taking more exercise and having a healthy diet may protect against bowel cancer, as well as weight gain and obesity, so we encourage people to do both.

(http://www.bbc.co.uk/news/health-12610236. Accessed 3-1-11)

Exercise, as tolerated, is always a good thing

If there is one thing that is consistently good for one's health, it is exercise. Of course, that does not mean participating in an Iron Man marathon or jogging across America. Common sense needs to be applied in most situations and extremes are to be avoided.

In my many years of medical research, exercise has been shown to decrease the risk of most major diseases, such as cancer, heart disease, strokes, obesity and diabetes.

Arguments continue over the mechanism by which exercise is helpful because, according to the teachings of the free radial theory, increased oxygen consumption during exercise should be uniformly harmful and even shorten one's life span. To the contrary, results of a study published in the Archives of Internal Medicine "clearly support the continued encouragement of physical activity, even among the oldest age groups. Indeed, it seems that it is never too late to start."

People even in their mid to late 80s can extend their life by a few years by getting four hours or more of exercise per week. Reportedly, "As little as four hours a week was as beneficial as more vigorous or prolonged activity." They also found that exercise had improvements even for previously sedentary 85-year-olds because their three-year survival rate was double that of inactive 85-year-old.

I believe that the most common denominators for the body's responses to exercise are the increases in oxygen consumption and oxygen utilization. Oxygen consumption increases up to 20 times during exercise, resulting in increased oxygen to most organs and tissues of the body. I believe that we should consider exercise to be a "medicine" and that each episode of exercise is equivalent to a substantial dose of oxygen and its subsequent metabolic products, which protect us from bacteria, fungi, viruses, protozoans and cancer.

Aerobic exercises are based on an oxygen boost to improve the immune system, improve overall health and aid in disease prevention. The importance of oxygen could not be more readily apparent. It is the essential sustaining and driving force for all aerobic cellular metabolism.

Routine exercise is widely recognized as one of the most important adjuncts for disease prevention and maintaining overall good health. Risk reduction for chronic degenerative diseases can even occur with low levels of exercise as was pointed out in consensus statements by the Centers for Disease Control and Prevention and the American College of Sports Medicine.

Combinations of a nutritious diet and regular exercise can be extremely important in maintaining health and in reducing overall risk of illness. So, take heart that at any age, even a little exercise can help maintain your health and extend your life. So, why is it so darned hard to do?

A 2011 study published in Proceedings of the National Academy of Sciences reports that, "Aerobic exercise seems to reduce brain atrophy in early-stage Alzheimer's patients, and that walking leads to slight improvement on mental tests among older people with memory problems."

Actually, a section of the brain involved in memory grew in size in older people who regularly took brisk walks for a year. One hundred twenty sedentary people, ages 55 to 80, were divided into two groups: Half began a program of walking for 40 minutes a day, three days a week to increase their heart rate. Among people who took part in the walking program, the hippocampus region of the brain grew in size by roughly 2 percent.

That is very impressive.

Exercise, with its associated increased oxygen consumption, is consistently seen as being good for overall health. Please remember that antioxidants have been shown to block some of the good effects of exercise. The importance of life-giving oxygen is readily apparent. It is drives all human aerobic cellular metabolism.

CHAPTER TWENTY THREE:

More current studies

Cancer cells know how to protect themselves

Lung cancer patients have higher GPx and lower SOD levels as determined by alterations of antioxidant activities in erythrocytes from patients with non-small cell lung carcinoma (NSCLC). In total, 189 cases of mostly advanced-stage IIIB or stage IV NSCLC and 202 healthy controls were studied. In subjects with lung cancer, there was similar catalase activity, **lower SOD activity** and **higher GPx** compared with controls. However, **more advanced disease (stage IV compared with stage IIIB) was associated with lower SOD activity.** Non-small cell lung carcinoma in Chinese subjects is associated with alterations in systemic antioxidant activities, which may play an important role in carcinogenesis and progression of cancer cell growth. (Ho et al, 2007).

I predicted that lung cancer patients would have higher GPx levels and lower SOD levels. The GPx would lead to an EMOD insufficiency and the low SOD would produce lowered amounts of tumoricidal peroxide. Both situations are conducive to allowing tumor growth. I feel that this goes hand in hand with the cancer cells to protect itself from EMOD induced apoptosis by having high levels of the antioxidants, vitamin C, lactate and glutathione.

Hypoxia (Oxygen) Threshold Levels

Hypoxia (defined as the fraction of measured O_2 partial pressures of <5 mmHg) is a statistically significant adverse prognostic factor of disease-free survival. Considerable data indicates that low O_2 in tumor cells is an adverse prognostic sign and this would be in direct contradiction to the free radical theory of aging and oxidative stress. In general, low tumor O_2 is associated with: increased aggressiveness of primary cancerous lesions, their ability to metastasize, and an increased resistance to treatments with irradiation, chemotherapeutics, and surgery.

Median O_2 partial pressures of less than 10 mmHg result in intracellular acidosis, ATP depletion, a drop in the energy supply and increasing levels of inorganic phosphate. Mitochondrial oxidative phosphorylation is limited at O_2 partial pressures of less than approximately 0.5 mmHg.

However, from this rather rudimentary summary of critical O_2 partial pressures for metabolic hypoxia, **there does not appear to be a single hypoxic threshold that is generally applicable**.

In general, a number of key findings have been described as follows: 1) **Most tumors have lower median O_2 partial pressures than their tissue of origin;** 2) many solid tumors contain areas of low O_2 partial pressure than cannot be predicted by clinical size, stage, grade, histology and site; 3) tumor-to-tumor variability in oxygenation is usually greater than intra-tumoral variability in oxygenation; and 4) **recurring tumors have a poorer oxygenation status than the corresponding primary tumors.**

Anoxia/hypoxia-induced proteome changes in neoplastic and stroma cells may lead to the arrest or impairment of neoplastic growth through molecular mechanisms, resulting in cellular quiescence, differentiation, apoptosis and necrosis. **Cells exposed to hypoxia are generally arrested at the G1/S-phase boundary.** (Giaccia, A.J. Hypoxic stress proteins: Survival of the fittest. Semin Radiat Oncol 1996; 6: 45-58). **Under anoxia, most cells are arrested immediately, regardless of their position in the cell cycle.**

Hypoxia can induce programmed (apoptotic) cell death in normal and neoplastic cells. The level of p53 in cells increases under hypoxic conditions, and **the increased level of p53 induces apoptosis by a pathway involving Apaf-1 and caspase-9 as downstream effectors.** (Soengas et al, 1999).

However, hypoxia also initiates p53-dependent apoptosis pathways involving hypoxia-inducible factor-1 (HIF-1), genes of the BCL-2 family, and other unidentified genes. (Shimizu et al, 1995). **Below a critical energy state, hypoxia/anoxia may result in necrotic cell death, a phenomenon seen in many human tumors** and experimental systems.

Hypoxia stimulates the transcription of glycolytic enzymes, glucose transporters (GLUT1 and GLUT3), angiogenic molecules, survival and growth factors (e.g. vascular endothelial growth factor [VEGF], angiogenin, platelet-derived growth factor-B, transforming growth factor-B, and insulin-like growth factor-II), enzymes, proteins involved in tumor invasiveness (e.g., urokinases-type plasminogen activator), chaperones, nuclear factor kB (NFkB) and other resistance-related proteins.

Hypoxia can drive progression of a malignant tumor which is a consequence of 1) an increasing neoplastic cell load, 2) microenvironment-induced (epigenetic) phenotypic changes in neoplastic and stroma cells and 3) genotypic changes and clonal selection of neoplastic cells. (Cheng et al, 1993).

It requires 3 times more radiation to kill cancer cells in the absence of O_2 than it does in the presence of normal levels of O_2. Hypoxia-associated resistance to photon radiotherapy is multifactorial. The presence of molecular oxygen increased DNA damage through the formation of oxygen free radicals, which occurs primarily after the interaction of radiation with intracellular water.

Tumor hypoxia

Adequate levels of oxygen are essential to effectively generate adequate tumoricidal EMOD levels and to kill a wide range of cancer cell types and tumor hypoxia can be a serious limiting factor in reducing the effectiveness of radiotherapy and some O_2-dependent cytotoxic agents, and photodynamic therapy. (Vaupel, Harrison, 2004).

Transient tumor hypoxia is associated with inadequate blood flow while chronic hypoxia is the consequence of the increased oxygen diffusion distance across an expanding tumor mass. However, many factors can result in tissue or cellular hypoxia such as anemia, poor oxygen absorption, decreased pulmonary function, etc. Both types of hypoxia are correlated with poor outcome for patients. Additionally, hypoxia also enhances chemoresistance of cancer cells. The delivery of chemotherapeutic drugs in hypoxic areas and their cellular uptake are affected by hypoxia and/or associated acidity. Many chemotherapeutic drugs require oxygen to generate EMODs that contribute to cytotoxicity. Hypoxia induces cellular adaptations that appears to compromise the efficacy of chemotherapy. In response to nutrient deprivation due to hypoxia, the rate of proliferation of cancer cells decreases but chemotherapeutic drugs are more effective against proliferating cells. In contrast, hypoxia induces adaptation by post-translational and transcriptional changes that promote cell survival and resistance to chemotherapy. Through these changes, hypoxia promotes angiogenesis, shift to glycolytic metabolism, expression of ABC transporters, cell survival by inducing the expression of genes encoding growth factors and the modulation of apoptotic process. (Cosse et al, 2008).

Mitochondria as targets for cancer chemotherapy

Heterogeneity of tumors dictates an individual approach to anticancer treatment. Despite their variability, **almost all cancer cells demonstrate enhanced uptake and utilization of glucose, a phenomenon known as the Warburg effect, whereas mitochondrial activity in tumor cells is suppressed.**

Considering the key role of mitochondria in cell death, **it appears that resistance of most tumors towards treatment can be, at least in part, explained by mitochondrial silencing in cancer cells.** This review is devoted to the role of mitochondria in cell death, and describes how targeting of mitochondria can make tumor cells more susceptible to anticancer treatment. (Gogvadze et al, 2009).

Ketones and lactate "fuel" tumor growth and metastasis: Evidence that epithelial cancer cells use oxidative mitochondrial metabolism

Previously, we proposed a new model for understanding the "Warburg effect" in tumor metabolism. In this scheme, cancer-associated fibroblasts undergo aerobic glycolysis and the resulting energy-rich metabolites are then transferred to epithelial cancer cells, where they enter the TCA cycle, resulting in high ATP production via oxidative phosphorylation. We have termed this new paradigm **"The Reverse Warburg Effect."** Here, we directly evaluate whether the end-products of aerobic glycolysis (3-hydroxy-butyrate and L-lactate) can stimulate tumor growth and metastasis, using MDA-MB-231 breast cancer xenografts as a model system. More specifically, we show that **administration of 3-hydroxy-butyrate (a ketone body) increases tumor growth by ~2.5-fold,** without any measurable increases in tumor vascularization/angiogenesis. **Both 3-hydroxy-butyrate and L-lactate functioned as chemo-attractants, stimulating the migration of epithelial cancer cells.** Although L-lactate did not increase primary tumor growth, it stimulated the formation of lung metastases by ~10-fold. Thus, we conclude that **ketones and lactate fuel tumor growth and metastasis, providing functional evidence to support the "Reverse Warburg Effect".** Moreover, we discuss the possibility that **it may be unwise to use lactate-containing i.v. solutions (such as Lactated Ringer's or Hartmann's solution) in cancer patients, given the dramatic metastasis-promoting properties of L-lactate.** Also, we provide evidence for the up-regulation of oxidative mitochondrial metabolism and the TCA cycle in human breast cancer cells in vivo, via an informatics analysis of the existing raw transcriptional profiles of epithelial breast cancer cells and adjacent stromal cells. Lastly, our findings may explain why diabetic patients have an increased incidence of cancer, due to increased ketone production, and a tendency towards autophagy/mitophagy in their adipose tissue. (Bonuccelli et al, 2010).

As was said by another researcher, "The so-called "Reverse Warburg Effect" doesn't disprove Warburg. In fact, no scientist or researcher has ever disproved the validity, correctness or applicability of Warburg's discoveries. At least three other Nobel Prizes came out of work based off of his own. These were men who worked with him and learned how to thoroughly research something. He never ever used the words "associated with" "seems to" "possibly" "could" and "more research is needed". His methods were so precise, rigorous and demanding that he could and did conclude saying "proved unquestionably". Since then he has been attacked and his work shelved. His work and conclusions have been looked down on as naive and simplistic. However, this came out of disagreements with him and not his work or conclusions. Instead of doing there own work to disprove him, his opponents relied on data from the 1920's-1950's using tissue glycolysis results from COMBINATIONS of mixed cancer and non-cancerous cells instead of 100% cancer cells. It wasn't until 1950 that 100% cancer cells could be grown and transplanted."

Arguments against the hypoxia/cancer theory

Although cancer is considered to be a disease caused by DNA alterations, the high genetic variability of tumor cells makes it difficult to exploit these alterations for the treatment of cancer. The influence of non-genetic factors on cancer is increasingly being acknowledged and a growing line of research suggests that hypoxia (a decrease in normal oxygen levels) may play a fundamental role in the development of this disease. This line of research is supported by the fact that **tumors often have hypoxic areas, that hypoxia activates the hypoxia-inducible factor 1 (HIF-1) and that HIF-1 activation plays a key role in cancer development.**

Evidence suggests, however, that **the idea of hypoxia playing a central role in cancer development has some drawbacks.** For instance, hypoxia has not been found in many tumors, HIF-1 activation has been observed in non-hypoxic tumor areas, and hypoxic tumor cells commonly have a reduced nutrient supply that restricts cell proliferation and tumor growth. **This article reviews the literature that does not support the idea of hypoxia playing a central role in cancer development and discusses a broader view in which the role of oxygen in cancer is not limited to a reduction in its normal levels.** According to this novel view, a deviation of the oxygen metabolism from the pathway that generates energy to the pathway that produces reactive oxygen species is crucial for cancer development. Interestingly, this switch in oxygen metabolism occurs under both hypoxic and normoxic conditions and may be exploited therapeutically. (Bonuccelli et al, 2010).

CHAPTER TWENTY FOUR:

Other EMOD prooxidant functions

Ischemic preconditioning blocked by antioxidants

Despite the very sensible notion that ROS are produced primarily with the reintro-duction of oxygen following ischemia, several investigators began to also observe ROS generation during ischemia. While seeming **paradoxical** at first, there is much literature to support this observation.

With ischemia the respiratory cytochromes become redox-reduced allowing them to directly transfer (i.e. "leak") electrons to oxygen. **Oxidants can also be protective**—not simply injurious. Much insight into this came out of work in preconditioning. In the late 1980s Murry et al. described ischemic preconditioning wherein **a brief non-lethal episode of ischemia conferred both short and longer-term protection to tissues against an ensuing lethal ischemic in-sult.** (Murry et al, 1998).

Another important lesson is contained (and was almost overlooked) within this seminal description of preconditioning, that antioxidants abolished the precondi-tioning protection. In other words, **treatment with antioxidants interfered with preconditioning protection and made the injury worse.**

Vanden **Hoek et al. demonstrated the loss of preconditioning protection with antioxidants clearly in cardiomyocytes.** (Vanden Hoek et al, 2000). Thus, antioxidants can also block other important functions of EMODs.

ACE Inhibitors have Antioxidant Effect

Teramoto examined the effects of angiotensin-converting enzyme (ACE) inhibi-tors on spontaneous or stimulated generation of reactive oxygen species (ROS) by bronchoalveolar lavage (BAL) cells prepared from 6 patients with chronic obstruc-tive pulmonary disease (COPD) and from age-matched control subjects without COPD. The application of **ACE inhibitors into culture media containing BAL cells inhibited spontaneous and stimulated generation of ROS** by BAL cells from COPD patients and control subjects in an ambroxol-concentration-dependent manner. Alacepril, an ACE inhibitor bearing SH-group, inhibited the oxy-gen radical production and generation by BAL cells from COPD patients in a dose-dependent fashion. Approximately 0.6-0.7 mM of alacepril inhibited 50% of the ROS production by BAL cells from COPD patients, whereas a slightly higher concentration (3 mM) of lisinopril, an ACE inhibitor not bearing an SH-group, was necessary to inhibit the production of ROS. These results suggest that **an ACE inhibitor may act as an pulmonary antioxidant in patients with COPD.** (Teramoto et al, 2000).

I believe that the antioxidant aspect of ACE inhibitors contribute to their dangerous properties. The same thing happened with cyclooxygenase inhibitors and with antioxidant vitamins, i.e., inhibition of EMOD production repeatedly leads to adverse effects in man.

Reactive oxygen species (ROS) play important roles in the pathogenesis of cardiovascular disease. **Surprisingly, large clinical trials have shown that ROS scavenging by antioxidant vitamins is ineffective or harmful.** Therefore, prevention of ROS formation, by targeting specific sources of superoxide anion and other ROS, might prove beneficial. Potential targets include the NADPH oxidases (Nox enzymes), xanthine oxidase, endothelial nitric oxide synthase and mitochondrial oxidases. Nox enzymes play a central role because they can regulate other enzymatic sources of ROS. Statins, angiotensin-converting enzyme inhibitors and angiotensin receptor antagonists block upstream signaling of Nox activation, which contributes to their clinical effectiveness. Here, we discuss novel possibilities where drugs that directly inhibit Nox activation could successfully inhibit oxidative stress (Guzik, Harrison, 2006)

I am astounded with disbelief-responses of some authors concerning the studies which show that antioxidants are ineffective and/or harmful. Today's scientists have been so indoctrinated into believing in the validity of the Free Radi-Crap theory, that they can not see the truth. EMODs are of low toxicity and are crucial for normal cellular functioning to occur. Carelessly blocking EMODs is obviously going to have harmful consequences. The antioxidants are ineffective because EMODs are not causing the many pathophysiologies that have been attributed to them in the past.

ACE inhibitor drugs, which block EMODs, linked to birth defects

Some blood pressure drugs previously thought to be safe when taken early in pregnancy now appear to substantially raise the risk of major birth defects. Babies whose **mothers took ACE inhibitors in their first trimester were more than twice as likely to be born with serious heart and brain problems** than those not exposed to any pressure-lowering medicines, a large study in

Tennessee found. Other types of blood pressure drugs did not raise the risk to babies.

The research raises troubling questions about the lack of safety data for many drugs prescribed to pregnant women. About 8% of pregnant women develop high blood pressure, which can lead to a heart attack or stroke.

A national survey found the number of ACE inhibitor prescriptions given to women of childbearing age increased from 1.4 million in 1995 to 2.7 million in 2002, the latest data available. ACE inhibitors already carry a strong Food and Drug Administration "black box" warning about their dangers in the later stages of pregnancy, and the label says the drugs should be discontinued when pregnancy is detected. But little has been known about their early effects.

Based on the new findings, taking these drugs during early pregnancy "cannot be considered safe and should be avoided," lead researcher Dr. William Cooper, a Vanderbilt University pediatrician, said in 6/7/06 New England Journal of Medicine.

Doctors said expectant mothers should not stop treatment, **because uncontrolled high blood pressure can harm them and the fetus, but should immediately switch to other** drugs. ACE inhibitors have been on the market for 25 years, but little research has been done on their effects during early pregnancy with the exception of animal experiments and small human studies. The drugs work by relaxing blood vessels and increasing blood flow to the heart. Last year, U.S. sales of ACE inhibitors topped $3.8 billion, with about 150 million prescriptions filled, according to IMS Health, a pharmaceutical information company. The top-sellers include Lotrel, Altace and Lisinopril.

In the study, researchers studied Medicaid records on 29,507 Tennessee infants born between 1985 and 2000. Of those, 411 had mothers who took a blood pressure drug at least once during their first trimester, including 209 who took ACE inhibitors.

About 7% of babies exposed to ACE inhibitors developed major birth defects compared with about 2% whose mothers took no drugs or other blood pressure medication, such as water pills, calcium channel blockers or beta blockers. The most common defects included holes in the heart and neurological and kidney problems.

"It's a sobering finding," said Dr. Robyn Barst, a pediatric cardiologist at Columbia University and spokeswoman for the American Heart Association. "It highlights our lack of data on many drugs that we think are perfectly safe." The study was partly funded by the FDA. Three co-authors reported receiving support or fees from Novartis AG or Pfizer Inc. Novartis makes Lotrel. Pfizer makes the calcium blocker Norvasc.

In an accompanying editorial, Friedman of the University of British Columbia said the ACE inhibitor study points to a larger problem about the lack of safety data available on most new drugs when they receive government approval. "The only way to discover (risks) is through long-term use. That's a little uncomfortable. It means you only learn about what drugs do to pregnancies after the drug's been used for a long time," Temple said.

In the early 1990s, the FDA required pharmaceutical companies to put warning stickers on ACE inhibitors after the agency received a few reports from women whose babies were harmed. **The label warned that ACE inhibitors can cause skull deformities, kidney failure, lung problems and even fetal death when taken in the last two-thirds of pregnancy.**

I believe that this demonstrates the danger of altering redox balance or status of the cell and the dangers of inhibiting prooxidant protective EMODs.

Antioxidant peroxiredoxin prevents programmed cell death in L. donovani

Leishmania promastigote cells transmitted by the insect vector get phagocytosed by macrophages and convert into the amastigote form. During development and transformation, the parasites are exposed to various concentrations of reactive oxygen species, which can induce **programmed cell death (PCD).** They show that **a mitochondrial peroxiredoxin (LdmPrx) protects Leishmania donovani from PCD.** Whereas this peroxiredoxin is restricted to the kinetoplast area in promastigotes, it covers the entire mitochondrion in amastigotes, accompanied by dramatically increased expression. A similar change in the expression pattern was observed during the growth of Leishmania from the early to the late logarithmic phase. Recombinant LdmPrx shows typical **peroxiredoxin-like enzyme activity. It is able to detoxify organic and inorganic peroxides** and prevents DNA from hydroxyl radical-induced damage. Most notably, **Leishmania parasites over-expressing this peroxiredoxin are protected from hydrogen peroxide-induced PCD.** This protection is also seen in promastigotes grown to the late logarithmic phase, also characterized by high expression of this peroxiredoxin. Apparently, the physiological role of this **peroxiredoxin is stabilization of the** mitochondrial membrane potential and, as a consequence, inhibition of PCD through removal of peroxides. (Harder et al, 2006).

I believe that this illustrates the dangers of antioxidants being used or given to patients with protozoan diseases or cancer.

Parasite develops antioxidant enzyme defense against EMOD kill

To defend themselves against oxygen-mediated killing mechanisms of host, parasites have developed antioxidant enzyme systems. S. mansoni superoxide dismutase, SOD, glutathione peroxidase, GPX, glutathione reductase, GR, and glutathione-s-transferase, GST, are major antioxidant enzymes that are involved in detoxification processes. (Callahan et al, 1988) (Mkoji et al, 1988a) (Mkoji et al, 1988b) (Nare et al, 1990) (O'Leary et al, 1991) (O'Leary et al, 1992) (James, 1994).

These schistosome oxidant-detoxicating systems play a role in protecting the parasite from damage as a result of ROS (EMODs). (Callahan et al, 1988) (Brody et al, 1992) (Mei et al, 1995) (James, 1994). I believe that this is an incredible example of nature assisting the survival of a parasite by the development of an antioxidant system to perpetuate its survival and help protect it against an EMOD-induced death.

It appears to me that cancer cells tend to do the same thing by having high levels of antioxidants, such as glutathione, vitamin C and lactic acid.

Microfilariae killed by H2O2 and singlet oxygen

The toxicity of the active oxygen species hydrogen peroxide, superoxide radical, hydroxyl radical and singlet oxygen to microfilariae (mf) has been studied in vitro, using active oxygen-generating systems and scavengers/inhibitors. Mf viability was monitored by uptake of the radiolabel, [3H]2-deoxy-D-glucose. **Hydrogen peroxide and singlet oxygen, but not superoxide radical or hydroxyl radical, are toxic for mf.** Hydrogen peroxide was toxic for mf within 2 h at concentrations as low as **5 microM, an amount eosinophils have been shown to release in vitro (Weiss et al. 1986). Catalase and thiourea, but not inactivated catalase, superoxide dismutase (SOD), singlet oxygen scavengers, or hydroxyl radical scavengers, protected mf.** Mf have relatively high levels of endogenous SOD but no measurable glutathione peroxidase and low levels of catalase when compared with other parasites. The low levels of hydrogen peroxide-scavenging enzymes correlate well with mf sensitivity to hydrogen peroxide and the protective effect of exogenous catalase. (Callahan et al, 1990). Again, **these data indicate potential harm caused by antioxidants which would block the ability of EMODs to kill pathogens.**

Malaria killed by H2O2

The murine malaria parasite Plasmodium yoelii was killed in vitro when incubated with glucose and glucose oxidase, a system generating hydrogen peroxide, or with xanthine and xanthine oxidase, a system which produces the superoxide anion and subsequently other products of the oxidative burst. **Catalase blocked the killing in both cases**; superoxide dismutase and scavengers of hydroxyl radicals or singlet oxygen were ineffective in the xanthine oxidase system. Thus, **hydrogen peroxide appears to be the main reactive oxygen species killing P. yoelii.** (Dockrek, Playfair, 1984).

Regular intake of supplements containing beta-carotene may increase cancer incidence and cancer deaths among smokers, according to a systematic review and meta-analysis published in 2008. The same report also showed that selenium supplementation may have cancer-fighting effects in men, while vitamin E supplementation had no effect on cancer incidence and mortality. (Bardia et al, 2008).

CHAPTER TWENTY FIVE:

Can Other Dietary Supplements Interfere with Cancer Treatment

Can Other Dietary Supplements Interfere with Cancer Treatment

Note: Review of *J Clin Oncol.* 2004;22(12):2489-503.

http://www.caring4cancer.com/go/cancer/nutrition/questions/can-dietary-supplements-interfere-with-cancer-treatment.htm

A study in the *Journal of Clinical Oncology* looked at the 15 best-selling herbal remedies that are used in the United States today. The researchers studied whether or not these remedies are likely to interact with medications that are used to treat cancer. This study suggests that **of the 15 most popular herbal remedies in the United States, nine may pose a risk of negative interactions with specific anti-cancer medications, including the popular remedies echinacea, ginseng and St John's wort.** Along with talking to the medical care team about dietary supplement use, taking time to learn more about which common herbs can interact with cancer treatments will help people who are diagnosed with cancer to make more informed choices about their own health care.

It is hoped that this type of research will help us understand which dietary supplements and herbs may interact with different types of medications, so that these products can be used more safely in the future.

Background

Surveys tell us that one-third of adults in the United States use complementary and alternative medicine (CAM), including herbs, on a regular basis. Using CAM is even more common among people who are being treated for cancer. **Studies tell us that up to 80% of people with cancer use CAM** and up to 63% take herbal remedies. Many health experts worry that some of these herbs may interact with other medications. This is a particular concern for people who are being treated for cancer because **many cancer medications have a very small 'window' in which they work. In other words, you have to have just the right amount of these medications in your body in order for them to fight the cancer most effectively. Having too much can cause toxic reactions. Having not enough means that the cancer is not being treated effectively.**

A 2004 study in the *Journal of Clinical Oncology* looked at the 15 best-selling herbs that are used in the United States today to try to determine whether or not these remedies are likely to interact with cancer medications.

What The Researchers Studied

For this study, the researchers looked at 15 top-selling herbs in the United States for the year 2002. These top selling herbs are:

Herbal Remedy	Rank Based on Sales	Typically Used To Treat
Garlic	1	High Cholesterol
Ginkgo	2	Memory Loss/Dementia
Echinacea	3	Infection Prevention (e.g. common cold)
Soy Supplements*	4	Menopause Symptoms
Saw Palmetto	5	Enlarged Prostate
Ginseng	6	Physical & Mental Fatigue
St. John's Wort	7	Mild Depression
Black Cohosh	8	Menopause Symptoms
Cranberry	9	Bladder Infections
Valerian	10	Insomnia & Stress
Milk Thistle	11	Liver problems due to hepatitis & alcohol use
Evening primrose	12	Premenstrual Syndrome (PMS)
Kava	13	Anxiety
Bilberry	14	Loss of Eyesight Due to Diabetes
Grape Seed	15	Allergies (e.g. hay fever)

*This refers to soy supplements, not whole soy foods.

Researchers used all of the detailed information that has been published on how these products work in our bodies to study whether or not they are likely to interact with different cancer medications. One way to understand how this works is to think about how the body actually uses and then excretes or 'gets rid of' different medications.

Sometimes, the medications that you take AND herbs that you take are processed by the same factory. If this is true, this can affect how both the medication and the herb work.

What The Study Found

After reviewing all of the information that is available on how the different cancer medications and the different herbs work in the body, the researchers reached some conclusions.

Of the 15 top selling herbs in the United States, 9 of them may have problems by interacting negatively with certain cancer medications. The following table summarizes the information on which herbs may interact with different types of cancer medications. Often, one drug will be called several different names.

Herb	AVOID Taking With The Following Cancer Medications*	May Interact Negatively With The Following Cancer Medications
Garlic	Decarbazine	Use with caution with other types of chemotherapy; research is inconclusive
Gingko	Alkylating Agents; Antitumor Antibiotics; Platinum Analogues	Use caution with Camptothecins, Cyclophosphamide, EGFR-TK inhibitors, Epipodophyllotoxins, Taxanes, and Vinca Alkaloids; research is inconclusive
Echinacea	Campothecins; Cyclophosphamide; EGFR-TK inhibitors; Epipodophyllotoxins; Taxanes; Vinca Alkaloids	None listed
Soy Supplements**	Tamoxifen; Avoid in women with estrogen positive breast cancer or endometrial cancer	None listed
Ginseng	Avoid in women with estrogen positive breast cancer or endometrial cancer	Use caution with Camptothecins, Cyclophosphamide, EGFR-TK inhibitors, Epipodophyllotoxins, Taxanes, and Vinca Alkaloids; research is inconclusive

St. John's Wort	Avoid with ALL types of chemotherapy; St John's Wort interacts with multiple medications through many different pathways	Avoid with ALL types of chemotherapy
Valerian	None listed	Use caution with Tamoxifen, Cyclophosphamide and Teniposide; research is inconclusive
Kava	Avoid if you have liver disease; do not take with cancer drugs that are toxic to the liver	Use caution with Camptothecins, Cyclophosphamide, EGFR-TK inhibitors, Epipodophyllotoxins, Taxanes, and Vinca Alkaloids; research is inconclusive
Grape Seed	None listed	Use caution with Camptothecins, Cyclophosphamide, EGFR-TK inhibitors, Epipodophyllotoxins, Taxanes, Vinca Alkaloids, Alkylating Agents, Antitumor Antibiotics and Platinum Analogues; research is inconclusive

Based on the research that is available today, **this study tells us that some popular herbs may interact negatively if taken with medications that are used to treat cancer.** This is important to keep in mind if you are currently undergoing treatment for cancer.

This research review does have some weaknesses. Some of the interactions are not proven, they are just suspected to be problems. Researchers may have incomplete information on how a particular herb works in the body. They may come up with a 'best guess' as to whether or not a certain herb will interact negatively with a particular medication. Sometimes, further studies will prove that a particular herb and drug do not interact negatively, even though early research suggested they could.

Subhuti Dharmananda, Ph.D., Director, Institute for Traditional Medicine, Portland, Oregon, states that, "The utilization of Chinese roots, leaves, and fruits (e.g., astragalus, gynostemma, ligustrum, and lycium), and several mushrooms (e.g., coriolus, ganoderma, cordyceps, and lentinus) for cancer patients is now a routine procedure when these patients visit acupuncturists, naturopathic physicians, and others offering adjunctive cancer health care."

He said, "Within the past couple of years, however, an increasing number of patients have been told by their oncologists to avoid herbs, and to more generally avoid supplements (such as vitamins), or, even more broadly, simply avoid *anything* with antioxidant potential while they are undergoing cancer therapies. The admonition itself is difficult to interpret, since all foods contain antioxidants and vitamins, and they also contain most of the other substances offered in dietary supplements. Most fruits, vegetables, beans, and nuts differ only slightly from herbs. A more specific recommendation is needed."

Dharmananda then discusses the work of Dr. David Golde, Physician-in-Chief at Memorial Sloan-Kettering Cancer Center, who said, "that taking large amounts of vitamin C could interfere with the effects of chemotherapy or even radiation therapy. These therapies often kill cells, in part, by using oxidative mechanisms. it's conceivable then, that vitamin C might make cancer treatment less effective, and it is reasonable that cancer patients undergoing chemotherapy avoid taking large amounts of this vitamin."

However, research from University of Tubingen, School of Medicine in Germany suggests caution in applying this knowledge to all antioxidants in all types of malignancies. Examination of the modulation of drug-induced cytotoxicity and clonogenic cell death of glioma cells by three structurally unrelated antioxidants revealed that these antioxidants inhibit acute cytotoxicity and clonogenic cell death induced by cisplatin. However, they had little effect on the toxicity of other cancer drugs including BCNU, doxorubicin, vincristine, cytarabine, or camptothecin.

Please remember the adomonitions of Dr. Blazek, "**Any drug that is taken during cancer radiotherapy or chemotherapy should be tested to prove that it does not protect the tumor cells, defeating the intended effect of the treatment.**"

Dr. Keith Bruninga, gastroenterologist at Rush-Presbyterian-St. Luke's has now looked to see how much protection vitamins E and C actually offer patients irradiated for prostate, cervical or endometrial cancer. Bruninga concluded, "**Our study showed that we can harness the potent antioxidant properties of the vitamins to repair cell damage and bring relief to many people who suffer from the persistent, lifestyle-altering symptoms of chronic** radiation proctitis," from a paper published in the April 2002 issue of The American Journal of Gastroenterology.

Blacks may need special considerations

Even **as overall cancer death rates continue a downward trend among black Americans, the community still bears the biggest brunt of cancer-related deaths in the United States**, a new report shows.

The **American Cancer Society** report released on **2-1-11** noted that as recently **as 2007, cancer fatalities among black men remained 32 percent higher than that of white men, while the cancer death rate among black women hovered at 16 percent above that of white women.**

The findings also showed that, **for most cancers, blacks face the shortest cancer survival prognosis compared with all other races and ethnicities.**

Breast and colorectal cancer deaths make up the bulk of excess deaths for black women, while higher fatalities among black men were due to prostate, lung and colorectal cancers.

However, the report does feature some bright spots: **the overall gap between black and whites in terms of cancer deaths has narrowed in recent years due to the faster decline in the rate of death among blacks (relative to whites) for both lung cancer (and other smoking-related cancers) and prostate cancer.**

In fact, **lung cancer fatality rates have actually evened out among younger blacks and whites**, the report noted.

Yet, the news is not equally good for all cancers, the cancer society cautioned. For example, **the race gap appears to have widened for deaths among women with breast cancer and for both men and women with colorectal cancer.**

"While the factors behind these racial disparities are multifaceted, **there is little doubt socioeconomic status plays a critical role**," Dr. Otis W. Brawley, chief medical officer for the cancer society, said in a news release. "Black Americans are disproportionately represented in lower socioeconomic groups. **For most cancers, the lower the socioeconomic status, the higher the risk.**"

Among the report's other findings:

- **Nearly 169,000 black Americans will be diagnosed with cancer each year, and more than 65,000 will succumb to their disease**.

- **Black men are most likely to face a prostate cancer diagnosis, with this cancer accounting for 40 percent of all cases among black American men.** Lung cancer is the second most prevalent, affecting 15 percent of all cancer cases, followed by colon and rectum cancer (9 percent).

- **Among black American women, breast cancer is the biggest concern, accounting for 34 percent of all cancer cases among black women.** As with black men, lung cancer is the second-most common diagnosis among black women (13 percent), followed by colon and rectum cancer (11 percent).

Dr. Alfred I. Neugut, co-director of cancer prevention at New York Presbyterian Hospital in New York City, stressed that **"there's no easy answer" to explain the race-based fatality gap. I believe that it is due to antioxidant stacking. The ingest more antioxidant-rich fried foods.**

"Everything plays a role," he noted. "To me, the term 'disparity' implies something pejorative, or an injustice of society, and some of this is about that. **But also some of it is biological, as with prostate cancer, which is not about disparity. It's simply a difference**."

"So, I would say delays in getting a diagnosis is a factor, but also much of it is treatment-related and some is differences in lifestyle," Neugut suggested. "But **what's most important is the access to care part,** because that's the part that should be the most easily remediable, and that's the part that's the most disturbing and constitutes a real disparity. And that's where I think we should focus our energies."

Dr. Basir U. Tareen, the physician-in-charge of urologic oncology at Beth Israel Medical Center in New York City, agreed **that prevention is key**.

"From my perspective, I would have said **that in terms of prostate cancer, for example, one of the things that we know is that it occurs at a much higher incidence among African-American men, and they also tend to have a more aggressive form of the cancer**," Tareen said. "So with this cancer, actually being black is one of the risk factors for the disease, and as a result **we**

actually start screening African-American men five years earlier than white men, just for that reason."

"But clearly, **people have various theories as to what is actually behind this,** depending on the particular cancer," Tareen added. "Whether there are socio-economic factors at play or genetic factors, or both. And so these numbers clearly show that we need to explore this further, in order to see whether there are pre-ventable factors here that we can do something about."

Most men die with prostate cancer, not from prostate cancer. The cost of the unnecessary treatment is measured in billions of dollars and in millions of men who have lost their virility/manhood unnecessarily.

Reportedly, **blacks produce more testosterone** and use/process it in the body differently than whites. They may also eat more greasy meats and meals which lead to more testosterone production. **I believe that the testosterone is adding to their antioxidant stacking.**

There are several clinical trials underway investigating Vitamin D3 supplementation for the prevention and treatment of Prostate Cancer. Reportedly, Black people require more sun exposure than do White people to get an adequate amount of natural Vitamin D3 absorption. This is most true for those living in the northern half of the country with longer winters and less sun exposure.

Vitamin D3 supplements are inexpensive and have been proven safe up to 10,000 IU's per day. **I believe that the prooxidant vitamin D3 is helping correct their EMOD insufficiency.**

Thus, blacks may need special considerations for cancer prevention and treatment.

CHAPTER TWENTY SIX:

Conclusions

**The disciplined and virtuous life
is an honored life.**
R. M. Howes, M.D., Ph.D.
9/7/09

What's the best advice to give to cancer patients on this issue? Simply acknowledge the truth. Acknowledge the scientific data. Stop denying the truth. Stop ingoring studies showing the ineffectiveness of the antioxidants and their harmful potential. Present patietns with the scientific data. Then, patients can then make up their own minds and make informed decisions as to which way to go.

There is still a great deal to learn about the interactions between cancer treatments and antioxidants. So, in the interim, play it safe. Whether or not an antioxidant can be helpful, harmful, or neutral theoretically depends, in part, on the specific antioxidant (and its dose and isomeric form used), the chemotherapeutic drugs being used, the types of cancer being treated, and the types of diet the patients are consuming (in addition to a host of other confounding factors). Considerable caution is recommended for both the taking of antioxidants by cancer patients and the making of categorical and sweeping statements that antioxidants should always be taken along with standard cancer therapy to reduce adverse effects.

However, **since there is a solid theoretical basis and potential for harm, people who are undergoing cancer therapy should exercise extreme caution before supplementing themselves with antioxidants**.

Some opponents of my studies may argue that my studies "ignore the broad totality of evidence that comes to largely opposite conclusions." This statement's authors also noted that intake of antioxidants from foods or supplements has been shown to reduce the risk of cardiovascular disease, some types of cancer, eye disease, and neurodegenerative diseases (as well as strengthen the immune system). However, my work shows that there is no consistency or predictability to the data and there have been no cases whereby antioxidants have been proven to prevent or cure *any* disease (none, zippo, nada), other than a simple deficiency state. Also, their lack of safety has been clearly identified.

We must strive to make the "cure" breakthroughs and I believe this can be accomplished via in depth knowledge of EMOD biochemistry.

It is believed by some that many cancers spontaneously regress. This must be exploited.

We must then turn our attention to cancer prevention.

We generate our crucial energy requirements by "oxidative phosphorylation," not reductive phosphorylation. We are oxygen dependent aerobes, not reduction dependent aerobes. In doing so, we generate therapeutic doses of EMODs to fight pathogens and cancer. Oxidation is absolutely critical for our well being and overall health. It is anything but the "enemy within," as it has been characterized by **outdated theories and outmoded thinking.** Stop ignoring the data.

We must be cautious of interrupting crucial complex intracellular and intercellular cross talk by the injudicious use of antioxidants and of blocking EMOD-messaging and induced apoptosis for controlling cancer. We must not let "antioxidant stacking" protect or shield neoplastic cells and prevent them from being exposed to the therapeutic EMODs generated during normal metabolism, chemo, PDT and radiation therapy. We must not help cancer to thrive. An overall cancer cure may still be a long time coming.

The bottom line:

In years gone by, the theoretical use of antioxidants seemed to be a good idea but study after study (i.e., hundreds of studies) have failed to show any **consistent measurable benefit** from taking antioxidant supplements. Ergo, the free radical theory has failed to meet the requirements of the scientific method and is no longer valid. I have endeavored to find more advanced and improved replacement theories.

The theory behind the use of antioxidants is plausible only if the free radical theory is sound. But it has been nullified. This is why there is no reproducibility of data in this area. **The theory has been wrong** and that is the reason that the antioxidant supplements available to us lack effectiveness and produce adverse effects. The free radical theory is passé!

Whatever the explanation, the American Heart Association's advisory statement is sound. There is no good reason, at this point, to spend your money on antioxidant supplements. Amen.

Proponents of antioxidant supplements suggest that increasing your antioxidant intake can help prevent chronic diseases, including <u>heart disease</u> and cancer. But, **antioxidants have proven to be neither safe nor effective.** While research shows that a diet high in antioxidant-rich fruits and vegetables can help protect against disease, it is clear that antioxidant supplements are equally ineffective in disease prevention. What is perhaps of more importance is that **over 80 studies indicate that antioxidant supplements pose considerable health risks.**

All sides of the argument

In this book, I have endeavored to present both sides of the argument, even though it was difficult at times to repeat some of the nonsense/nonscience that is out there. I presented you with their strongest arguments for the use of antioxidants by cancer survivors and pointed out their weakness in light of the overwhelming scientific evidence stacked up against them. Still, I informed you of their old fashioned and potentially dangerous notions.

Let me be clear

As was pointed out in an article entitled, *Antioxidants not heaven sent*, by Stefan Andrei Anghel in the Harvard Science Review, Spring 2010, **"It may come as a surprise that the current scientific consensus is that there is no health benefit to taking antioxidant supplements**. Even more unexpected news came this year when an article announced that **antioxidants may actually prevent the health-promoting effects of physical exercise....** If the model proposed by the authors of the study is correct, then **it may turn out that we have been systematically "poisoning" ourselves, increasing our disease risk and shortening our lifespan through antioxidant supplements."**

It was especially gratifying that Anghel cited one of my papers entitled, The Free Radical Fantasy, as the first reference in The Harvard Review and cited it two other times in the article.

On January 25, 2011, Sharon Begley noted in an article entitled, *Antioxidants fall from grace*, in *Newsweek* magazine that, "Now the research is challenging an even more fundamental tenet of the antioxidant craze. Many of the free radicals that are neutralized by antioxidants perform valuable functions in the body. The most important: fighting toxins (white blood cells churn out free radicals by the battalion to fight bacterial infection) and fighting cancer. Maybe it's not such a fabulous idea to flood the body with something that neutralizes these warriors of the immune system." And David Bradley said, "Suffice to say that taking antioxidant supplements ...

may not necessarily be good for your health if you already have health problems," especially cancer or an infection."

Begley said, "In 2009, 108 new food products with antioxidants touted on the label reached store shelves in the United States." Yes, Luke, the force is strong….the marketing force that is.

But at last, the antioxidant craze is dying down. People are becoming aware of their ineffectiveness and of their harm. In short, people are waking up to the fact that they have been victims of clever marketing campaigns, all of which were based on the profit motive and an invalidated theory.

Most of the dialogue concerning antioxidants is all about marketing and not about science.

Stop being a victim.

Wise up, folks!

In the end, the choice is yours.

Choose wisely!

**In trying to turn opinion on disease allowance
and coexistence,
I appear to be a petite Louisiana blue crab pushing
furiously against the bow of the lumbering QE2,
trying frantically to change its direction….
to keep it from hitting the upcoming shoals of misinforma-
tion.
By the tested laws of physics,
I can amend its course
but it is going to require that my
diminutive flippers move faster than
a redox electron.
In other words,
I've got to swim like hell.**
R. M. Howes, M.D., Ph.D.
9/20/09

I lived another day.
I breathed another day.
I shared another wondrous day of living
with my beautiful chemical cohort,
oxygen.
R. M. Howes, M.D., Ph.D.
2/22/11

I have presented approximately 106 studies showing **EMODs** are responsible for induction of apoptosis.

I have presented approximately 50 studies showing that antioxidants can block **EMOD** induced apoptosis.

There are 26 studies showing that antioxidants increased the risk of cancer and 2 showing they increased the mortality in cancer patients.

<u>Antioxidants increased the risk of the following cancers:</u>

- lung cancer, **(7 studies)** (up to 28% in smokers)
- prostate cancer, **(5 studies)**
- doubled the risk of adenoma recurrence,
- squamous cell skin cancer **(2 studies)**
- melanoma
- higher rate of second primary cancers(head and neck), local recurrence of the head and neck tumor tended to be higher, (2 studies)
- esophageal cancer, **(2 studies)**
- oral pre-malignant lesions,
- stomach cancer
- urinary bladder cancer
- breast cancer

<u>SUMMARY</u> of antioxidants causing various cancers include the following: lung cancer, breast cancer, prostate cancer, stomach cancer, esophageal cancer, head and neck cancer, bladder cancer, melanoma, adenomas, oral premalignant lesions.

Antioxidants increased the mortality in the following cancer patient groups (2 studies):

- 1) increase overall mortality in gastrointestinal cancer patients,
- 2) esophageal cancer deaths increased 14% in patients, (2 studies)

26 STUDIES SHOWING RELATIONSHIP OF HARMFUL EFFECTS OF ANTIOXIDANTS TO CANCER:

1) **Alpha-Tocopherol and beta-carotene supplements and lung cancer incidence in the alpha-tocopherol, beta-carotene cancer prevention study: effects of base-line characteristics and study compliance.** (Albanes et al, 1996) (#29,133 men, smokers) Supplementation with alpha-tocopherol or beta-carotene does not prevent lung cancer in older men who smoke. *beta-Carotene supplementation at pharmacologic levels may modestly increase lung cancer incidence in cigarette smokers.* The incidence of lung cancer was 18% higher among men who took the beta-carotene supplement and *eight percent more men in this group died, as compared to those receiving other treatments or placebo.* (Albanes et al, 1996). Smokers should avoid high-dose beta-carotene supplementation.

2) **The b-Carotene and Retinol Efficacy Trial (CARET) (Omenn et al, 1996) (#14,254 heavy smokers and 4,060 asbestos workers) (total #18,314 men and women); randomized, double-blind, placebo-controlled intervention; Duration of Treatment Years: 4; Daily Dose: 30 mg b-carotene, 25,000 IU retinol (as retinyl palmitate);** *28% increase in lung cancer; 26% increase in CVD (nonsignificant); 17% increase in total mortality* **among treatment group. This study was stopped 21 months earlier than planned.**

3) **Energy, nutrient intake and prostate cancer risk: a population-based case-control study in Sweden.** (Andersson et al. 1996) (#1,062). *In age-adjusted analyses, there were positive associations of prostate cancer (all stages combined) risk with total energy intake as well as intake of total fat (saturated and monounsaturated), protein, retinol and zinc.* The **positive association with energy intake was stronger for advanced cancer, with an excess risk of 70% for the highest quartile vs. the lowest.** *After adjustment for energy intake, there was no apparent association of prostate cancers (all stages combined) with any of the investigated nutrients. However, a weak positive association between intake of retinol and advanced cancer was ob-*

served. We conclude that our results provide some evidence that **total energy intake is a risk factor for prostate cancer**.

4) **Randomized Trial of Supplemental ß-Carotene to Prevent Second Head and Neck Cancer** (**Mayne et al, 2001**) (#264 patients who had been curatively treated for a recent early-stage squamous cell carcinoma of the oral cavity, pharynx, or larynx.); randomized, placebo-controlled, double-blinded clinical trial; 50 mg of ß-carotene per day; **Supplemental ß-carotene had no significant effect on second head and neck cancer or lung cancer**. Whereas none of the effects were statistically significant, the **point estimates suggested a possible decrease in second head and neck cancer risk** *but a possible increase in lung cancer risk.*

5) **Selenium and vitamin E supplements for prostate cancer: evidence or embellishment?** (Moyad et al. 2002) (# not available). **Selenium supplements provided a benefit only for those individuals who had lower levels of baseline plasma selenium.** *Other subjects, with normal or higher levels, did not benefit and may have an increased risk for prostate cancer. Vitamin E supplements in higher doses (> or =100 IU) were also associated with a higher risk of aggressive or fatal prostate cancer in nonsmokers from a past prospective study.*

6) **Vitamins E & A fail to reduce incidence or mortality of lung cancer: Cochrane Database Syst Rev. 2003.** (**Caraballoso et al., 2003**) (#109,394 participants); **When beta-carotene was combined with retinol, data from a single study showed that there was a statistically significant,** *increased risk of lung cancer incidence and mortality* **in people with risk factors for lung cancer who took both vitamins.**

7) **Neoplastic and Antineoplastic Effects of Beta Carotene on Colorectal Adenoma Recurrence: Results of a Randomized Trial** (Baron et al, 2003) (#864 subjects who had had an adenoma removed and were polyp-free); *For participants who smoked cigarettes and also drank more than one alcoholic drink per day, beta carotene doubled the risk of adenoma recurrence.*

8) **Selenium supplementation and secondary prevention of nonmelanoma skin cancer in a randomized trial.** (Duffield-Lillico, 2003) (#1,312). **Results from the Nutritional Prevention of Cancer Trial conducted among individuals at high risk of nonmelanoma skin cancer continue to demonstrate that selenium supplementation is ineffective at preventing basal cell carcinoma and that** *it increases the risk of squamous cell*

carcinoma and total nonmelanoma skin cancer. Selenium supplementation was associated with statistically significantly elevated risk of squamous cell carcinoma. (Duffield-Lillico, 2003).

9) **Use of multivitamins and prostate cancer mortality in a large cohort of US men.** (Stevens et al, 2005) (#475,726 men who were cancer-free). **The death rate from prostate cancer was marginally higher among men who took multivitamins regularly** (> or =15 times/month) **compared to non-users; this risk was statistically significant only for those multivitamin users who used no additional (vitamin A, C, or E) supplements.** In addition, risk was greatest during the initial four years of follow-up. CONCLUSIONS: *Regular multivitamin use was associated with a small increase in prostate cancer death rates.*

10) **A randomized trial of antioxidant vitamins to prevent second primary cancers in head and neck cancer patients.** (Bairati et al, 2005 Apr 6) (#540 patients with stage I or II head and neck cancer treated by radiation therapy). *Patients receiving alpha-tocopherol supplements had a higher rate of second primary cancers during the supplementation period but a lower rate after supplementation was discontinued.* Similarly, *the rate of having a recurrence or second primary cancer was higher during but lower after supplementation with alpha-tocopherol.* The proportion of participants free of second primary cancer overall after 8 years of follow-up was similar in both arms. CONCLUSIONS: *alpha-Tocopherol supplementation produced unexpected adverse effects on the occurrence of second primary cancers and on cancer-free survival.* (Bairati et al, 2005 Apr 6).

Note: *Patients taking an antioxidant were 1.65 times more likely to suffer a return of their original cancer during the three years they were on the supplement. The risk was highest among those taking only vitamin E (1.86 times higher).* Five years after they stopped taking the supplement, their recurrence risk had fallen to the same level as those in the placebo group. **Although suggestive of harm, these results were not statistically significant.**

11) **Randomized trial of antioxidant vitamins to prevent acute adverse effects of radiation therapy in head and neck cancer patients** (Bairati et al, 2005 Aug 20) (#540 patients with stage I or II head and neck cancer treated by radiation therapy) A randomized trial. During the course of the trial, **supplementation with beta-carotene was discontinued because of ethical concerns. Quality of life was not improved by the supplementation.** *The rate of local recurrence of the head and neck tumor tended to be higher in the*

supplement arm of the trial. CONCLUSION: Supplementation with high doses of alpha-tocopherol and beta-carotene during radiation therapy could reduce the severity of treatment adverse effects. However, **this trial suggests that use of high doses of antioxidants as adjuvant therapy might compromise radiation treatment efficacy.**

Note: *Researchers were concerned to find that the rate of local recurrence (that is, a return of the original cancer) was 54 percent higher among patients on the combination pill than those on placebo.* There was a smaller but still worrisome increase among those on vitamin E only.

NCI COMMENT: "This is a large, well-done study with good compliance from the participants," said Eva Szabo, M.D., of the National Cancer Institute's Division of Cancer Prevention. "The results demonstrate that the use of vitamin E supplementation is not beneficial to patients with stage I or II head and neck cancer, either as a chemoprevention agent or to enhance quality of life during radiation therapy."

12) **Smoking, alcohol drinking, green tea consumption and the risk of esophageal cancer in Japanese men.** (Ishikawa et al, 2006) (#9,008 men in Cohort 1 and 17,715 men in Cohort 2) *Cigarette smoking, alcohol drinking and green tea consumption were significantly associated with an increased risk of esophageal cancer. The population attributable fractions of esophageal cancer incidence that was attributable to smoking, alcohol drinking and green tea consumption were 72.0%, 48.6%, and 22.1%, respectively.*

CONCLUSIONS: Among the variables studied, *smoking has the largest public health impact on esophageal cancer incidence in Japanese men, followed by alcohol drinking and green tea drinking* (Ishikawa et al, 2006).

13) **Multivitamin Use and Risk of Prostate Cancer in the National Institutes of Health–AARP Diet and Health Study** (Lawson et al, 2007) (#295,344 men); investigated the association between multivitamin use and prostate cancer risk; *use of multivitamins more than seven times per week, when compared with never use, was associated with a doubling in the risk of fatal prostate cancer* (The study of Lawson et al. is observational, and therefore confounding by indication and other confounding cannot be excluded. But the sample studied is very large, which reduces random errors, and the study seems well conducted.)

14) **Health Professionals Follow-up Study (2007): Effect of vitamins C, E, A and carotenoids and the occurrence of oral pre-malignant lesions.** (Maserejian et al, 2007) (#42,340 men enrolled in the Health Professionals

Follow-up Study) (#207 found with oral premalignant lesions); researchers found no clear relationship with beta-carotene, lycopene, or lutein/zeaxanthin. **A trend** *for increased risk of oral pre-malignant lesions was observed with vitamin E, especially among current smokers and with vitamin E supplements. Beta-carotene also increased the risk among current smokers.* However, **dietary vitamin C was significantly associated with a reduced risk of oral premalignant lesions**: those with the highest intake had a 50 percent reduction in risk compared to those with the lowest intake.

15) **Antioxidant Supplementation Increases the Risk of Skin Cancers in Women but Not in Men.** (Hercberg et al, 2007) (#French adults, 7,876 women and 5,141 men. Total # = 13,017). *In women, the incidence of SC was higher in the antioxidant group.* **Conversely, in men, incidence did not differ between the 2 treatment groups.** Despite the small number of events, *the incidence of melanoma was also higher in the antioxidant group for women.*

16) **National Institutes of Health State-of-the-Science Conference Statement: Multivitamin/Mineral Supplements and Chronic Disease Prevention (NIH State-of-the Science Panel. 2007).** There is evidence, however, that certain ingredients in MVM supplements can produce adverse effects, including **reports from RCTs that noted excess lung cancer occurring in asbestos workers and smokers consuming b-carotene**. In addition, *esophageal cancer excess was found with long-term follow-up of older Chinese patients (the Linxian study by Blot et al.) treated with selenium, b-carotene, and vitamin E supplements* (Blot et al, 1993) (NIH State-of-the Science Panel. 2007).

17) **Systematic review: primary and secondary prevention of gastrointestinal cancers with antioxidant supplements.** (Bjelakovic, Nikolova, Simonette and Gludd, 2008 Sept) (#211,818 participants). We identified 20 randomized trials (211,818 participants) assessing beta-carotene, vitamin A, vitamin C, vitamin E, and selenium. **The antioxidant supplements were without a significant effect on the occurrence of gastrointestinal cancers. Antioxidant supplements had no significant effect on mortality in a random-effects model meta-analysis** but *significantly increased mortality in a fixed-effect model meta-analysis.* CONCLUSIONS: **There was no evidence that the studied antioxidant supplements prevented gastrointestinal cancers. On the contrary,** *they seem to increase overall mortality.*

18) **Long-term use of supplemental multivitamins, vitamin C, vitamin E, and folate does not reduce the risk of lung cancer. VITAL (VITamins And Lifestyle) study (2008)** (Slatore et al, 2008) (#77,721 men and women);

There was no inverse association with any supplement. *Supplemental vitamin E was associated with a small increased risk of lung cancer.* This risk of supplemental vitamin E was largely confined to current smokers and was greatest for non–small cell lung cancer.

19) **Efficacy of Antioxidant Supplementation in Reducing Primary Cancer Incidence and Mortality: Systematic Review and Meta-analysis.** (Bardia et al, 2008) (#104,196 participants). *Beta carotene supplementation was associated with an increase in the incidence of cancer among smokers and with a trend toward increased cancer mortality.*

20) **Total and Cancer Mortality After Supplementation With Vitamins and Minerals: 10 year Follow-up of the Linxian General Population Nutrition Intervention Trial. (Qiao et al, 2009) (#29,584 adult participants)** The General Population Nutrition Intervention Trial was a randomized primary esophageal and gastric cancer prevention trial. Treatment with **"factor D," a combination of 50 µg selenium, 30 mg vitamin E, and 15 mg beta-carotene** showed *esophageal cancer deaths increased 14% among those aged 55 years or older. Vitamin A and zinc supplementation was associated with increased total and stroke mortality.*

21) **Long-term use of beta-carotene, retinol, lycopene, and lutein supplements and lung cancer risk: results from the VITamins And Lifestyle (VITAL) study.** (Satia et al, 2009) (#77,126 (VITAL) cohort Study in Washington State). *Longer duration of use of individual beta-carotene, retinol, and lutein supplements* (but not total 10-year average dose) *was associated with statistically significantly elevated risk of total lung cancer and histologic cell types.*

22) **Folic acid and risk of prostate cancer: results from a randomized clinical trial.** (Figueiredo et al, 2009) (#643 randomly assigned men). Among the **643 men who were randomly assigned** to placebo or **supplementation with folic acid,** *the estimated probability of being diagnosed with prostate cancer over a 10-year period was 9.7% in the folic acid group and 3.3% in the placebo group.*

23) **Green tea consumption and risk of stomach cancer: a meta-analysis of epidemiologic studies** (Myung, Int J Cancer. et al, 2009) (#13 epidemiologic studies) *In the meta-analyses of the recent cohort studies, the highest green tea consumption was shown to significantly increase stomach cancer risk using the crude data,* but no significant association between them was seen when using the adjusted data. (Myung, Int J Cancer. et al, 2009).

24) **Green tea (Camellia sinensis) for the prevention of cancer. Chochrane Database Syst Rev. 2009 Jul 8;(3):CD005004.** (Boehm et al, 2009) (#Fifty-one studies with more than 1.6 million participants were included) **There was limited to moderate evidence that the consumption of green tea reduced the risk of lung cancer, especially in men, and** *urinary bladder cancer or that it could even increase the risk of the latter.* **There is insufficient and conflicting evidence to give any firm recommendations regarding green tea consumption for cancer prevention.**

25) **Multivitamin use and breast cancer incidence in a prospective cohort of Swedish women.** (Larsson et al, 2010) (#35,329 cancer-free women). *Multivitamin use was associated with a statistically significant increased risk of breast cancer. Use of multivitamins was linked to a statistically significant 19 per cent increased risk of breast cancer.*

Other research has found that *women who take multivitamins have increased breast density, which is linked to a relatively higher risk of breast cancer* (Berube et al, 2008). **The widespread use of multiviamins points out an important public health concern.**

26) **Daily intake of antioxidants in relation to survival among adult patients diagnosed with malignant glioma.** (DeLorenze et al. 2010). *For patients diagnosed with Grade II and Grade III histology, moderate (915.8-2118.3 mcg) intake of fat-soluble lycopene was associated with poorer survival* **when compared to low intake (0.0-914.8 mcg), for self-reported cases only.** *In Grade IV patients, moderate/high intake of cryptoxanthin and high intake of secoisolariciresinol were associated with poorer survival among all cases.* **Among Grade II patients,** moderate intake of water-soluble folate was associated with greater survival for all cases; *high intake of vitamin C and genistein and the highest level of the antioxidant index were associated with poorer survival for all cases.*

Total number of participants in the above studies totals 3,129,215. Note: one study on green tea did not give the number of participants but it did include 13 epidemiologic studies.

SECTION SEVEN:

CHRONOLOGICAL LIST OF ANTIOXIDANT/CANCER STUDIES

One hundred eighteen (118) studies showed antioxidant ineffectiveness in cancer treatment and thirty nine (39) of these studies showed harmful effects. (partially taken from *Death in small doses?* and from *Antioxidant Overkill*).

Total 118 studies below on cancer only. Total number of participants for these studies is over 11,127,347. **Some of these participants may have been repeats in follow up or parallel studies.** Studies ranged in size from less than 100 to over 1.6 million. Some studies did not have the number of participants available. One study was a murine study, i.e., (Fang et al, 2008).

There are 26 studies showing that antioxidants increased the risk of cancer. Total number of participants in these 26 studies totals 2,851,586. Note: one study on green tea did not give the number of participants but it did include 13 epidemiologic studies. Thus, this number is a low approximation.

SUMMARY of antioxidants causing various cancers include the following: lung cancer, breast cancer, prostate cancer, stomach cancer, esophageal cancer, head and neck cancer, bladder cancer, melanoma, adenomas, oral premalignant lesions.

Antioxidants increased the mortality in the following cancer patients (2 studies):

- 1) increase overall mortality in gastrointestinal cancer patients,

- 2) esophageal cancer deaths increased 14% in patients, (2 studies)

The following are studies in which the antioxidant vitamins either had no effect or had a harmful effect: (part taken from *Death in small doses?* and part from *Antioxidant Overkill*). Some new studies were also added.

Circa 1979

Failure of high-dose vitamin C (ascorbic acid) therapy to benefit patients with advanced cancer. A controlled trial. (Creagan et al, 1979) (#159 patients with advanced cancer) **One hundred and fifty patients with advanced cancer** participated in a **controlled double-blind study** to evaluate the effects of high-dose vitamin C on symptoms and survival. Patients were divided randomly into a group that **received vitamin C (10 g per day)** and one that received a comparably flavored lactose placebo. Sixty evaluable patients received vitamin C and 63 received a placebo. Both groups were similar in age, sex, site of primary tumor, performance score, tumor grade and previous chemotherapy. The two groups showed no appreciable difference in changes in symptoms, performance status, appetite or weight. The median survival for all patients was about seven weeks, and the survival curves essentially overlapped. In this selected group of patients, **we were unable to show a therapeutic benefit of high-dose vitamin C treatment.** (Creagan et al, 1979).

Circa 1985

High-dose vitamin C versus placebo in the treatment of patients with advanced cancer who have had no prior chemotherapy. A randomized double-blind comparison. (Moertel et al , 1985) (#100 patients with advanced colorectal cancer)

It has been claimed that high-dose vitamin C is beneficial in the treatment of patients with advanced cancer, especially patients who have had no prior chemotherapy. In a **double-blind study 100 patients with advanced colorectal cancer** were **randomly** assigned to treatment with either **high-dose vitamin C (10 g daily)** or placebo. Overall, these patients were in very good general condition, with minimal symptoms. None had received any previous treatment with cytotoxic drugs. Vitamin C therapy showed no advantage over placebo therapy with regard to either the interval between the beginning of treatment and disease progression or patient survival. Among patients with measurable disease, none had objective improvement. On the basis of this and our previous randomized study, it can be concluded that **high-dose vitamin C (10 g daily) therapy is not effective against advanced malignant disease regardless of whether the patient has had any prior chemotherapy.**

Circa 1990

Skin Cancer Prevention Study (Greenberg et al, 1990) (#1,805 men and women with recent nonmelanoma skin cancer); "A clinical trial of beta carotene to prevent basal-cell and squamous-cell cancers of the skin. The Skin Cancer Prevention Study Group." a **randomized, double-blind, placebo-controlled**

intervention; men and women with recent nonmelanoma skin cancer; b-carotene; No effect on occurrence of new nonmelanoma skin cancers.

Circa 1992

Diet in the Epidemiology of Postmenopausal Breast Cancer in the New York State Cohort (Graham et al, 1992) (#18,586 postmenopausal women); **did not associate a greater vitamin E intake with a reduced risk of developing breast cancer.**

Women's Health Study (WHS) (Buring and Hennekens, 1992) (#39,876 healthy women); randomized, double-blind; placebo-controlled intervention; 600 IU of natural-source vitamin E taken every other day provided no overall benefit for major cardiovascular events or cancer, did not affect total mortality, and decreased cardiovascular mortality in healthy women. These data do not support recommending vitamin E supplementation for cardiovascular disease or cancer prevention among healthy women. The WHS data suggest that **vitamin E provides no protection against cancer in women.** In addition, **vitamin E offered no overall protection against CVD.**

Isotretinoin-Basal Cell Carcinoma Study Group (Tangrea et al, 1992, 1993) (#981 patients with two or more previously treated basal cell carcinomas) randomly assigned; **low-dose regimen of isotretinoin not only is ineffective in reducing the occurrence of basal cell carcinoma at new sites in patients with two or more previously treated basal cell carcinomas but *also is associated with significant adverse systemic effects.*** The **toxicity associated with the long-term administration of isotretinoin, even at the low dose** (10 mg/day) **used in this trial, must be weighted in planning future prevention trials.** Isotretinoin is a modified vitamin A molecule used to treat severe <u>acne vulgaris</u>.

(adverse mucocutaneous effects and serum triglyceride elevations)

Circa 1993

Prospective Study of the Intake of Vitamins C, E, and A and the Risk of Breast Cancer (Hunter et al, 1993) (#89,494 women); prospective study; **Large intakes of vitamin C or E did not protect women in our study from breast cancer. 000** *A low intake of vitamin A may increase the risk of this disease.*

Serum micronutrients and the subsequent risk of cervical cancer in a population-based nested case-control study. (Batieha et al, 1993) (#15,161 women) A nested case-control study was conducted in Washington County, MD, to determine whether low serum micronutrients are related to the subsequent risk of cervical cancer. Among the **15,161 women** who donated blood for future cancer research during a serum collection campaign in 1974, **18 developed invasive cervical cancer and 32 developed carcinoma in situ** during the period January 1975 through May 1990. For each of these 50 cases, two matched controls were selected from the same cohort. The frozen sera of the cases and their matched controls were analyzed for a number of nutrients. The mean serum levels of total carotenoids, alpha-carotene, beta-carotene, cryptoxanthin, and lycopene were lower among cases than they were among controls. **When examined by tertiles, the risk of cervical cancer was significantly higher among women in the lower tertiles of total carotenoids, alpha-carotene, and beta-carotene as compared to women in the upper tertiles and the trends were statistically significant.** Cryptoxanthin was significantly associated with a lower risk of cervical cancer when examined as a continuous variable. **Retinol, lutein, alpha- and gamma-tocopherol, and selenium were not related to cervical cancer risk. 000** Smoking was also strongly associated with cervical cancer. These findings are suggestive of a protective role for total carotenoids, alpha-carotene and beta-carotene in cervical carcinogenesis and possibly for cryptoxanthin and lycopene as well.

Circa 1994

a-Tocopherol, b-Carotene Cancer Prevention Study (ATBC study) (Heinonen et al, **1994) (#29,133 men); randomized, double-blind, placebo-controlled intervention; no effect of vitamin E on lung cancer.** Men with known <u>coronary artery disease</u> given 50 mg of a synthetic vitamin E **had no reduction in fatal heart attacks.** *50% increase in hemorrhagic stroke deaths among vitamin E group; 11% increase in ischemic heart disease deaths among b-carotene group; 18% increase in lung cancer among b-carotene group.*

This study was stopped 21 months earlier than planned.

The incidence of lung cancer was 18% higher among men who took the beta-carotene supplement and eight percent more men in this group died, as compared to those receiving other treatments or placebo. (Albanes et al, 1996).

The negative (and harmful) results of the 2 beta carotene intervention trials were completely **unexpected and counterintuitive**, according to predominant thinking of the time, which was based totally on the free radical theory.

However, results from the **Alpha-Tocopherol Beta Carotene Prevention Study** (Heinonen et al, 1994) and the **Carotene and Retinol Efficiency Trial (CARET)** (Omenn et al, 1996) **showed an increase in lung cancer** among smokers or asbestos-exposed workers after beta carotene supplementation. **The Physician's Health Study**, in which only a small percentage of subjects were smokers (11%), showed no significant effect of beta carotene supplementation on lung cancer (Hennekens et al, 1996).

Polyp Prevention Study (Greenberg et al, 1994) (#864); randomized, double-blind, placebo-controlled intervention; There was no evidence that either beta carotene or vitamins C and E reduced the incidence of adenomas. CONCLUSION. The lack of efficacy of these vitamins argues against the use of supplemental beta carotene and vitamins C and E to prevent colorectal cancer.

CIRCA 1995

Dietary factors and risk of prostate cancer: a case-control study in Ontario, Canada. (Rohan et al. 1995) (#414)

The relationship between risk of prostate cancer and dietary intake of energy, fat, vitamin A, and other nutrients was investigated in a case-control study conducted in Ontario, Canada. Cases were men with a recent, histologically confirmed diagnosis of adenocarcinoma of the prostate notified to the Ontario Cancer Registry between April 1990 and April 1992. Controls were selected randomly from assessment lists maintained by the Ontario Ministry of Revenue, and were frequency-matched to the cases on age. The study included **207 cases (51.4 percent of those eligible) and 207 controls** (39.4 percent of those eligible), and information on dietary intake was collected from them by means of a quantitative diet history. There was a positive association between energy intake and risk of prostate cancer, such that men at the uppermost quartile level of energy intake had a 75 percent increase in risk. In contrast, there was no clear association between the non-energy effects of total fat and monounsaturated fat intake and prostate cancer risk. There was some evidence for an inverse association with saturated fat intake, although the dose-response pattern was irregular. There was a weak (statistically nonsignificant) positive association between polyunsaturated fat intake and risk of prostate cancer. Relatively high levels of retinol intake were associated with reduced risk, but **there was essentially no association between dietary be-ta-carotene intake and (prostate cancer) risk. There was no alteration in risk in association with dietary fiber, cholesterol, and vitamins C and E.** Although these patterns were evident both overall and within age-strata, and persisted after adjustment for a number of potential confounding factors, **they could reflect (in particular) the effect of non-respondent bias**.

Circa 1996

The b-Carotene and Retinol Efficacy Trial (CARET) (Omenn et al, 1996) (#14,254 heavy smokers and 4,060 asbestos workers) (total #18,314 men and women**); randomized, double-blind, placebo-controlled intervention; Duration of Treatment Years: 4; Daily Dose: 30 mg b-carotene, 25,000 IU retinol (as retinyl palmitate);** *28% increase in lung cancer; 26% increase in CVD (nonsignificant); 17% increase in total mortality* **among treatment group. This study was stopped 21 months earlier than planned.**

RMH Note: A 6-year follow-up of a large, randomized trial in people with a history of smoking has found that the overall harm associated with beta-carotene supplementation on cardiovascular disease mortality disappeared quickly after participants stopped taking the supplements. However, the risk of lung cancer may persist, especially in females and former smokers, according to the study in the December 1, 2004 issue of the Journal of the National Cancer Institute. Gary E. Goodman, M.D., of the Fred Hutchinson Cancer Research Center in Seattle, and colleagues followed the more than 18,000 participants in CARET for 6 years after the trial was stopped, until the end of 2001. **The increased risk of cardiovascular disease mortality quickly disappeared after participants stopped taking the supplements.** However, women had a higher risk of death from cardiovascular disease or from any cause than men. In addition, *the incidence of lung cancer and deaths from all causes decreased but did not disappear completely after the supplementation ceased.* The excess risk of lung cancer was restricted primarily to females and former smokers.

"When chemoprevention agents are administered to large, healthy populations, it is necessary to document long-term safety, efficacy and, importantly, the duration of the beneficial (or adverse) effect," the authors write. "**This is especially true when the basic underlying molecular and genetic mechanism of the agent is unclear.** The results of CARET and ATBC emphasize that chemoprevention trials require careful monitoring of all disease endpoints ... even after the study intervention is discontinued." (Goodman et al, 2004).

Based on the free radical theory, beta carotene was known to be an effective antioxidant and a precursor of vitamin A, and was therefore believe to be a plausible mechanism to block lung cancer. However, a series of beta carotene intervention trials were conducted that **categorically dispelled the notion that supplemental beta carotene could effectively reduce lung cancer risk** (Hennekens et al, 1996) **(**Heinonen et al, **1994)** (Omenn et al, NEJM. 1996).

The lessons from the beta-carotene studies in relation to chronic disease include the possibility that antioxidants may have surprising short and long term health consequences, even if generally regarded as safe, which could be important in determining the balance of benefits and risks for the individual.

Physicians' Health Study (PHSI) (Hennekens et al, 1996) (#22,071 US Physicians and Malignant Neoplasms or CVD**); randomized, double-blind, placebo-controlled intervention;** b-carotene in US Physicians and Malignant Neoplasms or CVD; among healthy men, 12 years of supplementation with **beta carotene produced neither benefit nor harm in terms of the incidence of malignant neoplasms, cardiovascular disease, or death from all causes.**

The Nutritional Prevention of Cancer Trial (Clark et al. 1996) (#1,312 **men and women with a history of basal or squamous cell carcinoma**) A multicenter, double-blind, randomized, placebo-controlled cancer prevention trial. **Selenium treatment did not protect against development of basal or squamous cell carcinomas of the skin.**

Daily Dose: 200 pg selenium; Primary Disease Outcome: Skin cancer, prostate cancer; Results: No effect on incidence of skin cancer; 63% reduction in prostate cancer incidence; reduction in total cancer mortality and total cancer incidence (this result has not been duplicated by other recent studies). Reference to this particular study was included, even though it did not test vitamins A, C or E, due to the antioxidant claims of selenium. This unbelievable decrease in prostate is not supported by other studies.

RMH Note: **Intakes of dietary or supplemental antioxidants were not associated with a decreased risk of prostate cancer among men in the Prostate (CaP), Lung, Colorectal, and Ovarian (PLCO) Cancer Screening Trial**, according to a study in the February 15, 2006 issue of the *Journal of the National Cancer Institute*. Kirsh and Hayes, at the National Cancer Institute, and colleagues assessed the risk of prostate cancer for **29,361 men ages** 55 to

74 enrolled in the PLCO Cancer Screening Trial, based on their daily intake of beta-carotene, vitamin E, and vitamin C. The researchers looked at intake of antioxidants from both dietary sources and from supplements. The authors found that, **overall, dietary or supplemental intake of vitamin E, vitamin C, or beta-carotene was not associated with prostate cancer incidence** in this group of PLCO trial participants. **In short,** in the 29,361 men in the trial, 1,338 cases of CaP were identified over the 8 years of follow-up. In general, **there was no clear CaP risk reduction resulting from dietary or supplemental intake of vitamins E and C or b-carotene** (Kirsh et al, 2006).

Energy, nutrient intake and prostate cancer risk: a population-based case-control study in Sweden. (Andersson et al. 1996) (#1,062). The role of diet in the etiology of prostate cancer remains unclear, because results from several case-control and cohort studies on fat intake and risk of prostate cancer have been inconsistent; few of the studies have adjusted the results for caloric intake. To examine the relationship between energy, intake of several nutrients and risk of prostate cancer (all stages combined and advanced stages separately), we conducted a population-based case-control study in Orebro County, Sweden, from 1989 through 1994. A total of **526 patients with newly diagnosed prostate cancer and 536 controls, (total 1,062) randomly** selected from the population register and frequency-matched by age, were included in the analyses. Information about dietary intake was obtained from a self-administered semi-quantitative food frequency questionnaire. Odds ratios with 95% confidence intervals were estimated by unconditional logistic regression. *In age-adjusted analyses, there were positive associations of prostate cancer (all stages combined) risk with total energy intake as well as intake of total fat (saturated and monounsaturated), protein, retinol and zinc.* The **positive association with energy intake was stronger for advanced cancer, with an excess risk of 70% for the highest quartile vs. the lowest.** *After adjustment for energy intake, there was no apparent association of prostate cancers (all stages combined) with any of the investigated nutrients. However, a weak positive association between intake of retinol and advanced cancer was observed.* We conclude that our results provide some evidence that **total energy intake is a risk factor for prostate cancer.**

Effects of selenium supplementation for cancer prevention in patients with carcinoma of the skin. A randomized controlled trial. Nutritional Prevention of Cancer Study Group. (Clark et al. 1996) (#1,312 patients)

OBJECTIVE: To determine whether a nutritional supplement of selenium will decrease the incidence of cancer. **DESIGN:** A multicenter, double-blind, randomized, placebo-controlled cancer prevention trial. **SETTING:** Seven dermatology clinics in the eastern United States. **PATIENTS:** A total of 1312 patients (mean age, 63 years; range, 18-80 years) with a history of basal cell or squamous cell carcinomas of the skin were randomized from 1983 through 1991. Patients were treated for a mean (SD) of 4.5 (2.8) years and had a total follow-up of 6.4 (2.0) years. **INTERVENTIONS:** Oral administration of 200 microg of selenium per day or placebo.

MAIN OUTCOME MEASURES: The primary end points for the trial were the incidences of basal and squamous cell carcinomas of the skin. The secondary end points, established in 1990, were all-cause mortality and total cancer mortality, total cancer incidence, and the incidences of lung, prostate, and colorectal cancers.

RESULTS: After a total follow-up of 8271 person-years, selenium treatment did not significantly affect the incidence of basal cell or squamous cell skin cancer. There were 377 new cases of basal cell skin cancer among patients in the selenium group and 350 cases among the control group, and 218 new squamous cell skin cancers in the selenium group and 190 cases among the controls. Analysis of secondary end points revealed that, compared with controls, patients treated with selenium had a nonsignificant reduction in all-cause mortality (108 deaths in the selenium group and 129 deaths in the control group and significant reductions in total cancer mortality (29 deaths in the selenium treatment group and 57 deaths in controls, total cancer incidence (77 cancers in the selenium group and 119 in controls, and incidences of lung, colorectal, and prostate cancers. Primarily because of the apparent reductions in total cancer mortality and total cancer incidence in the selenium group, the blinded phase of the trial was stopped early. No cases of selenium toxicity occurred.

CONCLUSIONS: Selenium treatment did not protect against development of basal or squamous cell carcinomas of the skin. However, results from secondary end-point analyses support the hypothesis that **supplemental selenium may reduce the incidence of, and mortality from, carcinomas of several sites.** These effects of selenium **require confirmation** in an independent trial of appropriate design before new public health recommendations regarding selenium supplementation can be made. (Clark et al. 1996).

Alpha-Tocopherol and beta-carotene supplements and lung cancer incidence in the alpha-tocopherol, beta-carotene cancer prevention study: effects of base-line characteristics and study compliance. (Albanes et al, 1996) (#29,133 men, smokers)

Experimental and epidemiologic investigations suggest that alpha-tocopherol (the most prevalent chemical form of vitamin E found in vegetable oils, seeds, grains, nuts, and other foods) and beta-carotene (a plant pigment and major precursor of vitamin A found in many yellow, orange, and dark-green, leafy vegetables and some fruit) might reduce the risk of cancer, particularly lung cancer. The initial findings of the Alpha-Tocopherol, Beta-Carotene Cancer Prevention Study (ATBC Study) indicated, however, that lung cancer incidence was increased among participants who received beta-carotene as a supplement. Similar results were recently reported by the Beta-Carotene and Retinol Efficacy Trial (CARET), which tested a combination of beta-carotene and vitamin A.

PURPOSE: We examined the effects of alpha-tocopherol and beta-carotene supplementation on the incidence of lung cancer across subgroups of participants in the ATBC Study defined by base-line characteristics (e.g., age, number of cigarettes smoked, dietary or serum vitamin status, and alcohol consumption), by study compliance, and in relation to clinical factors, such as disease stage and histologic type. Our primary purpose was to determine whether the pattern of intervention effects across subgroups could facilitate further interpretation of the main ATBC Study results and shed light on potential mechanisms of action and relevance to other populations.

METHODS: A total of **29,133 men aged 50-69 years who smoked five or more cigarettes** daily were **randomly assigned** to receive **alpha-tocopherol (50 mg), beta-carotene (20 mg), alpha-tocopherol and beta-carotene, or a placebo daily for 5-8 years** (median, 6.1 years). Data regarding smoking and other risk factors for lung cancer and dietary factors were obtained at study entry, along with measurements of serum levels of alpha-tocopherol and beta-carotene. Incident cases of lung cancer (n = 894) were identified through the Finnish Cancer Registry and death certificates. Each lung cancer diagnosis was independently confirmed, and histology or cytology was available for 94% of the cases. Intervention effects were evaluated by use of survival analysis and proportional hazards models. All P values were derived from two-sided statistical tests.

RESULTS: No overall effect was observed for lung cancer from alpha-tocopherol supplementation. *beta-Carotene supplementation was associated with increased lung cancer risk.* The beta-carotene effect appeared stronger, but not substantially different, in participants who smoked at least 20 cigarettes daily compared with those who smoked five to 19 cigarettes daily and in those with a higher alcohol intake compared with those with a lower intake.

CONCLUSIONS: Supplementation with alpha-tocopherol or beta-carotene does not prevent lung cancer in older men who smoke. *beta-Carotene supplementation at pharmacologic levels may modestly increase lung cancer incidence in cigarette smokers*, and this effect may be associated with heavier smoking and higher alcohol intake.

IMPLICATIONS: While the most direct way to reduce lung cancer risk is not to smoke tobacco, **smokers should avoid high-dose beta-carotene supplementation.** (Albanes et al, 1996).

Circa 1997

No effect of supplementation with vitamin E, ascorbic acid, or coenzyme Q10 on oxidative DNA damage estimated by 8-oxo-7,8-dihydro-2'-deoxyguanosine excretion in smokers. (Priemé et al. 1997) (#142 smoking men). The protective effect of fruit and vegetables against cancer has been related to their high antioxidant content. However, **results from intervention trials have not been conclusive on the protective effect of antioxidant supplementation.** In a randomized placebo-controlled trial we investigated the effect of dietary supplementation with antioxidants on a biomarker of oxidative DNA damage with mechanistic relation to carcinogenesis. One hundred forty-two smoking men aged 35-65 y were randomly assigned to one of the following seven treatments for 2 mo: 100 mg D-alpha-tocopheryl acetate plus 250 mg slow-release ascorbic acid twice a day (n = 20), 100 mg D-alpha-tocopheryl acetate twice a day (n = 20), 250 mg ascorbic acid twice a day (n = 21), 250 mg slow-release ascorbic acid twice a day (n = 21), 30 mg coenzyme Q10 in oil three times a day (n = 20), 30 mg coenzyme Q10 as granulate three times a day (n = 20), or placebo twice a day (n = 20). The trial outcome was the urinary excretion rate of 8-oxo-7, 8-dihydro-2'-deoxyguanosine (8-oxodG)-a repair product of oxidative DNA damage. **Two months of supplementation did not result in significant changes in the urinary excretion rate of 8-oxodG in any group. The lack of effect of antioxidant supplementation on the excretion rate of 8-oxodG, despite substantial increases in plasma antioxidant concentrations, agrees with the results from recent large intervention studies with cancer as an endpoint. The cancer-protective effect of fruit and vegetables seems to rely not on the effect of single antioxidants but rather on other anticarcinogenic compounds or on a concerted action of several micronutrients present in these foods** (Priemé H, Loft S, Nyyssönen K, Salonen JT, Poulsen HE. No effect of supplementation with vitamin E, ascorbic acid, or coenzyme Q10 on oxidative DNA damage estimated by 8-oxo-7,8-dihydro-2'-deoxyguanosine excretion in smokers. Am J Clin Nutr. 1997 Feb;65(2):503-7). 000

Preformed Vitamin A Study Showed No Trend to Reduce Breast Cancer Risk. (Longnecker, 1997) (#3,543 cases and 9,406 controls**)** Intake of fruits, vegetables, vitamin A, and related compounds are associated with a decreased **risk of breast cancer** in some studies, but additional data are needed. To estimate intake of beta-carotene and vitamin A, the authors included nine questions on food and supplement use in a population-based case-control study of breast cancer risk conducted in Maine, Massachusetts, New Hampshire, and Wisconsin in 1988-1991. Multivariate-adjusted models were fit to data for **3,543 cases and 9,406 controls**. Eating carrots or spinach more than twice weekly, compared with no intake, was associated with an odds ratio of 0.56. **Estimated intake of preformed vitamin A from all evaluated foods and supplements showed no trend or monotonic decrease in (breast cancer) risk across categories of intake.** These data do not allow us to distinguish among several potential explanations for the protective association observed between intake of carrots and spinach and risk of breast cancer. The findings are, however, consistent with a diet rich in these foods having a modest protective effect.

The majority of epidemiological studies have failed to find significant associations between retinol intake and breast cancer risk in women.

Circa 1998

SUVIMAX (Vasquez et al, 1998) (#13,017 French adults); take either a daily capsule containing **120 milligrams of ascorbic acid, 30 milligrams of vitamin E, six milligrams of beta carotene, 100 micrograms of selenium, and 20 milligrams of zinc**; or a placebo capsule; researchers found **no differences between the antioxidant and placebo group in terms of cancer incidence, or in cardiovascular disease incidence, or all-cause death.**

The Nurses' Health Study and Folic Acid and Colon Cancer (Giovannucci et al, 1998) (#88,756 women taking vitamin C and B-carotene, for 8 years); **No benefit with respect to colon cancer after 4 years of use and had no significant risk reductions after 5 to 9 or 10 to 14 years of use. Long-term use of over 15 years of multivitamins may substantially reduce risk for colon cancer.** This **effect may be related to the folic acid** contained in multivitamins.

Dr. Andy Ness, of Bristol University, reported in the British Medical Journal in Dec. 2004, that *there is the **possibility of increased risk of breast cancer in women taking folic acid supplements throughout pregnancy**. The researchers followed up **2,928 pregnant women** who had taken part in a supplemental trial in the

1960s. **The risk of death from breast cancer was much higher in women who had received high doses of the supplement than in those who had been given a placebo.** However, Godfrey Oakley and Jack Mandel, of Emory University, said other research studies indicate that more folic acid is likely to prevent breast cancer rather than cause it. **This is another glaring example of the contradictory and dangerous nature of the vitamin studies.**

Relationships of serum carotenoids, retinol, alpha-tocopherol, and selenium with breast cancer risk: results from a prospective study in Columbia, Missouri (United States). (Dorgan et al, 1998) (#105 cases of histologically confirmed breast cancer) To evaluate relationships of serum carotenoids, alpha-tocopherol, selenium, and retinol with breast cancer prospectively, we conducted a case-control study nested in a cohort from the Breast Cancer Serum Bank in Columbia, Missouri (United States). Women free of cancer donated blood to this bank in 1977-87. **During up to 9.5 years of follow-up** (median = 2.7 years), **105 cases of histologically confirmed breast cancer** were diagnosed. For each case, two women alive and free of cancer at the age of the case's diagnosis and matched on age and date of blood collection were selected as controls. A nonsignificant gradient of decreasing risk of breast cancer with increasing serum beta-cryptoxanthin was apparent for all women. Serum lycopene also was associated inversely with risk, and among women who donated blood at least two years before diagnosis, a significant gradient of decreasing breast cancer risk with increasing lycopene concentration was evident. A marginally significant gradient of decreasing risk with increasing serum lutein/zeaxanthin also was apparent among these women. **They did not observe any evidence for protective effects of alpha- and beta-carotene, alpha-tocopherol, retinol, or selenium for breast cancer.** Results of this study suggest that **the carotenoids beta-cryptoxanthin, lycopene, and lutein/zeaxanthin may protect against breast cancer**.

Two prospective studies did not observe significant associations between blood retinol levels and subsequent risk of developing breast cancer, i.e., Hulten and Dorgan.

The effects of antioxidant supplementation during Percoll preparation on human sperm DNA integrity (Hughes et al, 1998) (#150 patients) The integrity of sperm DNA is crucial for the maintenance of genetic health. A major source of damage is reactive oxygen species (ROS) generation; therefore, antioxidants may afford protection to sperm DNA. The objectives of the study were, first, to measure the effects of antioxidant supplementation in vitro on endogenous DNA damage in spermatozoa using the single cell gel electrophoresis (comet) assay and, second, to assess the effect of antioxidant supplementation given prior to X-ray irradiation on induced DNA damage. Spermatozoa from **150 patients** were prepared by Percoll centrifugation in the presence of **ascorbic acid (300, 600 microM), alpha tocopherol (30, 60 microM), urate (200, 400 microM), or acetyl cysteine (5, 10 microM).** DNA damage was induced by 30 Gy X-irradiation. DNA strand breakage was measured using the comet assay. **Sperm DNA was protected from DNA damage by ascorbic acid (600 microM), alpha tocopherol (30 and 60 microM) and urate (400 microM).** These antioxidants provided protection from subsequent DNA damage by X-ray irradiation. *In contrast, acetyl cysteine or ascorbate and alpha tocopherol together induced further DNA damage to human sperm.* Supplementation in vitro with the antioxidants ascorbate, urate and alpha tocopherol separately has beneficial effects for sperm DNA integrity.

Circa 1999

Women's Health Study (Lee et al., 1999) (#39,876 healthy women); 50 mg b-carotene (alternate days); No effect on incidence of cancer, CVD, or total mortality; no benefit or harm from beta-carotene supplementation after a median of 4.1 years on the incidence of cancer and of cardiovascular disease.

The beta-carotene part of the study was **stopped early,** *in 1996, when other studies showed no protection and even a possible risk of cancer.*

Beta carotene supplementation in prevention of basal-cell and squamous-cell carcinomas of the skin (Green et al, 1999) (#1,383 participants) **There was no beneficial or harmful effect on the rates of either type of skin cancer, as a result of beta carotene supplementation.**

Vitamins A, C and E and the Risk of Breast Cancer: results from a case-control study in Greece. (Bohlke et al, 1999) (#820 patients with breast cancer plus 1,548 controls) Although several dietary compounds are hypothesized to have anticarcinogenic properties, the role of specific micronutrients in the development of breast cancer remains unclear. To address this issue, **they assessed intake of retinol, b-carotene, vitamin C and vitamin E in relation to breast cancer risk** in a case–control study in Greece. **Eight hundred and twenty women with histologically confirmed breast cancer were compared with 1548 control women.** Dietary data were collected through a 115-item semiquantitative food frequency questionnaire. Data were modelled by logistic regression, with adjustment for total energy intake and established breast cancer risk factors, as well as mutual adjustment among the micronutrients. **Among post-menopausal women, there was no association between any of the micronutrients evaluated and risk of breast cancer.**

Among premenopausal women, beta-carotene, vitamin C and vitamin E were each inversely associated with breast cancer risk, but after mutual adjustment among the three nutrients only beta-carotene remained significant; the odds ratio (OR) for a one-quintile increase in beta-carotene intake was 0.84. The inverse association observed with beta-carotene intake, however, is slightly weaker than the association previously observed with vegetable intake in these data, raising the possibility that the observed beta-carotene effect is accounted for by another component of vegetables.

The effect of ascorbate and alpha-tocopherol supplementation in vitro on DNA integrity and hydrogen peroxide-induced DNA damage in human spermatozoa (Donnelly et al, <u>Mutagenesis</u>. 1999) (#Semen samples with normozoospermic and asthenozoospermic profiles (n = 15 for each control and antioxidant group) The aim of this study was to determine the effects of **supplementation with ascorbate and alpha-tocopherol, both singly and in combination**, during sperm preparation on subsequent sperm DNA integrity, induced DNA damage and reactive oxygen species (ROS) generation. Semen samples with normozoospermic and asthenozoospermic profiles (n = 15 for each control and antioxidant group) were prepared by Percoll density centrifugation where the medium had been supplemented with these antioxidants to a number of different concentrations, all within physiological levels. Controls were included which had no ascorbate or alpha-tocopherol added. DNA damage was induced using hydrogen peroxide (H_2O_2) and DNA integrity was determined using a modified alkaline single cell gel electrophoresis (Comet) assay, while ROS generation was measured using chemiluminescence. Addition of ascorbate to sperm preparation medium did not affect baseline DNA integrity but did provide sperm with complete protection against H_2O_2-induced DNA damage. Generation of H_2O_2-induced ROS was also significantly reduced after treatment with ascorbate, although baseline levels were unaffected by this antioxidant. Supplementation of sperm preparation medium with alpha-tocopherol did not influence baseline DNA integrity but provided sperm with dose-dependent protection against H_2O_2-induced DNA damage. Generation of H_2O_2-induced ROS was significantly reduced after treatment with alpha-tocopherol, although baseline ROS levels were unaffected by this antioxidant. **Addition of *both ascorbate and alpha-tocopherol in combination to sperm preparation medium actually induced DNA damage and intensified the damage induced by H_2O_2*, however, H_2O_2-induced ROS production was significantly**

reduced in a dose-dependent manner by supplementation with both vitamins.

Circa 2000

A randomized, 12-year primary-prevention trial of beta carotene supplementation for nonmelanoma skin cancer in the physician's health study. (Frieling et al, 2000) (#22,071)

Although basic research provides plausible mechanisms for benefits of beta carotene supplementation on nonmelanoma skin cancer (NMSC) primarily consisting of basal cell carcinoma (BCC) and squamous cell carcinoma (SCC), observational studies are inconsistent. Randomized trial data are limited to 1 trial of secondary prevention that showed no effect of beta carotene on the incidence of NMSC after 5 years.

OBJECTIVE: To test whether supplementation with beta carotene reduces the risk for development of a first NMSC, including BCC and SCC.

DESIGN: Randomized, double-blind, placebo-controlled trial with 12 years of beta carotene supplementation and follow-up. **SETTING:** Physicians' Health Study in the United States. **PARTICIPANTS:** Apparently healthy male physicians aged 40 to 84 years in 1982 **(N = 22,071). INTERVENTION:** Beta carotene, 50 mg, on alternate days.

MAIN OUTCOME MEASURE: Relative risk (RR) and 95% confidence interval (CI) for a first NMSC, BCC, and SCC. **RESULTS:** After adjusting for age and randomized aspirin assignment, there was no effect of beta carotene on the incidence of a first NMSC, BCC, or SCC. There was also no significant evidence of beneficial or harmful effects of beta carotene on NMSC by smoking status (current, past, or never).

CONCLUSION: This large-scale, randomized, primary prevention trial among apparently healthy well-nourished men indicates that an **average of 12 years of supplementation with beta carotene does not affect the development of a first NMSC, including BCC and SCC.** (Frieling et al, 2000).

Circa 2001

Dietary antioxidant vitamins, retinol, and breast cancer incidence in a cohort of Swedish women. (Michels et al, 2001) (#59,036 women free of cancer) Dietary antioxidant vitamins and retinol have been proposed to be protective against breast cancer on the basis of their ability to reduce oxidative DNA damage and their role in cell differentiation. Epidemiologic studies have not been convincing in supporting this hypothesis, but women with high exposure to free radicals and oxidative processes have not been specifically considered. They explored these issues in the Swedish Mammography Screening Cohort, a large population-based prospective cohort study in Sweden that comprised **59,036 women**, 40-76 years of age, who were free of cancer at baseline and who had answered a validated 67-item food frequency questionnaire. During 508,267 person-years of follow-up, 1,271 cases of invasive breast cancer were diagnosed. **There was no overall association between intake of ascorbic acid, beta-carotene, retinol or vitamin E and breast cancer incidence**. High intake of ascorbic acid was inversely related to breast cancer incidence among overweight women and women with high consumption of linoleic acid. Among women with a body mass index of 25 or below, the hazard ratio for breast cancer incidence was 1.27, comparing the highest to the lowest quintile of ascorbic acid intake. Consumption of foods high in ascorbic acid may convey protection from breast cancer among women who are overweight and/or have a high intake of linoleic acid.

Randomized Trial of Supplemental ß-Carotene to Prevent Second Head and Neck Cancer (Mayne et al, 2001) (#264 patients who had been curatively treated for a recent early-stage squamous cell carcinoma of the oral cavity, pharynx, or larynx.); randomized, placebo-controlled, double-blinded clinical trial; 50 mg of ß-carotene per day; After a median follow-up of 51 months, there **was no difference between the two groups** in the time to failure [second primary tumors plus local recurrences. **Supplemental ß-carotene had no significant effect on second head and neck cancer or lung cancer**. Whereas none of the effects were statistically significant, the **point estimates suggested a possible decrease in second head and neck cancer risk** *but a possible increase in lung cancer risk*.

Vitamin C and Vitamin E Supplement Use and Colorectal Cancer Mortality in a large American Cancer Society cohort. (Cancer Prevention Study II cohort - CPS-II) (Jacobs, 2001) (#711,891 men and women in U.S.A.)

Some recent epidemiological studies have suggested that use of vitamin C or vitamin E supplements, both of which are important antioxidants, may substantially reduce the risk of colon or colorectal cancer. They examined the association between colorectal cancer mortality and use of individual vitamin C and E supplements in the American Cancer Society's Cancer Prevention Study II cohort. We used proportional hazards modeling to estimate rate ratios among **711,891 men and women** in the United States who completed a self-administered questionnaire at study enrollment in 1982, had no history of cancer, and were followed for mortality through 1996. During the 14 years of follow-up, 4404 deaths from colorectal cancer occurred. After adjustment for multiple colorectal cancer risk factors, regular use of vitamin C or E supplements, even long-term use, was not associated with colorectal cancer mortality. The combined-sex rate ratios were 0.89 for 10 or more years of vitamin C use and 1.08) for 10 or more years of vitamin E use. In subgroup analyses, use of vitamin C supplements for 10 or more years was associated with decreased risk of colorectal cancer mortality before age 65 years and decreased risk of rectal cancer mortality at any age. **Our results do not support a substantial effect of vitamin C or E supplement use on overall colorectal cancer mortality.**

Risk of Ovarian Carcinoma and Consumption of Vitamins A, C and E and Specific Carotenoids: a prospective analysis. (Fairfield et al, 2001) (#80,326 women)

Antioxidant vitamins may decrease risk of cancer by limiting oxidative DNA damage leading to cancer initiation. Few prospective studies have assessed relations between antioxidant vitamins and ovarian carcinoma. METHODS: The authors prospectively assessed consumption of vitamins A, C, and E and specific carotenoids, as well as fruit and vegetable intake, in relation to ovarian carcinoma risk among Women reported on **known and suspected ovarian carcinoma risk 80,326 participants in the Nurses' Health Study who had no history of cancer other than nonmelanoma skin carcinoma.** factors including reproductive factors, smoking, and use of vitamin supplements on biennial mailed questionnaires from 1976 to 1996. Food frequency questionnaires were included in 1980, 1984, 1986, and 1990. The authors confirmed 301 incident cases of invasive epithelial ovarian carcinoma during 16 years of dietary follow-up (1980-1996). Pooled logistic regression was used to control for age, oral contraceptive use, body mass index, smoking history, parity, and tubal ligation. RESULTS: The authors observed no association between ovarian carcinoma risk and antioxidant vitamin consumption from foods, or foods and supplements together. The multivariate relative risks (95% confidence intervals [CIs]) for ovarian carcinoma among women in the highest versus lowest quintile of intake were 1.04 for vitamin A from foods and supplements; 1.01 for vitamin C; 0.88 for vitamin E; and 1.10 for beta-carotene. **Among users of vitamin supplements, the authors found no evidence of an association between dose or duration of any specific vitamin and ovarian carcinoma risk**, although the authors had limited power to assess these relations. **No specific fruits or vegetables were associated significantly** with ovarian carcinoma risk. **The authors found no association between ovarian carcinoma and consumption of total fruits or vegetables, or specific subgroups including cruciferous vegetables, green leafy vegetables, legumes, or citrus fruits. Women who consumed at least 2.5 total servings of fruits and vegetables as adolescents had a 46% reduction in ovarian carcinoma risk** (relative risk, 0.54, 95% CI, 0.29-1.03; P value for trend 0.04). CONCLUSIONS: **These data do not support an important relation between consumption of antioxidant vitamins from foods or supplements, or intake of fruits and vegetables, and incidence of ovarian carcinoma in this cohort.** However, modest associations cannot be excluded, and the authors' finding of an inverse association for total fruit and vegetable intake during adolescence raises the possibility that the pertinent exposure period may be much earlier than formerly anticipated.

As of 2010, new studies may be exposing another "medical myth." Investigators, writing in the Journal of the National Cancer Institute, are now telling us that **fruits and vegetables do not dramatically lower the risk of common diseases, including cancer.** Since the early 1980s, the dietary guidelines for Americans, published jointly by the USDA and the DHHS, have reflected the accumulated scientific research concerning diet and health. Early 1980 guidelines pertaining to nutrition and cancer were to "eat a variety of foods" and "eat foods with adequate starch and fiber." In 1990, "eat a variety of foods" remained a guideline but "choose a diet with plenty of vegetables, fruits, and grain products" replaced the starch and fiber reference. This mirrored the growing data suggesting a lowered risk of cancer with increased vegetable and fruit consumption. But, in 1995, grain products were placed ahead of vegetables and fruit in the guidelines to better reflect the structure of the USDA food pyramid. Other recommendations included the 1989 National Research Council *Diet and Health* report supporting consumption of 5 fruit and vegetable servings per day and the 1991 National Cancer Institute–DHHS sponsorship of the 5-A-Day Program. Public health guidelines for food oriented toward high vegetable and fruit consumption continued up to the present. This scenario led to the rising popularity of vitamin supplements from the 1980s until today, but there have been huge problems with these trends. First, the vitamin supplements were shown to lack the effect of vitamins acquired through the diet and second, vitamins A (beta carotene) and E (alpha tocopherol) were shown to have particularly harmful potential. Yet, recommendations promoting vegetable and fruit consumption remained a center piece, until now. A study of 500,000 Europeans joins a growing body of evidence undermining the high hopes that pushing "five-a-day" might slash Western cancer rates and it estimated that only around 2.5% of cancers could be averted by increasing fruit and vegetable intake. In short, **research has failed to substantiate the suggestion that as**

many as 50% of cancers could be prevented by boosting the public's consumption of fruit and vegetables.

This latest study, which analyzed recruits from 10 countries to the highly-regarded **European Prospective Investigation into Cancer and Nutrition, confirms that the association between fruit and vegetable intake and reduced cancer risk is indeed weak.** The team, led by researchers from the Mount Sinai School of Medicine, in New York, calculated for lifestyle factors such as smoking and exercise before drawing their conclusions.

Carotenoids, Alpha-tocopherols, and Retinol in Plasma and Breast Cancer Risk in Northern Sweden. (Hulten et al, 2001) (#201 cases and 290 referents) Using a nested case-referent design we evaluated the relationship between plasma levels of six carotenoids, alpha-tocopherol, and retinol, sampled before diagnosis, and later breast cancer risk. **Methods:** In total, 201 cases and 290 referents were selected from three population-based cohorts in northern Sweden, where all subjects donated blood samples at enrolment. All blood samples were stored at -80 degrees C. Cases and referents were matched for age, age of blood sample, and sampling centre. Breast cancer cases were identified through the regional and national cancer registries. **Results:** Plasma concentrations of carotenoids were positively intercorrelated. In analysis of three cohorts as a group **none of the carotenoids was found to be significantly related to the risk of developing breast cancer. Similarly, no significant associations between breast cancer risk and plasma levels of alpha -tocopherol or retinol were found.** However, **in postmenopausal women from a mammography cohort with a high number of prevalent cases, lycopene was significantly associated with a decreased risk of breast cancer.** A significant trend of an inverse association between lutein and breast cancer risk was seen in premenopausal women from two combined population-based cohorts with only incident cases. A non-significant reduced risk with higher plasma alpha -carotene was apparent throughout all the sub-analyses. **Conclusion: No significant associations were found between plasma levels of carotenoids, alpha -tocopherol or retinol and breast cancer risk in analysis of three combined cohorts.** However, results from stratified analysis by cohort membership and menopausal status suggest that lycopene and other plasma-carotenoids may reduce the risk of developing breast cancer and that menopausal status has an impact on the mechanisms involved.

Dietary antioxidant vitamins, retinol, and breast cancer incidence in a cohort of Swedish women. (Michels, 2001) (#59,036 women free of cancer)

Dietary antioxidant vitamins and retinol have been proposed to be protective against breast cancer on the basis of their ability to reduce oxidative DNA damage and their role in cell differentiation. Epidemiologic studies have not been convincing in supporting this hypothesis, but women with high exposure to free radicals and oxidative processes have not been specifically considered. We explored these issues in the Swedish Mammography Screening Cohort, a large population-based prospective cohort study in Sweden that comprised 59,036 women, 40-76 years of age, who were free of cancer at baseline and who had answered a validated 67-item food frequency questionnaire. During 508,267 person-years of follow-up, 1,271 cases of invasive breast cancer were diagnosed. Cox proportional hazards models were used to obtain hazard ratios (HRs) and 95% confidence intervals (CIs). **There was no overall association between intake of ascorbic acid, beta-carotene, retinol or vitamin E and breast cancer incidence.**

High intake of ascorbic acid was inversely related to breast cancer incidence among overweight women (HR=0.61; 95% CI 0.45-0.82, for highest quintile of intake among women with body mass index>25 kg/m(2)) and women with high consumption of linoleic acid (HR=0.72; 95% CI 0.52-1.02, for highest quintile of ascorbic acid intake and average consumption of more than 6 grams of linoleic acid per day). Among women with a body mass index of 25 or below, the hazard ratio for breast cancer incidence was 1.27, comparing the highest to the lowest quintile of ascorbic acid intake. Consumption of foods high in ascorbic acid may convey protection from breast cancer among women who are overweight and/or have a high intake of linoleic acid. (Michels, 2001).

Circa 2002

Mega-dose vitamins and minerals in the treatment of non-metastatic breast cancer: an historical cohort study (Lesperance et al, 2002) (#90 patients with non-metastatic breast cancer who received conventional treatment) a historical cohort of 90 patients with non-metastatic breast cancer who received conventional treatment (e.g., surgery, chemotherapy, radiation therapy, and hormonal therapy) either alone or in combination with high doses of b-carotene, vitamin C, niacin, selenium, coenzyme Q10, and/or zinc. **Breast cancer–specific survival (ie, patients censored only at death from breast cancer) and *disease-free survival were shorter in the nutrient-supplemented group than in the non-supplemented group*, but the differences were not statistically significant.**

Investigators stated that, "**It is troubling that both** (Lesperance et al, 2002 and Ferreira et al, 2004**) reported results suggesting poorer survival with concurrent administration of antioxidants and cytotoxic therapy.**"

Vitamin C and Vitamin E Supplement Use and Bladder Cancer Mortality in a Large Cohort of US Men and Women (Cancer Prevention Study II (CPS-II) (Jacobs et al., 2002) (#991,522 US adults in the Cancer Prevention Study II (CPS-II) cohort.); CPS-II participants completed a self-administered questionnaire at enrollment in 1982 and were followed regarding mortality through 1998. Regular vitamin C supplement use (≥15 times per month) was not associated with bladder cancer mortality, regardless of duration. Regular vitamin E supplement use for ≥10 years was associated with a reduced risk of bladder cancer mortality, but **regular use of shorter duration was not. Subjects who regularly consumed a vitamin E supplement for longer than 10 years had a reduced risk of death from bladder cancer. No benefit was seen from vitamin C supplements.**

Supplemental Vitamin C & E and Multivitamin use and Stomach Cancer Mortality in U.S.A. (Cancer Prevention Study II cohort - CPS-II) (Jacobs et al. Jan. 2002) (#1,045,923 in U.S.A.) Supplementation with antioxidant vitamins has been associated with decreased risk of stomach cancer or regression of precancerous lesions in high-risk areas of China and Colombia. We examined the association between stomach cancer mortality and regular use (> or =15 times per month) of individual vitamin C supplements, individual vitamin E supplements, and multivitamins among **1,045,923 United States adults in the Cancer Prevention Study II (CPS-II) cohort.** CPS-II participants completed a questionnaire at enrollment in 1982 and were followed for mortality through 1998. During follow-up, there were 1,725 stomach cancer deaths (1,127 in men and 598 in women). After adjustment for multiple potential stomach cancer risk factors, **vitamin C use at enrollment was associated with reduced risk of stomach cancer mortality.** However, this reduction in risk was observed only among participants with short duration use at enrollment. **There was no association between stomach cancer mortality and regular use of vitamin E or multivitamins, regardless of duration of use.** Our results suggest that **the use of vitamin C, vitamin E, or multivitamin supplements may not substantially reduce risk of stomach cancer mortality in North American** populations in which stomach cancer rates are relatively low. Our results do not rule out effects of vitamin supplementation in areas in which stomach cancer rates are high and stomach cancer etiology may differ.

As in any observational study, the effects of potential confounding factors need to be considered, which is particularly true in analyses of vitamin supplement use because regular vitamin users are generally more likely to practice "health-conscious" behaviors. **At this time researchers cannot confidently recommend vitamin E supplements for the prevention of cancer because the evidence on this issue is inconsistent and limited.**

A prospective study on supplemental vitamin E intake and risk of colon cancer in women and men. (Wu et al, 2002) (#87,998 females from the Nurses' Health Study and 47, 344 males from the Health Professionals Follow-up Study) (#135,332 total participants) They conducted a prospective study on the association between supplemental vitamin E and colon cancer in **87,998 females from the Nurses' Health Study and 47, 344 males from the Health Professionals Follow-up Study.** There was some suggestion that men with supplemental vitamin E intake of 300 IU/day or more may be at lower risk for colon cancer when compared with never users [multivariate relative risk (RR), 300-500 IU/day versus never users, 0.73; >or=600 IU/day versus never users = 0.70, but CIs included 1. **In women, there was no evidence for an inverse association between vitamin E supplementation and risk of colon cancer. Our findings do not provide consistent support for an inverse association between supplemental vitamin E and colon cancer risk.** Considering the paucity of epidemiological data on this association, further studies of vitamin E and colon cancer are warranted. 000

Selenium and vitamin E supplements for prostate cancer: evidence or embellishment? (Moyad et al. 2002) (# not available) Selenium and vitamin E are probably 2 of the most popular dietary supplements considered for use in the reduction of prostate cancer risk. This enthusiasm is reflected in the initiation of the **Selenium and Vitamin E Chemoprevention Trial (SELECT).** Is there sufficient evidence to support the use of these supplements in a large-scale prospective trial for patients who want to reduce the risk of prostate cancer? Results from numerous laboratory and observational studies support the use of these supplements, and data from recent prospective trials also add partial support. However, a closer analysis of the data reveals some interesting and unique associations. **Selenium supplements provided a benefit only for those individuals who had lower levels of baseline plasma selenium.** *Other subjects, with normal or higher levels, did not benefit and may have an increased risk for prostate cancer.* The concept that supplements reduce prostate cancer risk only in those at a higher risk and/or those with lower plasma levels of these compounds is supported by trials examining beta-carotene supplements. Smokers may be the only individuals who benefit, as has also been shown with vitamin E supplementation. In 4 recent prospective studies, vitamin E was found to reduce the risk of prostate cancer in past/recent and current smokers and those with low levels of this vitamin. *Vitamin E supplements in higher doses (> or =100 IU) were also associated with a higher risk of aggressive or fatal prostate cancer in nonsmokers from a past prospective study.* The dose of vitamin E in the SELECT trial (400 IU/day) is 8 times higher than what has been suggested to be effective (50 IU/day) by the largest randomized prospective trial in which the incidence rate of prostate cancer was used as an endpoint. Recent research also suggests that dietary vitamin E may be associated with a lower risk of prostate cancer than the vitamin E supplement. Additionally, **recent results from all past cardiovascular prospective, randomized trials suggest that vitamin E shows little benefit for cardiovascular disease risk, especially at the dose being used in the SELECT trial.** Other intriguing positive findings from past prospective studies of supplements suggest that aspirin and other nonsteroidal anti-inflammatory drugs have a role in reducing the risk of prostate cancer or other types of cancer (e.g., colon cancer). It may be time to conduct a large costly trial to reconsider the use of selenium and vitamin E supplements for the reduction of prostate cancer risk. Some evidence for the use of these supplements exists, but **serious embellishment of study findings may be leading to an inappropriate use of these supplements in a clinical setting.**

Moyad et al had published an article entitled, "Selenium and vitamin E supplements for prostate cancer: evidence or embellishment?" (Moyad et al, 2002).

Prospective study of carotenoids, tocopherols, and retinoid concentrations and the risk of breast cancer. (Sato et al, 2002) (#590)

Previous prospective studies have raised the possibility that the antioxidant properties of carotenoids and vitamin E (alpha-tocopherol) and the role of vitamin A (retinol) in cellular differentiation may be associated with a reduced risk of subsequent breast cancer. To investigate the association between serum and plasma **concentrations of retinol, retinyl palmitate, alpha-carotene, beta-carotene, beta-cryptoxanthin, lutein, lycopene, total-carotenoids, alpha-tocopherol, and gamma-tocopherol with subsequent development of breast cancer,** a nested case control study was conducted among female residents of Washington County, Maryland, who had donated blood for a serum bank in 1974 or 1989. Cases (n = 295) and controls (n = 295) were matched on age, race, menopausal status, and date of blood donation, and the analyses were stratified by cohort participation. Median concentrations of beta-carotene, lycopene, and total carotene were significantly lower in cases compared with controls in the 1974 cohort (13.1, 12.5, and 7.9% difference; P = 0.01, 0.04, and 0.04, respectively) and for lutein in the 1989 cohort (6.7% difference; P = 0.02). The risk of developing breast cancer in the highest fifth was approximately half of that of women in the lowest fifth for beta-carotene [odds ratio (OR) = 0.41; 95% confidence interval (CI) 0.22-0.79; P trend = 0.007], lycopene (OR = 0.55; 95% CI 0.29-1.06; P trend = 0.04), and total carotene (OR = 0.55; 95% CI 0.29-1.03; P trend = 0.02) in the 1974 cohort. **There was generally a protective association for other micronutrients in both cohorts, although none reached statistical significance.** The results suggest that carotenoids may protect against the development of breast cancer. (Sato et al, 2002).

Circa 2003

Vitamins E & A fail to reduce incidence or mortality of lung cancer: Cochrane Database Syst Rev. 2003. (Caraballoso et al., 2003) (#109,394 participants); **The electronic databases MEDLINE (1966-july 2001), EMBASE (1974-july 2001) and the Cochrane Controlled Trial Register (CENTRAL, Issue 3/2001) and bibliographies were searched. Duration of treatment varied from 2 to 12 years and follow-up was from two to five years. When beta-carotene was combined with retinol, data from a single study showed that there was a statistically significant,** *increased risk of lung cancer incidence and mortality* **in people with risk factors for lung cancer who took both vitamins. There is currently no evidence to support recommending vitamins such as alpha-tocopherol, beta-carotene or retinol, alone or in combination, to prevent lung cancer. A harmful effect was found for beta-carotene with retinol at pharmacological doses in people with risk factors for lung cancer.**

The researchers call their findings **"especially concerning"** because beta carotene doses are commonly included in over-the-counter vitamin supplements and multivitamin supplements that have been advocated for widespread use.

The study says that using vitamin supplements that contain beta carotene should be "actively discouraged" because of the increase in the risk of death. They also **recommend discontinuing study of beta carotene supplements because of their risk.**

Despite the negative findings of most of the clinical trials, **manufacturers continue to promote antioxidants as though they have been proven beneficial "wonder drugs."** Many also hype mixtures of beta-carotene and other carotenoids, which, they suggest, may provide the same benefits as fruits and vegetables, which they know is not true. **The FDA will not permit any of these**

substances to be labeled or marketed with claims that they can prevent disease. The increased death rate from lung cancer in smokers who took beta carotene is evidence enough that high doses of vitamins and minerals are not necessarily harmless and may be fatal.

Neoplastic and Antineoplastic Effects of Beta Carotene on Colorectal Adenoma Recurrence: Results of a Randomized Trial (Baron et al, 2003) (#864 subjects who had had an adenoma removed and were polyp-free); the effect of beta carotene supplementation on colorectal adenoma recurrence among subjects in a multicenter double-blind, placebo-controlled clinical trial of antioxidants for the prevention of colorectal adenomas. Results: **Among subjects who neither smoked cigarettes nor drank alcohol, beta-carotene was associated with a marked decrease in the risk of one or more recurrent adenomas, but beta carotene supplementation conferred a modest increase in the risk of recurrence among those who smoked.** *For participants who smoked cigarettes and also drank more than one alcoholic drink per day, beta carotene doubled the risk of adenoma recurrence.*

In 2003, the **U.S. Preventive Services Task Force** (an independent panel sponsored by the Agency for Healthcare Research and Quality) concluded that **"the evidence is insufficient to recommend for or against the use of supplements of vitamins A, C, or E; multivitamins with folic acid; or antioxidant combinations for the prevention of cancer or cardiovascular disease."**

Selenium supplementation and secondary prevention of nonmelanoma skin cancer in a randomized trial. (Duffield-Lillico, 2003) (#1,312). The Nutritional Prevention of Cancer Trial was a double-blind, randomized, placebo-controlled clinical trial designed to test whether selenium as selenized yeast (200 microg daily) could prevent nonmelanoma skin cancer among 1312 patients from the Eastern United States who had previously had this disease. Results from September 15, 1983, through December 31, 1993, showed no association between treatment and the incidence of basal and squamous cell carcinomas of the skin. This report summarizes the entire blinded treatment period, which ended on January 31, 1996. The association between treatment and time to first nonmelanoma skin cancer diagnosis and between treatment and time to multiple skin tumors overall and within subgroups, defined by baseline characteristics, was evaluated. Although results through the entire blinded period continued to show that selenium supplementation was not statistically significantly associated with the risk of basal cell carcinoma (hazard ratio [HR] = 1.09, 95% confidence interval [CI] = 0.94 to 1.26), *selenium supplementation was associated with statistically significantly elevated risk of squamous cell carcinoma* and of total nonmelanoma skin cancer.

Results from the Nutritional Prevention of Cancer Trial conducted among individuals at high risk of nonmelanoma skin cancer continue to demonstrate that selenium supplementation is ineffective at preventing basal cell carcinoma and that *it increases the risk of squamous cell carcinoma and total nonmelanoma skin cancer.* (Duffield-Lillico, 2003).

Incidence of cancer and mortality following alpha-tocopherol and beta-carotene supplementation: a post intervention follow-up. (Virtamo et al, 2003) (#25,563 men). In the Finnish Alpha-Tocopherol, Beta-Carotene Cancer Prevention (ATBC) Study, alpha-tocopherol supplementation decreased prostate cancer incidence, whereas beta-carotene increased the risk of lung cancer and total mortality. Post intervention follow-up provides information regarding duration of the intervention effects and may reveal potential late effects of these antioxidants.

OBJECTIVE: To analyze post intervention effects of alpha-tocopherol and beta-carotene on cancer incidence and total and cause-specific mortality.

DESIGN, SETTING, AND PARTICIPANTS: Post intervention follow-up assessment of cancer incidence and cause-specific mortality (6 years [May 1, 1993-April 30, 1999]) and total mortality (8 years [May 1, 1993-April 30, 2001]) of **25,563 men.** In the ATBC Study, 29 133 male smokers aged 50 to 69 years received **alpha-tocopherol (50 mg), beta-carotene (20 mg), both agents, or placebo daily for 5 to 8 years.** End point information was obtained from the Finnish Cancer Registry and the Register of Causes of Death. Cancer cases were confirmed through medical record review.

MAIN OUTCOME MEASURES: Site-specific cancer incidence and total and cause-specific mortality and calendar time-specific risk for lung cancer incidence and total mortality.

RESULTS: Overall post trial relative risk (RR) for lung cancer incidence (n = 1037) was 1.06 among recipients of beta-carotene compared with non-recipients. For prostate cancer incidence (n = 672), the RR was 0.88 for participants receiving alpha-tocopherol compared with nonrecipients. **No late preventive effects on other cancers were observed for either supplement.** There were 7.261 individuals who died by April 30, 2001, during the post trial follow-up period; the RR was 1.01 for alpha-tocopherol recipients vs nonrecipients and 1.07 for beta-carotene recipients vs nonrecipients. Regarding duration of intervention effects and potential late effects, the excess risk for beta-carotene recipients was no longer evident 4 to 6 years after ending the intervention and was primarily due to cardiovascular diseases.

CONCLUSIONS: The beneficial and adverse effects of supplemental alpha-tocopherol and beta-carotene disappeared during post intervention follow-up. The preventive effects of alpha-tocopherol on prostate cancer require confirmation in other trials. **Smokers should avoid beta-carotene supplementation.** (Virtamo et al, 2003).

Circa 2004

Cochrane Database Syst Rev. 2004: Vitamins E & A fail to reduce incidence or mortality of gastrointestinal cancer. (Cochrane Database Syst Rev.) (Bjelakovic et al, 2004) (#170,525 participants); **14 randomized trials (170,525 participants), assessing beta-carotene (9 trials), vitamin A (4 trials), vitamin C (4 trials), vitamin E (5 trials), and selenium (6 trials). Neither the fixed effect nor random effects meta-analyses showed significant effects of supplementation with antioxidants on the incidences of gastrointestinal cancers.** 000

Among the seven high-quality trials reporting on mortality (131,727 participants), the fixed effect unlike the random effects meta-analysis showed that *antioxidant supplements significantly increased mortality. Beta-carotene and vitamin A and beta-carotene and vitamin E significantly increased mortality,* while beta-carotene alone only tended to do so. **Selenium showed significant beneficial effect on gastrointestinal cancer incidences.** *When the selenium trials were excluded, both analyses showed a statistically significant increase in mortality, which was particularly strong in patients taking beta carotene and vitamin A.*

No single antioxidant or combination of antioxidants significantly reduced the incidence of esophageal, gastric, colorectal, pancreatic, or hepatic cancer.

CONCLUSIONS: **They could not find evidence that antioxidant supplements prevent gastrointestinal cancers. On the contrary,** *they seem to increase overall mortality.*

SU.VI.MAX Study (2004) (Hercberg et al, 2004) (#A total of 13,017 French adults (7,876 women aged 35-60 years and 5,141 men aged 45-60 years); **All participants took a single daily capsule of a combination of 120 mg of ascorbic acid, 30 mg of vitamin E, 6 mg of beta carotene, 100 mug of selenium, and 20 mg of zinc,** or a placebo. Median follow-up time was 7.5 years. RESULTS: **No major differences were detected between the groups in total cancer**

incidence, ischemic cardiovascular disease incidence or all-cause mortality. However, unexplainably, after 7.5 years, low-dose antioxidant supplementation lowered total cancer incidence and all-cause mortality in men but not in women.

A review of the epidemiological evidence for the 'antioxidant hypothesis' by the British Nutrition Foundation (the Food Standards Agency). (Stanner et al, 2004) (British Nutrition Foundation independent review) (an independent review of the scientific literature on the role of antioxidants in chronic disease prevention). The British Nutrition Foundation was recently commissioned by the Food Standards Agency to conduct a review of the government's research program on Antioxidants in Food. Part of this work involved an independent review of the scientific literature on the role of antioxidants in chronic disease prevention, which is presented in this paper. BACKGROUND: There is consistent evidence that diets rich in fruit and vegetables and other plant foods are associated with moderately lower overall mortality rates and lower death rates from cardiovascular disease and some types of cancer. The 'antioxidant hypothesis' proposes that vitamin C, vitamin E, carotenoids and other antioxidant nutrients afford protection against chronic diseases by decreasing oxidative damage. RESULTS: Although scientific rationale and observational studies have been convincing, **randomized primary and secondary intervention trials have failed to show any consistent benefit from the use of antioxidant supplements on cardiovascular disease or cancer risk, with some trials even suggesting possible harm in certain subgroups.** These trials have usually involved the administration of single antioxidant nutrients given at relatively high doses. The results of trials investigating the effect of a balanced combination of antioxidants at levels achievable by diet are awaited. CONCLUSION: **The suggestion that antioxidant supplements can prevent chronic diseases has not been proved or consistently supported by the findings of published intervention trials.** Further evidence regarding the efficacy, safety and appropriate dosage of antioxidants in relation to chronic disease is needed. The most prudent public health advice remains to increase the consumption of plant foods, as such dietary patterns are associated with reduced risk of chronic disease.

Fruit, vegetable, and antioxidant intake and all-cause, cancer, and cardiovascular disease mortality in a community-dwelling population in Washington County, Maryland (CLUE) (Genkinger et al. 2004) (#6,151). Higher intake of fruits, vegetables, and antioxidants may help protect against oxidative damage, thus lowering cancer and cardiovascular disease risk. This Washington County, Maryland, prospective study examined the association of fruit, vegetable, and antioxidant intake with all-cause, cancer, and cardiovascular disease death.

CLUE participants who donated a blood sample in 1974 and 1989 and completed a food frequency questionnaire in 1989 (N = 6,151) were included in the analysis. Participants were followed to date of death or January 1, 2002. Compared with those in the bottom fifth, participants in the highest fifth of fruit and vegetable intake had a lower risk of all-cause, cancer, and cardiovascular disease mortality. Higher intake of cruciferous vegetables was associated with lower risk of all-cause mortality. **No statistically significant associations were observed between dietary vitamin C, vitamin E, and beta-carotene intake and mortality.** Overall, **greater intake of fruits and vegetables was associated with lower risk of all-cause, cancer, and cardiovascular disease death.** These findings support the general health recommendation to consume multiple servings of fruits and vegetables (5-9/day).

Dietary carotenoids and risk of lung cancer in a pooled analysis of seven cohort studies. (Mannisto et al, 2004) (#399,765 participants)

Intervention trials with supplemental beta-carotene have observed either no effect or a harmful effect on lung cancer risk. Because food composition databases for specific carotenoids have only become available recently, epidemiological evidence relating usual dietary levels of these carotenoids with lung cancer risk is limited. We analyzed the association between lung cancer risk and intakes of specific carotenoids using the primary data from seven cohort studies in North America and Europe. Carotenoid intakes were estimated from dietary questionnaires administered at baseline in each study. We calculated study-specific multivariate relative risks (RRs) and combined these using a random-effects model. The multivariate models included smoking history and other potential risk factors. During follow-up of up to 7-16 years across studies, 3,155 incident lung cancer cases were diagnosed among **399,765 participants. beta-Carotene intake was not associated with lung cancer risk** (pooled multivariate RR = 0.98; 95% confidence interval, 0.87-1.11; highest versus lowest quintile). **The RRs for alpha-carotene, lutein/ zeaxanthin, and lycopene were also close to unity. beta-Cryptoxanthin intake was inversely associated with lung cancer risk** (RR = 0.76; 95% confidence interval, 0.67-0.86; highest versus lowest quintile). **These results did not change after adjustment for intakes of vitamin C (with or without supplements), folate (with or without supplements), and other carotenoids and multivitamin use.** The associations generally were similar among never, past, or current smokers and by histological type. Although smoking is the strongest risk factor for lung cancer, greater intake of foods high in beta-cryptoxanthin, such as citrus fruit, may modestly lower the risk. (Mannisto et al, 2004).

Circa 2005

Use of multivitamins and prostate cancer mortality in a large cohort of US men. (Stevens et al, 2005) (#475,726 men who were cancer-free). Investigators assessed the association between the use of multivitamins and prostate cancer mortality. METHODS: A total of 5585 deaths from prostate cancer were identified during 18 years of follow-up of 475,726 men who were cancer-free and provided complete information on multivitamin use at enrollment in the Cancer Prevention Study II (CPS-II) cohort in 1982. Cox proportional hazards modeling was used to measure the association between multivitamin use at baseline and death from prostate cancer and to adjust for potential confounders. RESULTS: **The death rate from prostate cancer was marginally higher among men who took multivitamins regularly** (> or =15 times/month) **compared to non-users; this risk was statistically significant only for those multivitamin users who used no additional (vitamin A, C, or E) supplements.** In addition, risk was greatest during the initial four years of follow-up. CONCLUSIONS: *Regular multivitamin use was associated with a small increase in prostate cancer death rates* in our study, and this association was limited to a subgroup of users.

HOPE-TOO Extension (Lonn et al, 2005) (#3,994 original study enrollees) **The Heart Outcomes Prevention Evaluation (HOPE) investigators report an extension of the 9,541-patient HOPE Vitamin E trial. In the 2.5-year extension of HOPE (HOPE-TOO)** 174 of the original 267 centers continued an extended follow-up. From these centers, **3,994** of the 7,030 original study enrollees who were still alive elected to continue the randomized vitamin E/placebo drug assignment. **After a mean of 7.2 years of follow-up, vitamin E did not significantly reduce the relative risk (RR) of total cancer incidence, of cancer death, or a composite of cardiovascular events including cardiovascular death, nonfatal myocardial infarction, and stroke, or of individual components of this composite end point. These findings of lack of benefit from vitamin E (natural source, 400 IU a-tocopheryl acetate) during the extended study are consistent with the original HOPE report and with recent meta-analyses of** Vivekananthan and Miller. *Another subgroup finding in HOPE-TOO was a vitamin E–associated increased risk of heart failure incidence that appeared in a secondary end point analysis in the 4.5-year report and persisted in the 7-year extended follow-up, as did the risk of hospitalization for heart failure.*

An increased risk of heart failure was associated with vitamin E supplementation in multiple analyses, including a 19% increased risk of all heart failure events and a 40% increase in the risk of hospital admission due to heart failure.

CONCLUSION: **In patients with vascular disease or diabetes mellitus, long-term vitamin E supplementation does not prevent cancer or major cardiovascular events and** *may increase the risk for heart failure.*

Patients in *the vitamin E group had a higher risk of heart failure and hospitalization for heart failure.* Similarly, among patients enrolled at the centers participating in the HOPE-TOO trial, **there were no differences in cancer incidence, cancer deaths, and major cardiovascular events, but** *higher rates of heart failure and hospitalizations for heart failure.*

The National Cancer Institute (NCI) issued a statement following the HOPE-TOO study as follows: **"NCI has never recommended that people take vitamin E outside a clinical trial for the prevention of cancer."**

Recent attempts the validate the teachings of the free radical theory, in the prevention of cardiovascular disease and cancer have failed, as demonstrated with vitamin E and beta carotene. Data on millions of patients have resulted in antioxidant failure and ineffectiveness in the prevention of disease. Moreover, **previously unrecognized risks caused by nutrient toxicity and nutrient interactions have surfaced during intervention studies.** (Lichtenstein and Russell, 2005). **My studies on millions of participants have found a failure of vitamins E and beta carotene to prevent CVD or cancer.**

Vitamin E in the primary prevention of cardiovascular disease and cancer: the Women's Health Study: a randomized controlled trial. *(Lee et al. 2005) (#39,876 healthy women)* "Vitamin E in the Primary Prevention of Cardiovascular Disease and Cancer" Basic research provides plausible mechanisms and observational studies suggest that apparently healthy persons, who self-select for high intakes of vitamin E through diet or supplements, have decreased risks of cardiovascular disease and cancer. **Randomized trials do not generally support benefits of vitamin E,** but there are few trials of long duration among initially healthy persons. Objective: To test whether vitamin E supplementation decreases risks of cardiovascular disease and cancer among healthy women. Design, Setting, and Participants In the Women's Health Study conducted between 1992 and 2004, 39,876 apparently healthy US women aged at least 45 years were randomly assigned to receive vitamin E or placebo and aspirin or placebo, using a 2 x 2 factorial design, and were followed up for an average of 10.1 years. Intervention: Administration of 600 IU of natural-source vitamin E on alternate days. Main Outcome Measures: Primary outcomes were a composite end point of first major cardiovascular event (nonfatal myocardial infarction, nonfatal stroke, or cardiovascular death) and total invasive cancer. Results: During follow-up, there were 482 major cardiovascular events in the vitamin E group and 517 in the placebo group, a nonsignificant 7% risk reduction. **There were no significant effects on the incidences of myocardial infarction, as well as ischemic or hemorrhagic stroke.** For cardiovascular death, there was a significant 24% reduction. **There was no significant effect on the incidences of total cancer (1437 cases in the vitamin E group and 1428 in the placebo group); or breast, lung, or colon cancers.**

Cancer deaths also did not differ significantly between groups. There was no significant effect of vitamin E on total mortality. The Women's Health Study particularly focused on bleeding at multiple sites, and found no overall increased rate of bleeding *but a small significantly increased risk for epistaxis among patients treated with vitamin E.* Conclusions The data from this large trial indicated that 600 IU of natural-source vitamin E taken every other day provided no overall benefit for major cardiovascular events or cancer, did not affect total mortality, and decreased cardiovascular mortality in healthy women. **These data do not support recommending vitamin E supplementation for cardiovascular disease or cancer prevention among healthy women.**

Randomized controlled trials like the WHS are considered the gold standard in medical research and provide the most reliable results.

A randomized trial of antioxidant vitamins to prevent second primary cancers in head and neck cancer patients. (Bairati et al, 2005 Apr 6) (#540 patients with stage I or II head and neck cancer treated by radiation therapy). We conducted a multicenter, **double-blind, placebo-controlled, randomized** chemoprevention trial 540 patients with stage I or II head and neck cancer treated by radiation therapy. Although low dietary intakes of antioxidant vitamins and minerals have been associated with higher risks of cancer, results of trials testing antioxidant supplementation for cancer chemoprevention have been equivocal. We assessed whether supplementation with antioxidant vitamins could reduce the incidence of second primary cancers among patients with head and neck cancer. Supplementation with alpha-tocopherol (400 IU/day) and beta-carotene (30 mg/day). In the course of the trial, **beta-carotene supplementation was discontinued after 156 patients had enrolled because of ethical concerns.** After a median follow-up of 52 months, second primary cancers and recurrences of the first tumor were diagnosed in 113 and 119 participants, respectively. The effect of supplementation on the incidence of second primary cancers varied over time. Compared with patients receiving placebo, *patients receiving alpha-tocopherol supplements had a higher rate of second primary cancers during the* *supplementation period* **but a lower rate after supplementation was discontinued.** Similarly, *the rate of having a recurrence or second primary cancer was higher during but lower after supplementation with alpha-tocopherol.* The proportion of participants free of second primary cancer overall after 8 years of follow-up was similar in both arms. CONCLUSIONS: *alpha-Tocopherol supplementation produced unexpected adverse effects on the occurrence of second primary cancers and on cancer-free survival.* (Bairati et al, 2005 Apr 6).

Note: *Patients taking an antioxidant were 1.65 times more likely to suffer a return of their original cancer during the three years they were on the supplement. The risk was highest among those taking only vitamin E (1.86 times higher).* Five years after they stopped taking the supplement, their recurrence risk had fallen to the same level as those in the placebo group. **Although suggestive of harm, these results were not statistically significant.**

Randomized trial of antioxidant vitamins to prevent acute adverse effects of radiation therapy in head and neck cancer patients (Bairati et al, 2005 Aug 20) (#540 patients with stage I or II head and neck cancer treated by radiation therapy) A randomized trial was conducted to determine whether supplementation with antioxidant vitamins could reduce the occurrence and severity of acute adverse effects of radiation therapy and improve quality of life without compromising treatment efficacy. During the course of the trial, **supplementation with beta-carotene was discontinued because of ethical concerns. Quality of life was not improved by the supplementation.** *The rate of local recurrence of the head and neck tumor tended to be higher in the supplement arm of the trial.* CONCLUSION: Supplementation with high doses of alpha-tocopherol and beta-carotene during radiation therapy could reduce the severity of treatment adverse effects. However, **this trial suggests that use of high doses of antioxidants as adjuvant therapy might compromise radiation treatment efficacy.**

Note: *Researchers were concerned to find that the rate of local recurrence (that is, a return of the original cancer) was 54 percent higher among patients on the combination pill than those on placebo.* There was a smaller but still worrisome increase among those on vitamin E only.

NCI COMMENT: "This is a large, well-done study with good compliance from the participants," said Eva Szabo, M.D., of the National Cancer Institute's Division of Cancer Prevention. "The results demonstrate that the use of vitamin E supplementation is not beneficial to patients with stage I or II head and neck cancer, either as a chemoprevention agent or to enhance quality of life during radiation therapy."

At about this point in 2005, the followers of the free radical theory were scrambling to explain the repeated RCT failures. **Despite overwhelming evidence on the damaging consequences of oxidative stress and its role in experimental diabetes, large scale clinical trials with classic antioxidants failed to demonstrate any benefit for diabetic patients** (Johansen et al, 2005).

Vitamin K3 triggers human leukemia cell death through hydrogen peroxide generation and histone hyperacetylation (Lin, Kang, Zheng, 2005) (#)

Vitamin K3 (VK3) is a well-known anticancer agent, but its mechanism remains elusive. In the present study, VK3 was found to simultaneously induce cell death, reactive oxygen species (ROS) generation, including superoxide anion (O_2^*-) and hydrogen peroxide (H_2O_2) generation, and histone hyperacetylation in **human leukemia HL-60 cells** in a concentration- and time-dependent manner. Catalase (CAT), an antioxidant enzyme that specifically scavenges H_2O_2, could significantly diminish both histone acetylation increase and cell death caused by VK3, whereas superoxide dismutase (SOD), an enzyme that specifically eliminates O_2^*-, showed no effect on both of these, leading to the conclusion that H_2O_2 generation, but not O_2^*- generation, contributes to VK3-induced histone hyperacetylation and cell death. This conclusion was confirmed by the finding that enhancement of VK3-induced H_2O_2 generation by vitamin C (VC) could significantly promote both the histone hyperacetylation and cell death. Further studies suggested that histone hyperacetylation played an important role in VK3-induced cell death, since sodium butyrate, a histone deacetylase (HDAC) inhibitor, showed no effect on ROS generation, but obviously potentiated VK3-induced histone hyperacetylation and cell death. Collectively, **these results demonstrate a novel mechanism for the anticancer activity of VK3, i.e., VK3 induced tumor cell death through H2O2 generation, which then further induced histone hyperacetylation.** (Lin et al, 2005).

Fruits and vegetables and ovarian cancer risk in a pooled analysis of 12 cohort studies. (Koushik et al, 2005) (#560,441 women)

Because fruits and vegetables are rich in bioactive compounds with potential cancer-preventive actions, increased consumption may reduce the risk of ovarian cancer. **Evidence on the association between fruit and vegetable intake and ovarian cancer risk has not been consistent.** We analyzed and pooled the primary data from 12 prospective studies in North America and Europe. Fruit and vegetable intake was measured at baseline in each study using a validated food-frequency questionnaire. To summarize the association between fruit and vegetable intake and ovarian cancer, study-specific relative risks (RR) were estimated using the Cox proportional hazards model, and then combined using a random-effects model. Among **560,441 women**, 2,130 cases of invasive epithelial ovarian cancer occurred during a maximum follow-up of 7 to 22 years across studies. **Total fruit intake was not associated with ovarian cancer risk**-the pooled multivariate RR for the highest versus the lowest quartile of intake was 1.06 [95% confidence interval (95% CI), 0.92-1.21; P value, test for trend = 0.73; P value, test for between-studies heterogeneity = 0.74]. Similarly, results for total vegetable intake indicated no significant association (pooled multivariate RR, 0.90; 95% CI, 0.78-1.04, for the highest versus the lowest quartile; P value, test for trend = 0.06; P value, test for between-studies heterogeneity = 0.31). Intakes of botanically defined fruit and vegetable groups and individual fruits and vegetables were also not associated with ovarian cancer risk. Associations for total fruits and vegetables were similar for different histologic types. These results suggest that **fruit and vegetable consumption in adulthood has no important association with the risk of ovarian cancer.** (Koushik et al, 2005).

Circa 2006

Multivitamin/mineral supplements and prevention of chronic disease. (Huang et al, 2006 May) OBJECTIVES: To review and synthesize published literature on the efficacy of multivitamin/mineral supplements and certain single nutrient supplements in the primary prevention of chronic disease in the general adult population, and on the safety of multivitamin/mineral supplements and certain single nutrient supplements, likely to be included in multivitamin/mineral supplements, in the general population of adults and children. DATA SOURCES: All articles published through February 28, 2006, on MEDLINE, EMBASE, and the Cochrane databases. REVIEW METHODS: Each article underwent double reviews on title, abstract, and inclusion eligibility. Two reviewers performed data abstraction and quality assessment. **Differences in opinion were resolved through consensus adjudication.** RESULTS: Few trials have addressed the efficacy of multivitamin/ mineral supplement use in chronic disease prevention in the general population of the United States. One trial on poorly nourished Chinese showed supplementation with combined Beta-carotene, vitamin E and selenium reduced gastric cancer incidence and mortality, and overall cancer mortality. In a French trial, combined vitamin C, vitamin E, Beta-carotene, selenium, and zinc reduced cancer risk in men but not in women. No cardiovascular benefit was evident in both trials. **Multivitamin/ mineral supplement use had no benefit for preventing cataract.** Zinc/ antioxidants had benefits for preventing advanced age-related macular degeneration in persons at high risk for the disease. **With few exceptions, neither Beta-carotene nor vitamin E had benefits for preventing cancer, cardiovascular disease, cataract, and age-related macular degeneration.** *Beta-carotene supplementation increased lung cancer risk in smokers and persons* *exposed to asbestos.* **Folic acid alone or combined with vitamin B12 and/ or vitamin B6 had no significant effects on cognitive function.** Selenium may confer benefit for cancer prevention but not cardiovascular disease prevention. Calcium may prevent bone mineral density loss in postmenopausal women, and may reduce vertebral fractures, but not non-vertebral fractures. The evidence suggests dose-dependent benefits of vitamin D with/without calcium for retaining bone mineral density and preventing hip fracture, non-vertebral fracture and falls. **We found no consistent pattern of increased adverse effects of multivitamin/mineral supplements except for skin yellowing by Beta-carotene.** CONCLUSIONS: Multivitamin/mineral supplement use may prevent cancer in individuals with poor or suboptimal nutritional status. The heterogeneity in the study populations limits generalization to United States population. **Multivitamin/ mineral supplements conferred no benefit in preventing cardiovascular disease or cataract,** and may prevent advanced age-related macular degeneration only in high-risk individuals. The overall quality and quantity of the literature on the safety of multivitamin/mineral supplements is limited.

The Efficacy and Safety of Multivitamin and Mineral Supplement Use To Prevent Cancer and Chronic Disease in Adults: A Systematic Review for a National Institutes of Health State-of-the-Science Conference. (Huang et al, 2006 Sept)

BACKGROUND: Multivitamin and mineral supplements are the most commonly used dietary supplements in the United States. PURPOSE: To synthesize studies on the efficacy and safety of multivitamin/mineral supplement use in primary prevention of cancer and chronic disease in the general population. DATA SOURCES: English-language literature search of the MEDLINE, EMBASE, and Cochrane databases through February 2006 and hand-searching of pertinent journals and articles. STUDY SELECTION: **Randomized, controlled trials** in adults were reviewed to assess efficacy, and **randomized, controlled trials and observational studies in adults or children were reviewed to assess safety.** DATA EXTRACTION: Paired reviewers extracted data and independently assessed study quality. DATA SYNTHESIS: 12 articles from 5 randomized, controlled trials that assessed efficacy and 8 articles from 4 randomized, controlled trials and 3 case reports on adverse effects were identified. Study quality was rated fair for the studies on cancer, cardiovascular disease, cataracts, or age-related macular degeneration and poor for the studies on hypertension. **In a poorly nourished Chinese population, combined supplementation with beta-carotene, alpha-tocopherol, and selenium reduced the incidence of and mortality rate from gastric cancer and the overall mortality rate from cancer by 13% to 21%. In a French trial, combined supplementation with vitamin C, vitamin E, beta-carotene,**

selenium, and zinc reduced the rate of cancer by 31% in men but not in women. Multivitamin and mineral supplements had no significant effect on cardiovascular disease or cataracts, except that combined beta-carotene, selenium, alpha-tocopherol, retinol, and zinc supplementation reduced the mortality rate from stroke by 29% in the Linxian study and that a combination of 7 vitamins and minerals stabilized visual acuity loss in a small trial. **Combined zinc and antioxidants slowed the progression of advanced age-related macular degeneration in high-risk persons.** No consistent adverse effects of multivitamin and mineral supplements were evident. LIMITATIONS: Only randomized, controlled trials were considered for efficacy assessment. Special nutritional needs, such as use of folic acid by pregnant women to prevent birth defects, were not addressed. Findings may not apply to use of commercial multivitamin supplements by the general U.S. population. CONCLUSIONS: **Evidence is insufficient to prove the presence or absence of benefits from use of multivitamin and mineral supplements to prevent cancer and chronic disease.**

Antioxidants Vitamin C and Vitamin E for the Prevention and Treatment of Cancer (Coulter et al, 2006) (Thirty-eight studies); **The systematic review of the literature does not support the hypothesis that the use of supplements of vitamin C or vitamin E in the doses tested helps prevent and/ or treat cancer in the populations tested. The findings from randomized clinical trials were generally negative.**

Meta-analysis: antioxidant supplements for primary and secondary prevention of colorectal adenoma (2006) (Bjelakovic et al., 2006) (#17,620 participants); eight randomized trials **(17,620 participants). Neither fixed-effect nor random-effect model meta-analyses showed statistically significant effects of supplementation with beta-carotene, vitamins A, C, E and selenium alone or in combination. They found no convincing evidence that antioxidant supplements have significant beneficial effect on primary or secondary prevention of colorectal adenoma.**

Supplemental and dietary vitamin E, beta-carotene, and vitamin C intakes and prostate cancer risk (PLCO Trial) (Kirsh et al, 2006) (#29,361 men during up to 8 years of follow-up); the screening arm of the Prostate, Lung, Colorectal, and Ovarian Cancer Screening Trial; Overall, **there was no association between prostate cancer risk and dietary or supplemental intake of vitamin E, beta-carotene, or vitamin C. CONCLUSIONS: Our results do not provide strong support for population-wide implementation of high-dose antioxidant supplementation for the prevention of prostate cancer.** However, vitamin E supplementation in male smokers and beta-carotene supplementation in men with low dietary beta-carotene intakes were associated with reduced risk of this disease.

Intakes of vitamins A, C and E and folate and multivitamins and lung cancer: a pooled analysis of 8 prospective studies. (Cho et al, 2006) (#430,281 persons over a maximum of 6-16 years in the studies)

Intakes of **vitamins A, C and E and folate** have been hypothesized to reduce lung cancer risk. We examined these associations in a pooled analysis of the primary data from 8 prospective studies from North America and Europe. Baseline vitamin intake was assessed using a validated food-frequency questionnaire, in each study. We calculated study-specific associations and pooled them using a random-effects model. During follow-up of 430,281 persons over a maximum of 6-16 years in the studies, 3,206 incident lung cancer cases were documented. Vitamin intakes were inversely associated with lung cancer risk in age-adjusted analyses; the associations were greatly attenuated after adjusting for smoking and other risk factors for lung cancer. The pooled multivariate relative risks, comparing the highest vs. lowest quintile of intake from food-only, were 0.96 for vitamin A, 0.80 for vitamin C, 0.86 for vitamin E and 0.88 for folate. The association with vitamin C was not independent of our previously reported inverse association with beta-cryptoxanthin. Further, **vitamin intakes from foods plus supplements were not associated with a reduced risk of lung cancer in multivariate analyses, and use of multivitamins and specific vitamin supplements was not significantly associated with lung cancer risk.** The results generally did not differ across studies or by sex, smoking habits and lung cancer cell type. In conclusion, **these data do not support the hypothesis that intakes of vitamins A, C and E and folate reduce lung cancer risk.**

In discussing the role of micronutrients, Shenkin said, "Micronutrients play a central role in metabolism and in the maintenance of tissue function, but effects in preventing or treating disease which is not due to micronutrient deficiency cannot be expected from increasing the intake. **Provision of excess supplements to individuals who do not need them may be harmful.** Clinical benefit is most likely in those individuals who are severely depleted and at risk of complications, and is unlikely if this is not the case. Much more research is needed to characterize better markers of micronutrient status both in terms of metabolic effects and antioxidant effects (Shenkin, 2006).

In 2009, Park et al. said, "Older adults are particularly vulnerable to deficiencies of calcium, vitamin D, and vitamin B12. Although **MVM supplements have not been shown to prevent several major chronic diseases,** they do substantially

Prof Randolph M. Howes MD, PhD

increase vitamin and mineral intakes and blood concentrations, thus improving overall micronutrient status. (Park et al, 2008).

Dietary supplementation with different vitamin C doses: no effect on oxidative DNA damage in healthy people. (Herbert et al. 2006) (#160 volunteers). Antioxidants are believed to prevent many types of disease. Some previous studies suggest that dietary supplementation with vitamin C results in a decrease in the level of one of the markers of oxidative damage-8-oxoguanine in the DNA of peripheral blood mononuclear cells (PBMC). AIM OF TRIAL: To investigate the effect of different dose levels of dietary supplementation with vitamin C on oxidative DNA damage. METHODS: A **randomized double-blind placebo-controlled trial** was carried out using three different levels (80, 200 and 400 mg) of dietary vitamin C supplementation in a healthy population of **160 volunteers**; supplementation was for a period of 15 weeks followed by a 10 week washout period. Peripheral blood samples were obtained every 5 weeks from baseline to 25 weeks.

RESULTS: An increase in PBMC vitamin C levels was not observed following supplementation in healthy volunteers. **There was no effect found on 8-oxoguanine measured using HPLC with electrochemical detection for any of the three supplemented groups compared to placebo.** 8-oxoadenine levels were below the limit of detection of the HPLC system used here. CONCLUSIONS: **Supplementation with vitamin C had little effect on cellular levels in this group of healthy individuals,** suggesting their diets were replete in vitamin C. The dose range of vitamin C used did not affect oxidative damage in PBMC DNA.

Smoking, alcohol drinking, green tea consumption and the risk of esophageal cancer in Japanese men. (Ishikawa et al, 2006) (#9,008 men in Cohort 1 and 17,715 men in Cohort 2)

Although smoking and alcohol drinking are established risk factors of esophageal cancer, their public health impact is unclear. Furthermore, the effect of green tea is controversial.

METHODS: The present study was based on a pooled analysis of two prospective cohort studies. A self-administered questionnaire about health habits was distributed to **9,008 men in Cohort 1 and 17,715 men in Cohort 2**, aged 40 years or older, with no previous history of cancer. We identified 38 and 40 patient cases with esophageal cancer among the subjects in Cohort 1 (9.0 years of follow-up) and Cohort 2 (7.6 years of follow-up), respectively. Cox proportional hazards regression was used to estimate hazard ratios (HRs) of the risk of esophageal cancer incidence.

RESULTS: *Cigarette smoking, alcohol drinking and green tea consumption were significantly associated with an increased risk of esophageal cancer.* Compared with men who had never smoked, never drunk alcohol or green tea, the pooled multivariate HRs for men who were currently smoking > or =20 cigarettes/day, drinking alcohol daily, or drinking > or =5 cups green tea/day, respectively. *The population attributable fractions of esophageal cancer incidence that was attributable to smoking, alcohol drinking and green tea consumption were 72.0%, 48.6%, and 22.1%, respectively.*

CONCLUSIONS: Among the variables studied, *smoking has the largest public health impact on esophageal cancer incidence in Japanese men, followed by alcohol drinking and green tea drinking* (Ishikawa et al, 2006).

Intake of major carotenoids and the risk of epithelial ovarian cancer in a pooled analysis of 10 cohort studies. (Koushik et al, 2006) (#521,911 women)

Carotenoids, found in fruits and vegetables, have the potential to protect against cancer because of their properties, including their functions as precursors to vitamin A and as antioxidants. We examined the associations between intakes **of alpha-carotene, beta-carotene, beta-cryptoxanthin, lutein/zeaxanthin and lycopene and the risk of invasive epithelial ovarian cancer.** The primary data from 10 prospective cohort studies in North America and Europe were analyzed and then pooled. Carotenoid intakes were estimated from a validated food frequency questionnaire administered at baseline in each study. Study-specific relative risks (RR) were estimated using the Cox proportional hazards model and then combined using a random-effects model. Among 521,911 women, 2,012 cases of ovarian cancer occurred during a follow-up of 7-22 years across studies. **The major carotenoids were not significantly associated with the risk of ovarian cancer.** The pooled multivariate RRs (95% confidence intervals) were 1.00 (0.95-1.05) for a 600 microg/day increase in alpha-carotene intake, 0.96 for a 2,500 microg/day increase in beta-carotene intake, 0.99 for a 100 microg/day increase in beta-cryptoxanthin intake, 0.98 for a 2,500 microg/day increase in lutein/zeaxanthin intake and 1.01 for a 4,000 microg/day increase in lycopene intake. These associations did not appreciably differ by study (p-values, tests for between-studies heterogeneity >0.17). Also, the observed associations did not vary substantially by subgroups of the population or by histological type of ovarian cancer. **These results suggest that consumption of the major carotenoids during adulthood** does not play a major role in the incidence of ovarian cancer. (Koushik et al, 2006).

Circa 2007

Multivitamin Use and Risk of Prostate Cancer in the National Institutes of Health–AARP Diet and Health Study (Lawson et al, 2007) (#295,344 men); investigated the association between multivitamin use and prostate cancer risk; *use of multivitamins more than seven times per week, when compared with never use, was associated with a doubling in the risk of fatal prostate cancer* (The study of Lawson et al. is observational, and therefore confounding by indication and other confounding cannot be excluded. But the sample studied is very large, which reduces random errors, and the study seems well conducted.) **According to Victoria Stevens of the American Cancer Society, "There certainly is no evidence in healthy, relatively well-nourished people that vitamins or anti-oxidants protect against chronic diseases."**

The results are in accord with the results of systematic reviews and meta-analyses of randomized clinical trials (Vivekananthan et al., 2003) (Bjelakovic et al, Cochrane Database Syst Rev. 2004) (Stevens et al, 2005) (Bjelakovic et al, 2007) (Caraballoso et al., 2003).

Lawson et al. add to the growing evidence that questions the beneficial value of antioxidant vitamin pills in generally well-nourished populations and underscore the possibility that antioxidant supplements could have unintended consequences for our health.

Health Professionals Follow-up Study (2007): Effect of vitamins C, E, A and carotenoids and the occurrence of oral pre-malignant lesions. (Maserejian et al, 2007) (#42,340 men enrolled in the Health Professionals Follow-up Study) (#207 found with oral premalignant lesions); researchers found no clear relationship with beta-carotene, lycopene, or lutein/zeaxanthin. **A trend for** *increased risk of oral pre-malignant lesions was observed with vitamin E, especially among current smokers and with vitamin E supplements. Beta-carotene also increased the risk among current smokers.* However, **dietary vitamin C was significantly associated with a reduced risk of oral pre-malignant lesions**: those with the highest intake had a 50 percent reduction in risk compared to those with the lowest intake.

The role of vitamin E in the prevention of cancer: a meta-analysis of randomized controlled trials. (Alkhenizan and Hafez, 2007) (#167,025 subjects)

There are conflicting results in published randomized controlled trials (RCTs) on the role of vitamin E in the prevention of cancer. We conducted a meta-analysis of RCTs to evaluate the role of vitamin E in the prevention of cancer in adults. METHODS: We included RCTs in which the outcomes of the intake of vitamin E supplement alone or with other supplements were compared to a control group. The primary outcomes were total mortality, cancer mortality, total incidence of cancer, and incidence of lung, stomach, esophageal, pancreatic, prostate, breast and thyroid cancers. All identified trials were reviewed independently by the two reviewers to determine whether trials should be included or excluded. The quality of all included studies was scored independently by the two reviewers. RESULTS: Twelve studies, which included **167,025 participants**, met the inclusion criteria. There were no statistically significant differences in total mortality among the different groups of patients included in this meta-analysis. **Vitamin E was associated with a significant reduction in the incidence of prostate cancer, but it did not reduce the incidence of any other types of cancer.** CONCLUSIONS: **Vitamin E supplementation was not associated with a reduction in total mortality, cancer incidence, or cancer mortality,** but it **was associated with a statistically significant reduction in the incidence of prostate cancer.** Vitamin E can be used in the prevention of prostate cancer in men who are at high risk of prostate cancer. **This recently published meta-analysis of 12 randomized controlled trials concluded that vitamin E supplementation was not associated with overall cancer incidence, cancer mortality, or total mortality.**

Chemoprevention of Primary Liver Cancer: A Randomized, Double-Blind Trial in Linxian, China. (Qu et al, 2007) (#29,450 initially healthy adults) Primary liver cancer is a common malignancy with a dismal prognosis. New primary prevention strategies are needed to reduce mortality from this disease. They examined the effects of supplementation with four different combinations of vitamins and minerals on primary liver cancer mortality among **29,450** initially healthy adults from Linxian, China. Methods: Participants were randomly assigned to take either a vitamin–mineral combination ("factor") or a placebo daily for 5.25 years (March 1986–May 1991). **Four factors (at doses one to two times the US Recommended Daily Allowance)—retinol and zinc (factor A); riboflavin and niacin (factor B); ascorbic acid and molybdenum (factor C); and beta-carotene, alpha-tocopherol, and selenium (factor D)—were tested in a partial factorial design.** The study outcome was primary liver cancer death occurring from 1986 through 2001. Adjusted Cox proportional hazards models were used to calculate hazard ratios (HRs) and 95% confidence intervals (CIs) of liver cancer death with and without each factor. All P values are two-sided. Results: A total of 151 liver cancer deaths occurred during the analysis period. **No**

**statistically significant differences in liver cancer mortality were found
comparing the presence and absence of any of the four intervention factors.** However, **both factor A and factor B reduced liver cancer mortality
in individuals younger than 55 years at randomization but not in older individuals.** Factor C reduced liver cancer death, albeit with only borderline statistical significance in males but not in females. Cumulative risks of liver cancer death
were 6.0 per 1000 in the placebo arm, 5.4 per 1000 in the arms with two factors,
and 2.4 per 1000 in the arm with all four factors. Conclusion: **None of the factors tested reduced overall liver cancer mortality.**000 However, **three factors reduced liver cancer mortality in certain subgroups.**

As of 2007, no study had yet provided conclusive evidence of the beneficial effect
of antioxidant supplementation in critically ill patients. The clinical evidence provided so far showed that there are several factors which might determine the efficacy of antioxidant supplementation in critically ill patients. There may be a need
for large multi-center prospective randomized control trials to assess the effects
of different types and doses of antioxidant supplementation in selected groups
of patients with different types of critical illness. In critical illness, overwhelming
inflammatory mediator response to infective or non-infective stimuli results in excessive production of free radicals (Mishra, 2007). **I believe that the increased
production of EMODs during periods of illness are "a natural protective
response to illness."**

**Antioxidant Supplementation Increases the Risk of Skin Cancers in
Women but Not in Men.** (Hercberg et al, 2007) (#French adults, 7,876 women
and 5,141 men. Total # = 13,017). This research aimed to test whether supplementation with a combination of antioxidant vitamins and minerals could reduce
the risk of **skin cancers (SC).** It was performed within the framework of the
**Supplementation in Vitamins and Mineral Antioxidants study, a random-
ized, double-blinded, placebo-controlled, primary prevention trial** testing
the efficacy of nutritional doses of antioxidants in reducing incidence of cancer and
ischemic heart disease in the general population. French adults (7,876 women and
5,141 men) were randomized to take an oral daily capsule of antioxidants (120 mg
vitamin C, 30 mg vitamin E, 6 mg ß-carotene, 100 μg selenium, and 20 mg zinc) or
a matching placebo. The median time of follow-up was 7.5 y. A total of 157 cases of
all types of SC were reported, from which 25 were melanomas. Because the effect
of antioxidants on SC incidence varied according to gender, men and women were
analyzed separately. *In women, the incidence of SC was higher in the antioxidant group.* **Conversely, in men, incidence did not differ between the 2
treatment groups.** Despite the small number of events, *the incidence of melanoma was also higher in the antioxidant group for women.* The incidence of

nonmelanoma SC did not differ between the antioxidant and placebo groups. Our findings suggest that antioxidant supplementation affects the incidence of SC differentially in men and women. (Hercberg et al, 2007).

National Institutes of Health State-of-the-Science Conference Statement: Multivitamin/Mineral Supplements and Chronic Disease Prevention (NIH State-of-the Science Panel. 2007). At least half of American adults take a dietary supplement, the majority of which are multivitamin/multimineral (MVM) supplements. As more and more Americans seek strategies for maintaining good health and preventing disease, and as the marketplace offers an increasing number of products to fulfill that desire, **it is important that consumers have the best possible information to make their choices.** Assessing the available scientific evidence on the benefits of MVM supplement use for chronic disease prevention, identifying the gaps in the evidence, and recommending an appropriate research agenda to meet the shortfalls are subjects considered in this report.

Most people assume that the ingredients in MVM supplements are safe. There is evidence, however, that certain ingredients in MVM supplements can produce adverse effects, including **reports from RCTs that noted excess lung cancer occurring in asbestos workers and smokers consuming b-carotene.** In addition, *esophageal cancer excess was found with long-term follow-up of older Chinese patients (the Linxian study by Blot et al.) treated with selenium, b-carotene, and vitamin E supplements* (Blot et al, 1993) (NIH State-of-the Science Panel. 2007).

Tumor-targeted induction of oxystress for cancer therapy (Fang, Nakamura, Iyer, 2007) (#) Reactive oxygen species (ROS), such as superoxide anion radicals (O_2^{*-}) and hydrogen peroxide (H_2O_2) are potentially harmful by-products of normal cellular metabolism that directly affect cellular functions. ROS is generated by all aerobic organisms and it seems to be **indispensable for signal transduction pathways that regulate cell growth and reduction-oxidation (redox) status**. However, overproduction of these highly reactive oxygen metabolites can initiate lethal chain reactions, which involve oxidation and damage to structures that are crucial for cellular integrity and survival. In fact, **many antitumor agents, such as vinblastine, cisplatin, mitomycin C, doxorubicin, camptothecin, inostamycin, neocarzinostatin and many others exhibit antitumor activity via (EMOD) ROS-dependent activation of apoptotic cell death, suggesting potential use of ROS as an antitumor principle. Thus, a unique anticancer strategy named "oxidation therapy" has been developed by inducing cytotoxic oxystress for cancer treatment. This goal could be achieved mainly by two methods, namely, (i) inducing the generation**

of **ROS directly to solid tumors and (ii) inhibiting the antioxidative enzyme (defense) system of tumor cells.** Since 1950s, many strategies have been employed based on the first method, namely, administration of ROS per se (e.g. H_2O_2) or ROS generating enzyme to tumor bearing animals. However no successful and practical results were obtained probably because of the lack of tumor selective ROS delivery and hence resulting in subsequent induction of severe side effects. To overcome these obstacles, we developed polyethylene glycol (PEG) conjugated O_2^*- or H_2O_2-generating enzymes, xanthine oxidase (XO) and D-amino acid oxidase (DAO) (PEG-DAO) respectively. More recently, a pegylated (PEG) zinc protoporphyrin (PEG-ZnPP) and a highly water soluble micellar formulation of ZnPP based on amphiphilic styrene maleic acid (SMA) copolymer, SMA-ZnPP, are prepared, which are potent inhibitors of heme oxygenase-1 (HO-1). **HO-1 is a major antioxidative enzyme of tumors, that is different in mechanism of catalase or superoxide dismutase (SOD).** Consequently, both PEG-enzymes and PEG-ZnPP exhibited superior in vivo pharmacokinetics than their parental molecules, particularly in tumor delivery by taking advantage of the EPR effect of macromolecular nature, and thus showed remarkable antitumor effects suggesting the potentials of this anticancer therapeutic for clinical application. Furthermore, **it has been well known that many antioxidative enzymes such as catalase, SOD are down-regulated in most solid tumors in vivo.** On the contrary, **HO-1 is highly upregulated and it plays a very important role of antioxidation, because HO-1 generates biliverdin, which being converted to bilirubin exhibits a very potent antioxidative effect, and hence antiapoptosis in tumors.** Thus this oxidation therapy, by inhibiting this HO-1 dependent antioxidant (bilirubin) formation by ZnPP, and by enhancing ROS generation, is expected to offer a powerful therapeutic modality for future anticancer therapy. (Fang, Nakamura, Iyer, 2007).

I believe that a sufficiency of EMODs should be referred to as "prooxidant sufficiency" or bliss and avoidance of the old inaccurate term of "oxidative stress."

Diet and risk of ovarian cancer in the California Teachers Study cohort. 000 (Chang et al, 2007) (#97,275)

Dietary phytochemical compounds, including isoflavones and isothiocyanates, may inhibit cancer development but have not yet been examined in prospective epidemiologic studies of ovarian cancer. The authors have investigated the association between consumption of these and other nutrients and ovarian cancer risk in a prospective cohort study. Among **97,275 eligible women in the California Teachers Study cohort** who completed the baseline dietary

412

assessment in 1995-1996, 280 women developed invasive or borderline ovarian cancer by December 31, 2003. Multivariable Cox proportional hazards regression, with age as the timescale, was used to estimate relative risks and 95% confidence intervals; all statistical tests were two sided. **Intake of isoflavones was associated with lower risk of ovarian cancer.** Compared with the risk for women who consumed less than 1 mg of total isoflavones per day, the relative risk of ovarian cancer associated with consumption of more than 3 mg/day was 0.56 (95% confidence interval: 0.33, 0.96). **Intake of isothiocyanates or foods high in isothiocyanates was not associated with ovarian cancer risk, nor was intake of macronutrients, antioxidant vitamins, or other micronutrients. Although dietary consumption of isoflavones may be associated with decreased ovarian cancer risk, most dietary factors are unlikely to play a major role in ovarian cancer development** (Chang et al, 2007).

Dietary carotenoids and risk of colorectal cancer in a pooled analysis of 11 cohort studies. (Mannisto et al, 2007) (#702,647 participants)

Dietary carotenoids have been hypothesized to protect against epithelial cancers. The authors analyzed the associations between intakes of specific carotenoids (alpha-carotene, beta-carotene, beta-cryptoxanthin, lutein + zeaxanthin, and lycopene) and risk of colorectal cancer using the primary data from 11 cohort studies carried out in North America and Europe. Carotenoid intakes were estimated from food frequency questionnaires administered at baseline in each study. During 6-20 years of follow-up between 1980 and 2003, 7,885 incident cases of colorectal cancer were diagnosed among 702,647 participants. The authors calculated study-specific multivariate relative risks and then combined them using a random-effects model. In general, intakes of specific carotenoids were not associated with colorectal cancer risk. The pooled multivariate relative risks of colorectal cancer comparing the highest quintile of intake with the lowest ranged from 0.92 for lutein + zeaxanthin to 1.04 for lycopene; only for lutein + zeaxanthin intake was the result borderline statistically significant (95% confidence interval: 0.84, 1.00). The associations observed were generally similar across studies, for both sexes, and for colon cancer and rectal cancer. **These pooled data did not suggest that carotenoids play an important role in the etiology of colorectal cancer.** (Mannisto et al, 2007).

Circa 2008

Systematic review: primary and secondary prevention of gastrointestinal cancers with antioxidant supplements. (Bjelakovic, Nikolova, Simonette and Gludd, 2008 Sept) (#211,818 participants). The evidence on whether antioxidant

413

supplements prevent gastrointestinal cancers is contradictory. Using the Cochrane Collaboration methodology, we reviewed the randomized trials comparing antioxidant supplements with placebo or no intervention on the occurrence of gastrointestinal cancers. RESULTS: We identified 20 randomized trials (211,818 participants) assessing beta-carotene, vitamin A, vitamin C, vitamin E, and selenium. **The antioxidant supplements were without a significant effect on the occurrence of gastrointestinal cancers. Antioxidant supplements had no significant effect on mortality in a random-effects model meta-analysis** but *significantly increased mortality in a fixed-effect model meta-analysis.* CONCLUSIONS: **There was no evidence that the studied antioxidant supplements prevented gastrointestinal cancers. On the contrary,** *they seem to increase overall mortality.*

Vitamin E and selenium supplementation and risk of prostate cancer in the Vitamins and lifestyle (VITAL) study cohort (Peters et al, 2008) (#35,242 men) RESULTS: **A 10-year average intake of supplemental vitamin E was not associated with a reduced prostate cancer risk overall.** CONCLUSIONS: In this prospective cohort, **long-term supplemental intake of vitamin E and selenium were not associated with prostate cancer risk overall**; however, risk of clinically relevant advanced disease was reduced with greater long-term vitamin E supplementation.

Long-term use of supplemental multivitamins, vitamin C, vitamin E, and folate does not reduce the risk of lung cancer. VITAL (VITamins And Lifestyle) study (2008) (Slatore et al, 2008) (#77,721 men and women); explore the association of supplemental multivitamins, vitamin C, vitamin E, and folate with incident lung cancer; Prospective cohort; Cases were identified through the Seattle–Puget Sound **SEER (Surveillance, Epidemiology, and End Results)** cancer registry. **There was no inverse association with any supplement.** *Supplemental vitamin E was associated with a small increased risk of lung cancer.* This risk of supplemental vitamin E was largely confined to current smokers and was greatest for non–small cell lung cancer.

Conclusions: **Supplemental multivitamins, vitamin C, vitamin E, and folate were not associated with a decreased risk of lung cancer.** *Supplemental vitamin E was associated with a small increased risk of lung cancer.*

Patients should be counseled against using these supplements to prevent lung cancer.

The Institute of Medicine states that most North American adults get enough vitamin E from their normal diets to meet current recommendations.

The recent announcement of early termination of the Selenium and Vitamin E Cancer Prevention Trial's (SELECT) interventions because of lack of efficacy and observation of possible adverse events (i.e., small and not statistically significant increases in type 2 diabetes in those receiving selenium alone and in prostate cancer incidence in the vitamin E (alone) group) should serve as a reminder that the unexpected can happen in these well-designed trials (Lippman et al, 2009).

Efficacy of Antioxidant Supplementation in Reducing Primary Cancer Incidence and Mortality: Systematic Review and Meta-analysis. (Bardia et al, 2008) (#104,196 participants). Twelve eligible trials, 9 of high methodological quality, were identified (total subject population, 104,196). **Antioxidant supplementation did not significantly reduce total cancer incidence or mortality or any site-specific cancer incidence.** *Beta carotene supplementation was associated with an increase in the incidence of cancer among smokers and with a trend toward increased cancer mortality.* Selenium supplementation was associated with reduced cancer incidence in men but not in women and with reduced cancer mortality. **Vitamin E supplementation had no apparent effect on overall cancer incidence or cancer mortality.** CONCLUSION: *Beta carotene supplementation appeared to increase cancer incidence and cancer mortality among smokers,* **whereas vitamin E supplementation had no effect.** Selenium supplementation might have anticarcinogenic effects in men and thus requires further research.

Carotenoids and the risk of developing lung cancer: a systematic review. (Gallicchio et al, 2008) (Six randomized clinical trials & 25 prospective observational studies) Carotenoids are thought to have anti-cancer properties, but findings from population-based research have been inconsistent. OBJECTIVE: They aimed to conduct a systematic review of the associations between carotenoids and lung cancer. DESIGN: They searched electronic databases for articles published through September 2007. **Six randomized clinical trials examining the efficacy of beta-carotene supplements and 25 prospective observational studies** assessing the associations between carotenoids and lung cancer were analyzed by using random-effects meta-analysis. RESULTS: The pooled relative risk (RR) for the studies comparing beta-carotene supplements with placebo was 1.10. Among the observational studies that adjusted for smoking, the pooled RRs comparing highest and lowest categories of total carotenoid intake and of total carotenoid serum concentrations were 0.79 and 0.70, respectively. For beta-carotene, highest compared with lowest pooled RRs were 0.92 for dietary intake and 0.84 for serum concentrations. For other carotenoids, the RRs comparing highest and lowest categories of intake ranged from 0.80 for beta-cryptoxanthin to 0.89 for alpha-carotene and lutein-zeaxanthin; for serum concentrations, the RRs ranged from 0.71 for lycopene to 0.95 for lutein-zeaxanthin. CONCLUSIONS: **beta-Carotene supplementation is not associated with a decrease in the risk of developing lung cancer**. Findings from prospective cohort studies suggest inverse associations between carotenoids and lung cancer; however, **the decreases in risk are generally small and not statistically** significant. These inverse associations may be the result of carotenoid measurements' function as a marker of a healthier lifestyle (higher fruit and vegetable consumption) or of residual confounding by smoking.

Mistletoe therapy in oncology (Horneber et al, 2008) (#21 included studies, overall comprising 3,484 randomized cancer patients).

Mistletoe extracts are commonly used in cancer patients. It is claimed that they improve survival and quality of life (QOL) in cancer patients.

OBJECTIVES: To determine the effectiveness, tolerability and safety of mistletoe extracts given either as monotherapy or adjunct therapy for patients with cancer.

SEARCH STRATEGY: Search sources included the Cochrane Central Register of Controlled Trials (CENTRAL, Issue 3, 2007) Cochrane Complementary Medicine Field Registry of randomized clinical trials (RCTs) and controlled clinical trials, MEDLINE, EMBASE, HEALTHSTAR, INT. HEALTH TECHNOLOGY ASSESSMENT, SOMED, AMED, BIOETHICSLINE, BIOSIS, CancerLit, CATLINE, CISCOM (August 2007). For the search the Standard Operating Procedures of the Information System in Health Economics at the German Institute for Medical Documentation and Information (DIMDI) were utilized. Reference lists of relevant articles and authors extensive files were searched for additional studies. Manufacturers of mistletoe preparations were contacted.

SELECTION CRITERIA: We included RCTs of adults with cancer of any type. **The interventions were mistletoe extracts as sole treatments or given concomitantly with chemo- or radiotherapy.** The outcome measures were survival times, tumor response, QOL, psychological distress, adverse effects from antineoplastic treatment and safety of mistletoe extracts.

DATA COLLECTION AND ANALYSIS: Three review authors independently assessed trials for inclusion in the review. All review authors independently took part in the extraction of data and assessment of study quality and clinical relevance. Disagreements were resolved by consensus. Study authors were contacted where information was unclear. Methodological quality was narratively described and additionally assessed with the Delphi list and the Jadad score. High methodological quality was defined if six out of nine Delphi criteria, or four out of five Jadad criteria were fulfilled. Results were presented qualitatively.

MAIN RESULTS: Eighty studies were identified. Fifty-eight were excluded for various reasons, usually **as there was no prospective trial design with randomized treatment allocation.** Of the **21 included studies** 13 provided data on survival, 7 on tumor response, 16 on measures of QOL or psychological outcomes, or prevalence of chemotherapy-related adverse effects and 12 on side effects of mistletoe treatment; **overall comprising 3,484 randomized cancer patients.** Interventions evaluated were 5 preparations of mistletoe extracts from 5 manufacturers and one commercially not available preparation. The general reporting of RCTs was poor. Of the 13 trials investigating survival, 6 showed some evidence of a benefit, but none of them was of high methodological quality. The results of two trials in patients with melanoma and head and neck cancer gave some evidence that the used mistletoe extracts are not effective for improving survival. Of the 16 trials investigating the efficacy of mistletoe extracts for either improving QOL, psychological measures, performance index, symptom scales or the reduction of adverse effects of chemotherapy, 14 showed some evidence of a benefit, but only 2 of them including breast cancer patients during chemotherapy were of higher methodological quality. Data on side effects indicated that, depending on the dose, mistletoe extracts were usually well tolerated and had few side effects.

AUTHORS' CONCLUSIONS: The evidence from RCTs to support the view that the application of mistletoe extracts has impact on survival or leads to an improved ability to fight cancer or to withstand anticancer treatments is weak. Nevertheless, there is some evidence that mistletoe extracts may offer benefits on measures of QOL during chemotherapy for breast cancer, but these results need replication. Overall, more high quality, independent clinical research is needed to truly assess the safety and effectiveness of mistletoe extracts. Patients receiving mistletoe therapy should be encouraged to take part in future trails. (Horneber et al, 2008).

Mistletoes (*Viscum album*) are highly specialized angiosperms of the family Loranthaceae. The antioxidant activity of phenolics is mainly because of their redox properties, which allow them to act as reducing agents, hydrogen donors, free radical scavenger, singlet oxygen quenchers and metal chelators. This present study has verified that *V. album* extracts can act as primary and/or secondary antioxidants, being free radical scavengers and potent Fe chelators, and these properties of health benefit are host dependent. (Adedayo and Ganiyu, 2008).

Oxystress inducing antitumor therapeutics via tumor-targeted delivery of PEG-conjugated D-amino acid oxidase (Fang et al, 2008) (#)

We had developed a H(2)O(2) generating enzyme, polyethylene glycol conjugated D-amino acid oxidase (PEG-DAO), which exhibited potent antitumor activity by generating toxic reactive oxygen species, namely oxidation therapy, subsequently **showed remarkable antitumor effect on murine Sarcoma 180 solid tumor,** by taking advantage of the enhanced permeability and retention effect. Along this line, we report here the preparation of PEG-DAO by use of recombinant DAO and its antitumor activity by using various tumor cell lines and tumor models. Recombinant DAO (rDAO) was obtained from E. coli BL21 (DE3) carrying the porcine DAO expression vector with high yield (20 mg/l) and high enzyme activity (5.3 U/mg). Pegylated rDAO (PEG-rDAO) showed high stability against sonication, repeated freezing/thawing, lyophilization and exhibited superior in vivo pharmacokinetics. PEG-rDAO had a molecular size of 65 kDa and existed as nanoparticles in aqueous solution with mean particle diameter of 119 nm. In vitro experiments showed strong cytotoxicity of PEG-rDAO against various tumor cells, whereas less cytotoxicity was found against various normal cells. In vivo antitumor treatment was carried out **using 2 mice tumor models, namely colon 38 tumor and Meth A tumor model.** PEG-rDAO was administered i.v. and after an adequate lag time, D-proline (the substrate of DAO) was injected i.p. to the tumor-bearing mice. Consequently, preferential generation of H(2)O(2) in the tumor was successfully achieved, which **resulted in remarkable suppression of tumor growth without any visible side effects.** These findings suggest a potential of PEG-rDAO as a novel anticancer strategy toward clinical development. (Fang et al, 2008).

Circa 2009

Plasma carotenoids, retinol, and tocopherols and postmenopausal breast cancer risk in the Multiethnic Cohort Study: a nested case-control study. (Epplein et al, 2009) (#286 incident postmenopausal breast cancer cases were matched to 535 controls)

Assessments by the handful of prospective studies of the association of serum antioxidants and breast cancer risk have yielded inconsistent results. This multiethnic nested case-control study sought to examine the association of plasma carotenoids, retinol, and tocopherols with postmenopausal breast cancer risk. Methods: From the biospecimen subcohort of the Multiethnic Cohort Study, **286 incident post-menopausal breast cancer cases were matched to 535 controls** on age, sex, ethnicity, study location (Hawaii or California), smoking status, date/time of collection and hours of fasting. We measured prediagnostic circulating levels of individual carotenoids, retinol, and tocopherols. Conditional logistic regression was used to compute odds ratios and 95% confidence intervals. **Results: Women with breast cancer tended to have lower levels of plasma carotenoids and tocopherols than matched controls, but the differences were not large or statistically significant and the trends were not monotonic. No association was seen with retinol.** A sensitivity analysis excluding cases diagnosed within 1 year after blood draw did not alter the findings. Conclusions: **The lack of significant associations in this multiethnic population is consistent with previously observed results from less racially-diverse cohorts and serves as further evidence against a causal link between plasma micronutrient concentrations and postmenopausal breast cancer risk.**

Vitamins E and C in the prevention of prostate and total cancer in men: the Physicians' Health Study II randomized controlled trial (2009) (Gazziano et al, 2009) (#14,641 male physicians); evaluate whether long-term vitamin E or C supplementation decreases risk of prostate and total cancer events among men; a randomized, double-blind, placebo-controlled factorial trial of vitamins E and C that began in 1997 and continued until its scheduled completion on August 31, 2007. **Neither vitamin E nor vitamin C had a significant effect on prostate, colorectal, lung, or other site-specific cancers.** CONCLUSIONS: In this large, long-term trial of male physicians, in these **data neither vitamin E nor C supplementation reduced the risk of prostate or total cancer, provide no support for the use of these supplements for the prevention of cancer in middle-aged and older men.**

Advertisers suggest that taking certain vitamin or mineral supplements can lower prostate cancer risk. While some studies have found that there might be a protective benefit from some supplements, recent **results from 2 large studies didn't find any**. (Lippman et al, 2009) (Gaziano et al, 2009)

In 2001, researchers from the National Cancer Institute (NCI) and the Southwest Oncology Group (SWOG) launched the massive **SELECT study (short for Selenium and Vitamin E Cancer Prevention Trial)** to find out whether taking selenium and vitamin E supplements could protect men from prostate cancer. **In October 2008, researchers halted the trial after early analysis showed**

the supplements weren't working, and in fact, in some cases, may have been doing more harm than good.

In another large, long-term trial, called **the Physicians' Health Study II**, researchers from Brigham and Women's Hospital and Harvard Medical School studied whether taking vitamin E or vitamin C could reduce the risk of prostate cancer. Nearly **15,000 male doctors** participated in the trial. **After an average of 8 years, neither vitamin E nor vitamin C seemed to lower the risk of prostate cancer.**

Effect of selenium and vitamin E on risk of prostate cancer and other cancers: the Selenium and Vitamin E Cancer Prevention Trial (SELECT) (2009) (Lippman et al, 2009) (#35,533 men) **There were statistically nonsignificant increased risks of prostate cancer in the vitamin E group** but not in the selenium + vitamin E group. CONCLUSION: **Selenium or vitamin E, alone or in combination at the doses and formulations used, did not prevent prostate cancer in this population of relatively healthy men.** *The trial was stopped ahead of its original 12 year deadline because of a lack of any noticeable benefit.*

"**The largest prostate cancer prevention trial has found that selenium is no more effective than a placebo**," said David Schardt, a senior nutritionist. "Bayer is ripping people off when it suggests otherwise in these dishonest ads."

Multivitamin Use and Risk of Cancer and Cardiovascular Disease in the Women's Health Initiative Cohorts (Neuhouser et al, 2009) (#161,808 postmenopausal women taking part in the Women's Health Initiative clinical trials); **Conclusion:** After a median follow-up of 8.0 and 7.9 years in the clinical trial and observational study cohorts, respectively, the Women's Health Initiative study provided convincing evidence that **multivitamin use has little or no influence on the risk of common cancers, CVD, or total mortality in postmenopausal women.**

There was no evidence that multivitamins confer meaningful benefit or harm in relation to cancer or cardiovascular disease. The risk for invasive cancers of the breast, colon/rectum, endometrium, lung, bladder, and ovary was no different among women who used multivitamin compared with those who did not use multivitamins. Similarly, risk of myocardial infarction, stroke, venous thrombosis, and death from any cause was no different for multivitamin users than for nonusers. **Multivitamins do not appear to be effective for the prevention of cancer or cardiovascular disease.**

Neuhouser said: "To our surprise, we found that multivitamins did not lower the risk of the most common cancers and also had no impact on heart disease."

Thus, the largest multivitamin study shows that they do nothing to protect against cancer. Marian L. Neuhouser, the lead author and a nutritional epidemiologist with the Fred Hutchinson Cancer Research Center in Seattle, said, "**Consumers spend money on dietary supplements with the thought that they are going to improve their health, but there's no evidence for this.** Buying more fruits and vegetables might be a better choice."

In a separate statement, Neuhouser said: "Dietary supplements are used by more than half of all Americans, who spend more than 20 billion dollars on these products each year. However, scientific data are lacking on the long-term health benefits of supplements." Neuhouser suggested that women concentrate on getting their nutrients from food rather than supplements.

Researchers found the 41.5% of women who regularly took multivitamins were no more likely to avoid a range of cancers, heart disease, stroke or blood clots than those who didn't. In short, this large US study of over 160,000 postmenopausal women found no convincing evidence that long term use of multivitamins changed their risk of developing common cancers, cardiovascular disease or dying prematurely.

Effects of antioxidant supplements on cancer prevention: meta-analysis of randomized controlled trials (Myung et al, 2009) (#161,045 total subjects); searched Medline (PubMed), Excerpta Medica database, and the Cochrane Review in October 2007; Among 3327 articles searched, 31 articles on 22 randomized controlled trials, which included 161,045 total subjects, 88,610 in antioxidant supplement groups and 72,435 in placebo or no-intervention groups, were included in the final analyses. **In a fixed-effects meta-analysis of all 22 trials, antioxidant supplements were found to have no preventive effect on cancer. Conclusions:** The meta-analysis of randomized controlled trials indicated that **there is no clinical evidence to support an overall primary and secondary preventive effect of antioxidant supplements on cancer.**

MULTIVITAMINS: There was no evidence that multivitamins confer meaningful benefit or harm in relation to cancer or cardiovascular disease. The risk for invasive cancers of the breast, colon/rectum, endometrium, lung, bladder, and ovary was no different among women who used multivitamin compared with those who did not use multivitamins. Similarly, risk of myocardial infarction, stroke, venous thrombosis, and

death from any cause was no different for multivitamin users than for nonusers. Multivitamins do not appear to be effective for the prevention of cancer or cardiovascular disease.

Total and Cancer Mortality After Supplementation With Vitamins and Minerals: 10 year Follow-up of the Linxian General Population Nutrition Intervention Trial. (Qiao et al, 2009) (#29,584 adult participants) The General Population Nutrition Intervention Trial was a randomized primary esophageal and gastric cancer prevention trial conducted from 1985 to 1991, in which **29,584 adult participants** in Linxian, China, were given daily vitamin and mineral supplements. Treatment with **"factor D," a combination of 50 µg selenium, 30 mg vitamin E, and 15 mg beta-carotene,** led to decreased mortality from all causes, cancer overall, and gastric cancer. **Here, they present a 10-year follow-up after the end of active intervention.** Hazard ratios (HRs) and 95% confidence intervals (CIs) for the cumulative effects of four vitamin and mineral supplementation regimens were calculated using adjusted proportional hazards models. Results: **Participants who received factor D had lower overall mortality and gastric cancer mortality; reduction in cumulative gastric cancer mortality from 4.28% to 3.84%, than subjects who did not receive factor D.** Reductions were mostly attributable to benefits to subjects younger than 55 years. **Esophageal cancer deaths between those who did and did not receive factor D were not different overall;** however, decreased 17% among participants younger than 55 but *esophageal cancer deaths increased 14% among those aged 55 years or older. Vitamin A and zinc supplementation was associated with increased total and stroke mortality;* vitamin C and molybdenum supplementation, with decreased stroke mortality. Conclusion: The beneficial effects of selenium, vitamin E, and beta-carotene on mortality were still evident up to 10 years after the cessation of supplementation and were consistently greater in younger participants. Late effects of other supplementation regimens were also observed. **This study illustrates the confusion in the data, especially with the Linxian studies. They represent an exception to most of the other studies and should be viewed with caution.**

Long-term use of beta-carotene, retinol, lycopene, and lutein supplements and lung cancer risk: results from the VITamins And Lifestyle (VITAL) study. (Satia et al, 2009) (#77,126 (VITAL) cohort Study in Washington State) **High-dose beta-carotene supplementation in high-risk persons has been linked to increased lung cancer risk in clinical trials;** whether effects are similar in the general population is unclear. The authors examined associations of supplemental beta-carotene, retinol, vitamin A, lutein, and lycopene with lung cancer risk among participants, aged 50-76 years, in the VITamins And

Lifestyle (VITAL) cohort Study in Washington State. In 2000-2002, eligible persons (n = **77,126**) completed a 24-page baseline questionnaire, including detailed questions about supplement use (duration, frequency, dose) during the previous 10 years from multivitamins and individual supplements/mixtures. Incident lung cancers (n = 521) through December 2005 were identified by linkage to the Surveillance, Epidemiology, and End Results cancer registry. ***Longer duration of use of individual beta-carotene, retinol, and lutein supplements*** *(but not total 10-year average dose)* ***was associated with statistically significantly elevated risk of total lung cancer and histologic cell types.*** There was little evidence for effect modification by gender or smoking status. **Long-term use of individual beta-carotene, retinol, and lutein supplements should not be recommended for lung cancer prevention, particularly among smokers.**

Vitamin and mineral use and risk of prostate cancer: the case-control surveillance study. (Zhang et al. 2009) (#1,706 prostate cancer cases and 2,404 matched controls). ***Men who used zinc for ten years or more, either in a multivitamin or as a supplement, had an approximately two-fold increased risk of prostate cancer. The finding that long-term zinc intake from multivitamins or single supplements was associated with a doubling in risk of prostate cancer adds to the growing evidence for an unfavorable effect of zinc on prostate cancer carcinogenesis.***

Total dietary antioxidant index and survival in patients with glioblastoma multiforme. (Il'yasova et al. 2009) (#814 glioblastoma multiforme cases). **Overall, our results indicated no consistent, significant association of survival with dietary antioxidant intake or its combination with vitamin supplements. 000**

Glioblastoma multiforme (GBM') is the most common and most aggressive type of primary brain tumor in humans, involving glial cells and accounting for 52% of all parenchymal brain tumor cases and 20% of all intracranial tumors.

Associations between alpha-tocopherol, beta-carotene, and retinol and prostate cancer survival. (Watters et al. 2009) (#29,133). Previous studies suggest that carotenoids and tocopherols (vitamin E compounds) may be inversely associated with prostate cancer risk, yet little is known about how they affect prostate cancer progression and survival. We investigated whether serum alpha-tocopherol, beta-carotene, and retinol concentrations, or the alpha-tocopherol and beta-carotene trial supplementation, affected survival of men diagnosed with prostate cancer during the **alpha-Tocopherol, beta-Carotene Cancer Prevention Study, a randomized, double-blind, placebo-controlled primary**

prevention trial testing the effects of beta-carotene and alpha-tocopherol supplements on cancer incidence in adult male smokers in southwestern Finland (n = **29,133).** Prostate cancer survival was examined using the Kaplan-Meier method with deaths from other causes treated as censoring, and using Cox proportional hazards regression models with hazard ratios (HR) and 95% confidence intervals (CI) adjusted for family history of prostate cancer, age at randomization, benign prostatic hyperplasia, age and stage at diagnosis, height, body mass index, and serum cholesterol. As of April 2005, 1,891 men were diagnosed with prostate cancer and 395 died of their disease. **Higher serum alpha-tocopherol at baseline was associated with improved prostate cancer survival**, especially among cases who had received the alpha-tocopherol intervention of the trial and who were in the highest quintile of alpha-tocopherol at baseline or at the 3-year follow-up measurement. **Serum beta-carotene, serum retinol, and supplemental beta-carotene had no apparent effects on survival.** These findings suggest that higher alpha-tocopherol (and not beta-carotene or retinol) status increases overall prostate cancer survival. Further investigations, possibly including randomized studies, are needed to confirm this observation. (Watters et al. 2009).

Antioxidant Supplementation and Risk of Incident Melanomas. Results of a Large Prospective Cohort Study. (Asgari et al, 2009) (#69,671 men and women). **Objective** To examine whether *antioxidant supplement use is associated with melanoma risk in light of recently published data from the Supplementation in Vitamins and Mineral Antioxidants (SUVIMAX) study, which reported a 4-fold higher melanoma risk in women* randomized to receive a supplement with nutritionally appropriate doses of antioxidants. **Design:** Population-based prospective study (Vitamins and Lifestyle [VITAL] cohort). **Setting:** Western Washington State. **Participants** A total of **69,671 men and women** who self-reported (1) intake of multivitamins and supplemental antioxidants, including selenium and beta carotene, during the past 10 years and (2) melanoma risk factors on a baseline questionnaire. **Main Outcome Measure:** Incident melanoma identified through linkage to the Surveillance, Epidemiology, and End Results (SEER) cancer registry. **Results:** Cox proportional hazards regression models were used to estimate multivariable relative risks (RRs) and 95% confidence intervals (CIs) for multivitamin, supplemental selenium, and supplemental beta carotene use. **After adjusting for melanoma risk factors, we did not detect a significant association between multivitamin use and melanoma risk in women or in men.** Moreover, we **did not observe increased melanoma risk with the use of supplemental beta carotene** or selenium at doses comparable with those of the SUVIMAX study. **Conclusion: Antioxidants taken in nutritional doses do not seem to increase melanoma risk.**

Folic acid and risk of prostate cancer: results from a randomized clinical trial. (Figueiredo et al, 2009) (#643 randomly assigned men). Data regarding the association between folate status and risk of prostate cancer are sparse and conflicting. We studied prostate cancer occurrence in the Aspirin/Folate Polyp Prevention Study, a placebo-controlled randomized trial of aspirin and folic acid supplementation for the chemoprevention of colorectal adenomas conducted between July 6, 1994, and December 31, 2006. Participants were followed for up to 10.8 years and asked periodically to report all illnesses and hospitalizations. Aspirin alone had no statistically significant effect on prostate cancer incidence, but there were marked differences according to folic acid treatment. Among the **643 men who were randomly assigned** to placebo or **supplementation with folic acid, *the estimated probability of being diagnosed with prostate cancer over a 10-year period was 9.7% in the folic acid group and 3.3% in the placebo group*.** In contrast, baseline dietary folate intake and plasma folate in nonmultivitamin users were inversely associated with risk of prostate cancer, although these associations did not attain statistical significance in adjusted analyses. These findings highlight the potential complex role of folate in prostate cancer and the possibly different effects of folic acid-containing supplements vs natural sources of folate (Figueiredo et al, 2009).

Vitamins C and E and Beta Carotene Supplementation and Cancer Risk: Women's Antioxidant Cardiovascular Study (2009) A Randomized Controlled Trial (Lin et al, 2009) (#7,627 female health professionals); vitamin C (500 mg of ascorbic acid daily), natural-source vitamin E (600 IU of a-tocopherol every other day), and beta carotene (50 mg every other day). **There were no statistically significant effects of use of any antioxidant on total cancer incidence.** Conclusions: **Supplementation with vitamin C, vitamin E, or beta carotene offers no overall benefits in the primary prevention of total cancer incidence or cancer mortality.** Observational studies suggested that a diet high in fruits and vegetables, both of which are rich with antioxidants, may prevent cancer development. However, findings from randomized trials of the association between antioxidant use and cancer risk have been mostly negative. **Methods:** From 8,171 women who were randomly assigned in the **Women's Antioxidant Cardiovascular Study**, a double-blind, placebo-controlled 2 × 2 × 2 factorial trial of vitamin C (500 mg of ascorbic acid daily), natural-source vitamin E (600 IU of a-tocopherol every other day), and beta carotene (50 mg every other day), 7,627 women who were free of cancer before random assignment were selected for this study. Diagnoses and deaths from cancer at a specific site were confirmed by use of hospital reports and the National Death Index. Cox proportional hazards regression models were used to assess hazard ratios (represented as relative risks [RRs]) of common cancers associated with use of antioxidants, either individually or in combination. Subgroup analyses were conducted to determine if duration of use modified the association of supplement use with cancer risk. All statistical tests were two-sided. **Results** During an average 9.4 years of treatment, 624 women developed incident invasive cancer and 176 women died from cancer. **There were no statistically significant effects of use of any antioxidant on total cancer incidence. Similarly, no effects of these antioxidants were observed on cancer mortality. Duration and combined use of the three antioxidants also had no effect on cancer incidence and cancer death. Conclusions: Supplementation with vitamin C, vitamin E, or beta carotene offers no overall benefits in the primary prevention of total cancer incidence or cancer mortality** (Lin et al, 2005).

Green tea, black tea consumption and risk of lung cancer: a meta-analysis (Tang et al, 2009) (#meta-analysis included 22 studies**)**

Studies investigating the association of green tea and black tea consumption with lung cancer risk have reported inconsistent findings. To provide a quantitative assessment of this association, we conducted a meta-analysis on the topic. Studies were identified by a literature search in PubMed from 1966 to November 2008 and by searching the reference lists of relevant studies. Summary relative risk (RR) estimates and their corresponding 95% confidence intervals (CIs) were calculated based on random-effects model. Our meta-analysis included 22 studies provided data on consumption of green tea or black tea, or both related to lung cancer risk. **For green tea, the summary RR indicated a borderline significant association between highest green tea consumption and reduced risk of lung cancer.** Furthermore, **an increase in green tea consumption of two cups/ day was associated with an 18% decreased risk of developing lung cancer. For black tea, no statistically significant association was observe through the meta-analysis.** In conclusion, our data suggest that high or an increase in consumption of green tea but not black tea may be related to the reduction of lung cancer risk. (Tang et al, 2009).

Green tea consumption and risk of stomach cancer: a meta-analysis of epidemiologic studies (Myung, Int J Cancer. et al, 2009) **(#13 epidemiologic studies)**

This meta-analysis investigated the quantitative association between the consumption of green tea and the risk of stomach cancer in epidemiologic studies using crude data and adjusted data. We searched MEDLINE, EMBASE and the Cochrane Review in August 2007. All the articles searched were independently reviewed and selected by 3 evaluators according to predetermined criteria. A total of 13

epidemiologic studies were included. When all the case-control and cohort studies were pooled, the odds ratios (OR) [corrected] of stomach cancer for the highest level of green tea consumption when compared with the lowest level of consumption were shown to be 1.10 using the crude data and 0.82 using the adjusted data. In the meta-analyses of case-control studies, **no significant association was seen between green tea consumption and stomach cancer using the crude data, but green tea was shown to have a preventive effect on stomach cancer using the adjusted data.** *In the meta-analyses of the recent cohort studies, the highest green tea consumption was shown to significantly increase stomach cancer risk using the crude data,* but no significant association between them was seen when using the adjusted data. **Unlike the case-control studies, no preventive effect on stomach cancer was seen for the highest green tea consumption in the meta-analysis of the recent cohort studies.** Further clinical trials are needed (Myung, Int J Cancer. et al, 2009).

Green tea consumption and gastric cancer in Japanese: a pooled analysis of six cohort studies. (Inoue et al, 2009) (# 219,080 subjects, 3,577 cases of gastric cancer)

Previous experimental studies have suggested many possible anti-cancer mechanisms for green tea, but **epidemiological evidence for the effect of green tea consumption on gastric cancer risk is conflicting**.

OBJECTIVE: To examine the association between green tea consumption and gastric cancer.

METHODS: We analysed original data from six cohort studies that measured green tea consumption using validated questionnaires at baseline. Hazard ratios (HRs) in the individual studies were calculated, with adjustment for a common set of variables, and combined using a random-effects model.

RESULTS: During 2 285 968 person-years of follow-up for **a total of 219,080 subjects, 3,577 cases of gastric cancer were identified.** Compared with those drinking <1 cup/day, **no significant risk reduction for gastric cancer was observed with increased green tea consumption in men, even in stratified analyses by smoking status and subsite. In women, however, a significantly decreased risk was observed for those with consumption of > or =5 cups/day.** This decrease was also significant for the distal subsite. **In contrast, a lack of association for proximal gastric cancer was consistently seen in both men and women.**

CONCLUSIONS: Green tea may decrease the risk of distal gastric cancer in women (Inoue et al, 2009).

Green tea (Camellia sinensis) for the prevention of cancer. Chochrane Database Syst Rev. 2009 Jul 8;(3):CD005004. (Boehm et al, 2009) (#Fifty-one studies with more than 1.6 million participants were included)

Tea is one of the most commonly consumed beverages worldwide. Teas from the plant Camellia sinensis can be grouped into green, black and oolong tea. Cross-culturally tea drinking habits vary. **Camellia sinensis contains the active ingredient polyphenol, which has a subgroup known as catechins. Catechins are powerful antioxidants.** It has been suggested that green tea polyphenol may inhibit cell proliferation and observational studies have suggested that green tea may have cancer-preventative effects.

OBJECTIVES: To critically assess any associations between green tea consumption and the risk of cancer incidence and mortality.

SEARCH STRATEGY: We searched eligible studies up to January 2009 in the Cochrane Central Register of Controlled Trials (CENTRAL), MEDLINE, EMBASE, Amed, CancerLit, Psych INFO and Phytobase and reference lists of previous reviews and included studies.

SELECTION CRITERIA: We included all prospective, controlled interventional studies and observational studies, which either assessed the associations between green tea consumption and risk of cancer incidence or that reported on cancer mortality.

DATA COLLECTION AND ANALYSIS: At least two review authors independently applied the study criteria, extracted data and assessed methodological quality of studies. Due to the nature of included studies, which were mainly epidemiological, results were summarized descriptively according to cancer diagnosis.

MAIN RESULTS: Fifty-one studies with more than 1.6 million participants were included. Twenty-seven of them were case-control studies, 23 cohort studies and one randomized controlled trial (RCT). **Twenty-seven studies tried to establish an association between green tea consumption and cancer of the digestive tract, mainly of the upper gastrointestinal tract, five with breast cancer, five with prostate cancer, three with lung cancer, two with ovarian cancer, two with urinary bladder cancer one with oral cancer, three further studies included patients with various cancer**

diagnoses. The methodological quality was measured with the Newcastle-Ottawa scale (NOS). The 9 nested case-control studies within prospective cohorts were of high methodological quality, 13 of medium, and 1 of low. One retrospective case-control study was of high methodological quality and 21 of medium and 5 of low. **Results from studies assessing associations between green tea and risk of digestive tract cancer incidence were highly contradictory. There was limited evidence that green tea could reduce the incidence of liver cancer. The evidence for esophageal, gastric, colon, rectum, and pancreatic cancer was conflicting.** In prostate cancer, observational studies with higher methodological quality and the only included RCT suggested a decreased risk in men consuming higher quantities green tea or green tea extracts. **However, there was limited to moderate evidence that the consumption of green tea reduced the risk of lung cancer, especially in men, and *urinary bladder cancer or that it could even increase the risk of the latter.* There was moderate to strong evidence that green tea consumption does not decrease the risk of dying from gastric cancer. There was limited moderate to strong evidence for lung, pancreatic and colorectal cancer.**

AUTHORS' CONCLUSIONS: There is insufficient and conflicting evidence to give any firm recommendations regarding green tea consumption for cancer prevention. The results of this review, including its trends of associations, need to be interpreted with caution and their generalisability is questionable, as the majority of included studies were carried out in Asia (n = 47) where the tea drinking culture is pronounced. **Desirable green tea intake is 3 to 5 cups per day (up to 1200 ml/day), providing a minimum of 250 mg/day catechins. If not exceeding the daily recommended allowance, those who enjoy a cup of green tea should continue its consumption.** Drinking green tea appears to be safe at moderate, regular and habitual use (Boehm et al, 2009) (Boehm et al. Green tea.

Lack of genoprotective effect of phytosterols and conjugated linoleic acids on Caco-2 cells (and did not exhibit potential anti-carcinogenic activity) (Daly et al, 2009) (#)

Much interest has focused on the cholesterol-lowering effects of phytosterols (plant sterols) but limited data suggests they may also possess anti-carcinogenic activity. **Conjugated linoleic acids (CLA),** sourced from meat and dairy products of ruminant animals, has also received considerable attention as a potential anti-cancer agent. Therefore, the aims of this project were to (i) examine the effects of phytosterols and CLA on the viability and growth of **human intestinal Caco-2 cells** and (ii) determine their potential genoprotective (comet assay),

COX-2 modulatory (ELISA) and apoptotic (Hoechst staining) activities. **The Caco-2 cell line is a continuous line of heterogeneous human epithelial colorectal adenocarcinoma cells**, developed by the Sloan-Kettering Institute for Cancer Research through research conducted by Dr. Jorgen Fogh. Caco-2 cells were supplemented with the phytosterols campesterol, b-sitosterol, or b-sitostanol, or a CLA mixture, or individual CLA isomers (c10t12-CLA, t9t11-CLA) for 48 h. The three phytosterols, at the highest levels tested, were found to reduce both the viability and growth of Caco-2 cells while CLA exhibited isomer-specific effects. **None of the phytosterols protected against DNA damage.** At a concentration of 25 µM, both c10t12-CLA and t9t11-CLA enhanced ($P < 0.05$) oxidant-induced, but not mutagen-induced, DNA damage. Neither the phytosterols nor CLA induced apoptosis or modulated COX-2 production. In conclusion, **campesterol, b-sitosterol, b-sitostanol, c10t12-CLA, and t9t11-CLA were not toxic to Caco-2 cells, at the lower levels tested, and did not exhibit potential anti-carcinogenic activity** (Daly et al, 2009).

Pre-radiotherapy plasma carotenoids and markers of oxidative stress are associated with survival in head and neck squamous cell carcinoma patients: a prospective study (Sakhi et al, 2009) (#178 total; 78 HNSCC patients and 100 healthy controls).

The purpose of this study was to compare plasma levels of antioxidants and oxidative stress biomarkers in **head and neck squamous cell carcinoma (HNSCC)** patients with healthy controls. Furthermore, the effect of radiotherapy on these biomarkers and their association with survival in HNSCC patients were investigated.

METHODS: Seventy-eight HNSCC patients and 100 healthy controls were included in this study. Follow-up samples at the end of radiotherapy were obtained in 60 patients. **Fifteen antioxidant biomarkers (6 carotenoids, 4 tocopherols, ascorbic acid, total antioxidant capacity, glutathione redox potential, total glutathione and total cysteine) and four oxidative stress biomarkers (total hydroperoxides, gamma-glutamyl transpeptidase, 8-isoprostagladin F2alpha and ratio of oxidized/total ascorbic acid) were measured in plasma samples.** Analysis of Covariance was used to compare biomarkers between patients and healthy controls. Kaplan-Meier plots and Cox' proportional hazards models were used to study survival among patients.

RESULTS: Dietary antioxidants (carotenoids, tocopherols and ascorbic acid), **ferric reducing antioxidant power (FRAP)** and modified FRAP were lower in HNSCC patients compared to controls and **dietary antioxidants decreased**

during radiotherapy. **Total hydroperoxides (d-ROMs), a marker for oxidative stress**, were higher in HNSCC patients compared to controls and increased during radiotherapy. Among the biomarkers analyzed, **high levels of plasma carotenoids before radiotherapy are associated with a prolonged progression-free survival.** Additionally, **high relative increase in plasma levels of d-ROMs and high relative decrease in FRAP during radiotherapy are also positively associated with survival.**

CONCLUSIONS: Biomarkers of antioxidants and oxidative stress are unfavorable in HNSCC patients compared to healthy controls, and radiotherapy affects many of these biomarkers. **Increasing levels of antioxidant biomarkers before radiotherapy and increasing oxidative stress during radiotherapy may improve survival indicating that different factors/mechanisms may be important for survival before and during radiotherapy in HNSCC patients.** Thus, the therapeutic potential of optimizing antioxidant status and oxidative stress should be explored further in these patients. *I believe that this important study shows that increased plasma EMODs and lowered plasma antioxidants are associated with increased survival in HNSCC.* (Sakhi et al, 2009).

The protective effect of silibinin against mitomycin C-induced intrinsic apoptosis in human melanoma A375-S2 cells. (Jiang et al, 2009)

Silibinin, a natural flavonoid, is known for its hepatoprotective, anti-inflammatory, and anti-carcinogenic effects. We found that silibinin exhibited a protective effect against chemotherapeutic reagent mitomycin C-induced cell death in A375-S2 cells in a p53-dependent manner, which contradicted the findings of previous studies investigating the anti-neoplastic activity of silibinin and developing silibinin as a potential anti-neoplastic drug in clinical therapy. Mitomycin C administration triggered a time- and dose-dependent cell death in A375-S2 cells. Apoptotic morphology, DNA fragmentation, and caspase-3 activation demonstrated that the major cause of A375-S2 cell death by mitomycin C was apoptosis. This was associated with a marked increase of p53 level and changes in mitochondria associated proteins. However, preincubation with silibinin prior to mitomycin C treatment substantially suppressed cell apoptosis, attenuated the change of p53 and Bcl-2 expressions, blocked the translocation of Bax to mitochondrial outer membrane, and ameliorated the loss of mitochondrial membrane potential, but mitomycin C stimuli led to few changes in the protein levels of caspase 8, Fas ligand, and Fas-associated death domain protein, indicating that silibinin protected cells from mitomycin C-induced apoptosis mainly via suppressing the mitochondria-mediated intrinsic apoptosis pathway, but not in an extrinsic manner (Jiang et al, 2009).

Circa 2010

Multivitamin use and breast cancer incidence in a prospective cohort of Swedish women. (Larsson et al, 2010) (#35,329 cancer-free women). Many women use multivitamins in the belief that these supplements will prevent chronic diseases such as cancer and cardiovascular disease. However, whether the use of multivitamins affects the risk of breast cancer is unclear. **Objective:** They prospectively examined the association between multivitamin use and the incidence of invasive breast cancer in the **Swedish Mammography Cohort. Design:** In 1997, **35,329 cancer-free women** completed a self-administered questionnaire that solicited information on multivitamin use as well as other breast cancer risk factors. Relative risks (RRs) and 95% CIs were calculated by using Cox proportional hazard models and adjusted for breast cancer risk factors. **Results:** During a mean follow-up of 9.5 y, 974 women were diagnosed with incident breast cancer. *Multivitamin use was associated with a statistically significant increased risk of breast cancer.* The association did not differ significantly by hormone receptor status of the breast tumor. **Conclusions:** These results suggest that *multivitamin use is associated with an increased risk of breast cancer. Use of multivitamins was linked to a statistically significant 19 per cent increased risk of breast cancer* (after adjusting for lifestyle and risk factors like weight, diet, smoking, exercise, and family history of breast cancer.

Women and men use multivitamins in the belief that they will protect them from chronic diseases like cancer and heart disease but that is not proven. Please remember that in **February 2009, the *Archives of Internal Medicine* published details of a large US study of over 160,000 postmenopausal women that found no convincing evidence that long term use of multivitamins changed their risk of developing common cancers, cardiovascular disease or dying prematurely.**

Other research has found that *women who take multivitamins have increased breast density, which is linked to a relatively higher risk of breast cancer* (Berube et al, 2008). The widespread use of multiviamins points out an important public health concern.

Daily intake of antioxidants in relation to survival among adult patients diagnosed with malignant glioma. (DeLorenze et al. 2010). Geometric mean values for 11 fat-soluble and 6 water-soluble individual antioxidants, antioxidant index and 3 macronutrients were virtually the same when comparing all cases (n=748) to self-reported cases only (n=450). *For patients diagnosed with Grade II and Grade III histology, moderate (915.8-2118.3 mcg) intake of fat-soluble lycopene was associated with poorer survival* when compared to low intake

(0.0-914.8 mcg), for self-reported cases only. High intake of vitamin E and moderate/high intake of secoisolariciresinol among Grade III patients indicated greater survival for all cases. *In Grade IV patients, moderate/high intake of cryptoxanthin and high intake of secoisolariciresinol were associated with poorer survival among all cases.* **Among Grade II patients,** moderate intake of water-soluble folate was associated with greater survival for all cases; *high intake of vitamin C and genistein and the highest level of the antioxidant index were associated with poorer survival for all cases.*

CONCLUSIONS: The associations observed in our study suggest that the influence of some antioxidants on survival following a diagnosis of malignant glioma are inconsistent and vary by histology group.

Vitamin C: intravenous use by complementary and alternative medicine practitioners and adverse effects (Padayatty et al, 2010) (172 practitioners administered IV vitamin C to **11,233 patients**)

Investigators surveyed attendees at annual CAM Conferences in 2006 and 2008, and determined sales of intravenous vitamin C by major U.S. manufacturers/distributors. We also queried practitioners for side effects, compiled published cases, and analyzed FDA's Adverse Events Database. Of 199 survey respondents (out of 550), 172 practitioners administered IV vitamin C to **11,233 patients** in 2006 and 8876 patients in 2008. Average dose was 28 grams every 4 days, with 22 total treatments per patient. Estimated yearly doses used (as 25 g/50 ml vials) were 318,539 in 2006 and 354,647 in 2008. Manufacturers' yearly sales were 750,000 and 855,000 vials, respectively. Common reasons for treatment included infection, cancer, and fatigue. *Of 9,328 patients for whom data is available, 101 had side effects, mostly minor, including lethargy/fatigue in 59 patients, change in mental status in 21 patients and vein irritation/phlebitis in 6 patients. Publications documented serious adverse events, including 2 deaths in patients known to be at risk for IV vitamin C.* Due to confounding causes, the FDA Adverse Events Database was uninformative. Total numbers of patients treated in the US with high dose vitamin C cannot be accurately estimated from this study. **(RMH Note: Here are two more dead bodies!)**

CONCLUSIONS: High dose IV vitamin C is in unexpectedly wide use by CAM practitioners. **Other than the known complications of IV vitamin C in those with renal impairment or glucose 6 phosphate dehydrogenase deficiency**, high dose intravenous vitamin C appears to be **remarkably safe**. Physicians should inquire about IV vitamin C use in patients with cancer, chronic, untreatable, or intractable conditions and be observant of unexpected harm, drug interactions, or benefit (Padayatty et al, 2010).

Green Tea Drinking and Subsequent Risk of Breast Cancer in a Population to Based Cohort of Japanese Women/No effect. (Iwasaki et al, 2010) (#53,793).

Although many *in vitro* and animal studies have demonstrated a protective effect of green tea against breast cancer, findings from epidemiological studies have been inconsistent, and whether high green tea intake reduces the risk of breast cancer remains unclear.

Methods: In this Japan Public Health Center-based Prospective Study, **581 cases of breast cancer were newly diagnosed in 53,793 women during 13.6 years' follow-up** from the baseline survey in 1990 to 1994. After the five-year follow-up survey in 1995 to 1998, 350 cases were newly diagnosed in 43,639 women during 9.5 years' follow-up. The baseline questionnaire assessed the frequency of total green tea drinking while the five-year follow-up questionnaire assessed that of two types of green tea, *Sencha* and *Bancha/Genmaicha*, separately.

Results: Compared with women who drank less than one cup of green tea per week, the adjusted hazard ratio (HR) for women who drank five or more cups per day was 1.12 in the baseline data. Similarly, compared with women who drank less than one cup of *Sencha* or *Bancha/Genmaicha* per week, adjusted HRs for women who drank 10 or more cups per day were 1.02 for *Sencha* and 0.86 for *Bancha/Genmaicha*. No inverse association was found regardless of hormone receptor-defined subtype or menopausal status.

Conclusions: In this **population-based prospective cohort study in Japan we found no association between green tea drinking and risk of breast cancer** (Iwasaki et al, 2010). 000

Specifically, **(-)-epigallocatechin-3-gallate (EGCG), the most abundant and biologically active catechin in green tea, might play an important role in cancer prevention, but this is not supported by this study.**

Green tea consumption and breast cancer risk or recurrence: a meta-analysis. (Ogunleye et al, 2010) (#5,617 breast cancer cases). Green tea is a commonly consumed beverage in Asia and has been suggested to have anti-inflammatory and possible anti-carcinogenic properties in laboratory studies. We sought to examine the association between green tea consumption and risk of breast cancer incidence or recurrence, using all available epidemiologic evidence to date. We conducted a systematic search of five databases and performed a meta-analysis of studies of breast cancer risk and recurrence published between 1998 and 2009, encompassing 5,617 cases of breast cancer. Summary relative risks (RR) were calculated using a fixed effects model, and tests of heterogeneity across combined studies were conducted. We identified two studies of breast cancer recurrence and seven studies of breast cancer incidence. Increased green tea consumption (more than three cups a day) was inversely associated with breast cancer recurrence. An analysis of case-control studies of breast cancer incidence suggested an inverse association with a pooled RR of 0.81 while **no association was found among cohort studies of breast cancer incidence. Combining all studies of breast cancer incidence resulted in significant heterogeneity.** Available epidemiologic evidence supports the hypothesis that increased green tea consumption may be inversely associated with risk of breast cancer recurrence. **The association between green tea consumption and breast cancer incidence remains unclear based on the current evidence** (Ogunleye et al, 2010).

Long-Term Use of supplemental vitamin C, vitamin D and vitamin E does not reduce the risk of urothelial cell carcinoma of the bladder in the VITamins and Lifestyle Study. (Hotaling 2010) (#77,050 eligible VITAL participants). Urothelial carcinoma has the highest lifetime treatment cost of any cancer, making it an ideal target for preventative therapies. Previous work has suggested that certain vitamin and mineral supplements may reduce the risk of urothelial carcinoma. We used the prospective VITamins And Lifestyle cohort to examine the association of all commonly taken vitamin and mineral supplements as well as 6 common anti-inflammatory supplements with incident urothelial carcinoma in a United States population. **Long-Term Use of supplemental vitamin C, vitamin D and vitamin E does not reduce the risk of urothelial cell carcinoma of the bladder in the VITamins and Lifestyle Study. 000**

The vitamin C: vitamin K3 system - enhancers and inhibitors of the anticancer effect. (Lamson DW et al, 2010)

The oxidizing anticancer system of vitamin C and vitamin K_3 (VC:VK_3, producing hydrogen peroxide via superoxide) was combined individually with melatonin, curcumin, quercetin, or cholecalciferol (VD_3) to determine interactions. Substrates were LNCaP and **PC-3 prostate cancer cell lines.** Three of the tested antioxidants displayed differences in cell line cytotoxicity. **Melatonin combined with VC:VK_3 quenched the oxidizing effect,** while VC:VK_3 applied 24 hours after melatonin showed no quenching. With increasing curcumin concentrations, an apparent combined effect of VC:VK_3 and curcumin occurred in LNCaP cells, but not

PC-3 cells. Quercetin alone was cytotoxic on both cell lines, but demonstrated an additional 50-percent cytotoxicity on PC-3 cells when combined with VC:VK$_3$. **VD$_3$ was effective against both cell lines, with more effect on PC-3.** This effect was negated on LNCaP cells with the addition of VC:VK$_3$. In conclusion, **a natural antioxidant can enhance or decrease the cytotoxicity of an oxidizing anticancer system in vitro, but generalizations about antioxidants cannot be made.** (Lamson et al, 2010).

Age-related cataract in a randomized trial of vitamins E and C in men. (Christen et al. 2010) (#11,545). **OBJECTIVE:** To test whether supplementation with alternate-day vitamin E or daily vitamin C affects the incidence of age-related cataract in a large cohort of men.

METHODS: In a randomized, double-masked, placebo-controlled trial, **11,545 apparently healthy US male physicians** 50 years or older without a diagnosis of cataract at baseline were randomly assigned to receive **400 IU of vitamin E or placebo on alternate days and 500 mg of vitamin C** or placebo daily.

MAIN OUTCOME MEASURE: Incident cataract responsible for a reduction in best-corrected visual acuity to 20/30 or worse based on self-report confirmed by medical record review.

APPLICATION TO CLINICAL PRACTICE: Long-term use of vitamin E and C supplements has no appreciable effect on cataract.

RESULTS: After 8 years of treatment and follow-up, 1174 incident cataracts were confirmed. There were 579 cataracts in the vitamin E-treated group and 595 in the vitamin E placebo group. For vitamin C, there were 593 cataracts in the treated group and 581 in the placebo group.

CONCLUSION: Long-term alternate-day use of 400 IU of vitamin E and daily use of 500 mg of vitamin C had no notable beneficial or harmful effect on the risk of cataract. (Christen et al. 2010).

Circa 2011

Vitamin E and All-cause Mortality: A Meta-Analysis (Abner EL, et al, 2011) (#246,371 subjects and 29,295 all-cause deaths).

The current analysis reexamines the relationship between supplemental vitamin E and all-cause mortality. All **randomized, controlled trials** testing the treatment effect of vitamin E supplementation in adults for at least one year were sought. **MEDLINE, the Cochrane Library, and Biological Abstracts databases were searched using the terms "vitamin E," "alpha-tocopherol," "antioxidants," "clinical trial," and "controlled trial" for studies published through April 2010**; results were limited to English, German, or Spanish language articles. Studies were also obtained through reference mining. All randomized controlled trials using vitamin E, with a supplementation period of at least one year, to prevent or treat disease in adults were identified and abstracted independently by two raters. Mortality data from trials with a supplementation period of at least one year were pooled. The selected trials (n = 57) were published between 1988 and 2009. Sample sizes range from 28 to 39,876 (median = 423), **yielding 246,371 subjects and 29,295 all-cause deaths. Duration of supplementation for the 57 trials range from one to 10.1 years** (median = 2.6 years). A random effects meta-analysis produce an overall risk ratio of 1.00 (95% confidence interval: 0.98, 1.02); **additional analyses suggest no relationship between dose and risk of mortality. Based on the present meta-analysis, supplementation with vitamin E appears to have no effect on all-cause mortality at doses up to 5,500 IU/d.** (Abner et al, 2011).

Effect of vitamins C and E on antioxidant status of breast-cancer patients undergoing chemotherapy (Suhail et al, 2011) (#forty untreated breast-cancer patients (stage II) and compared with those of healthy controls).

Reactive oxygen/nitrogen species generated by chemotherapy. What is known and Objective: antineoplastic agents are prime suspects for the toxic side-effects of acute or chronic chemotherapy. The present study was undertaken to test whether **vitamins C and E (VCE) supplementation** protect against some of the harmful effects of treatment. In a commonly used anticancer drugs in breast-cancer patients. Methods: **randomized** 5-month study, the activity of various antioxidant enzymes (superoxide dismutase, catalase, glutathione-S-transferase and glutathione reductase) and the levels of malondialdehyde and reduced glutathione were measured in **forty untreated breast-cancer patients (stage II) and compared with those of healthy controls.** The degree of DNA damage was also assessed in the peripheral lymphocytes of the patients by alkaline single cell gel electrophoresis. The untreated patients were then randomly assigned to either mg/m(2) i.v. day 1, treatment with chemotherapy alone (5-fluorouracil 500 mg/m(2) i.v. day 1, mg/m(2) i.v. day 1 and cyclophosphamide 500 doxorubicin 50 weeks for six cycles) or to the same chemotherapy regimen supplemented every 3 mg gelatin capsule). On mg tablet and vitamin E 400 with VCE (vitamin C 500 completion of the treatments, both the groups were studied again for the levels The of the markers measured prior to treatment. **Results and Discussion: untreated group** showed significantly lower levels of antioxidant enzymes (P<0 001) and reduced glutathione (P<0 001), and more extensive lipid peroxidation (P<0 001) and DNA damage than healthy controls. Similar but less pronounced patterns were observed in the patients receiving chemotherapy alone. The group of patients receiving VCE supplementation had all the marker levels moving towards normal values. Activities of superoxide dismutase, catalase, glutathione-S-transferase and glutathione reductase, and the levels of reduced glutathione were significantly increased (P<0 01) while, **the levels of malondialdehyde and DNA damage were significantly (P<0 01) reduced in the VCE supplemented group relative to those of patients receiving chemotherapy alone as well as relative to the pretreatment levels.** What is new and Co-administration of VCE restored antioxidant status, lowered by treatment. **Conclusion:** the presence of breast-cancer and chemotherapy. **DNA damage was also reduced by VCE.** The results suggest that VCE should be useful in protecting against chemotherapy-related side-effects and a randomized control trial to evaluate the effectiveness of VCE in breast-cancer patients using clinical outcomes would be appropriate. (Suhail et al, 2011). **I believe that this shows that antioxidant supplementation restores harmful levels of antioxidants and this is verified by the reduced levels of DNA damage. In short, they are counteracting EMOD effects and apoptosis and protecting cancer cells.**

Long-Term Use of supplemental vitamins and minerals does not reduce the risk of urothelial cell carcinoma of the bladder in the VITamins and Lifestyle Study. (Hotaling et al, 2011) (#77,050 eligible VITAL participants)

Urothelial carcinoma has the highest lifetime treatment cost of any cancer, making it an ideal target for preventative therapies. Previous work has suggested that certain vitamin and mineral supplements may reduce the risk of urothelial carcinoma. We used the prospective VITamins And Lifestyle cohort to examine the association of all commonly taken vitamin and mineral supplements as well as 6 common anti-inflammatory supplements with incident urothelial carcinoma in a United States population.

Materials and Methods

A total of **77,050 eligible VITAL participants** completed a detailed questionnaire at baseline on supplement use and cancer risk factors. After 6 years of follow-up 330 incident urothelial carcinoma cases in the cohort were identified via linkage to the Seattle-Puget Sound SEER cancer registry. **We analyzed use of supplemental vitamins (multivitamins, beta-carotene, retinol, folic acid, and vitamins B1, B3, B6, B12, C, D and E), minerals (calcium, iron, magnesium,** zinc and selenium) and anti-inflammatory supplements (glucosamine, chondroitin, saw palmetto, ginkgo biloba, fish oil and garlic). For each supplement the hazard ratios (risk ratios) for urothelial carcinoma comparing each category of users to nonusers, and 95% CIs, were determined using Cox proportional hazards regression, adjusted for potential confounders.

Results: None of the vitamin, mineral or anti-inflammatory supplements was significantly associated with urothelial carcinoma risk in age adjusted or multivariate models.

Conclusions: The results of this study do not support the use of commonly taken vitamin or mineral supplements or 6 common anti-inflammatory supplements for the chemoprevention of urothelial carcinoma. (Hotaling et al, 2011).

The effect of supplemental vitamins and minerals on the development of prostate cancer: a systematic review and meta-analysis. (Stratton, Godwin, 2011) (#Fourteen articles were included) Vitamin supplementation is used for many purposes with mainly alleged benefits. One of these is the use of various vitamins for the prevention of prostate cancer.

METHODS: We conducted a systematic review and meta-analysis on this topic. Pubmed, Embase and the Cochrane Database were searched; as well, we hand searched the references in key articles. Randomized controlled trials (RCTs), cohort studies and case-control studies were included. The review assessed the effect of supplemental vitamins on the risk of prostate cancer and on disease severity and death in men with prostate cancer.

RESULTS: Fourteen articles were included in the final assessment. Individually, a few of these studies showed a relationship between the ingestion of supplemental vitamins or minerals and the incidence or severity of prostate cancer, especially in smokers. However, neither the use of multivitamin supplementation nor the use of individual vitamin/mineral supplementation affected the overall occurrence of prostate cancer or the occurrence of advanced/metastatic prostate cancer or death from prostate cancer when the results of the studies were combined in a meta-analysis. We also conducted several sensitivity analyses by running meta-analysis using just the higher quality studies and just the RCTs. There were still no associations found.

CONCLUSIONS: There is no convincing evidence that the use of supplemental multivitamins or any specific vitamin affects the occurrence or

severity of prostate cancer. There was high heterogeneity among the studies so it is possible that unidentified subgroups may benefit or be harmed by the use of vitamins (Stratton, Godwin, 2011).

The outcome of 5-ALA-mediated photodynamic treatment in melanoma cells is influenced by vitamin C and heme oxygenase-1. (Grimm et al, 2011) (#)

Photodynamic therapy (PDT) is an important clinical approach for cancer treatment. It involves the administration of a photosensitizer, followed by its activation with light and induction of cell death. **The underlying mechanism is an increased production of reactive oxygen species (ROS) leading to oxidative stress, which is followed by cell death. However, effectiveness of PDT is limited due to an initiation of endogenous rescue response systems like heme oxygenase-1 (HO-1) in tumor cells.** In recent years, **consuming of antioxidant supplements has become widespread,** but the effect of exogenously applied antioxidants on cancer therapy outcome remains unclear. Thus, this study was aimed to investigate if exogenous antioxidants might decrease ROS-induced cytotoxicity in photodynamic treatment. **Lycopene, b-carotene, vitamin C, N-acetylcysteine, trolox, and N-tert-butyl-a-phenylnitrone in different doses were administered to human melanoma cells prior exposure to photodynamic treatment. Supplementation with vitamin C resulted in a significant decrease of the cell death rate,** whereas the other tested antioxidants had no effect on cell viability and oxidative stress markers. **The simultaneous application of vitamin C with the HO-1 activity inhibitor zinc protoporphyrine IX (ZnPPIX) caused a considerable decrease of photodynamic treatment-induced cytotoxicity compared to ZnPPIX alone.** It can be summarized that exogenously applied antioxidants do not have a leading role in the protective response against photodynamic treatment. However, further studies are necessary to investigate more antioxidants and other substances, which might affect the outcome of photodynamic treatment in cancer therapy (Grimm et al, 2011).

The protective effects of nutritional antioxidant therapy on Ehrlich solid tumor-bearing mice depend on the type of antioxidant therapy chosen: histology, genotoxicity and hematology evaluations. (Miranda-Vilela AL, et al, 2011)

Strong evidence indicates that reactive oxygen species (ROS) play an important role in the initiation as well as the promotion phase of carcinogenesis. **Studies support the role of ROS in cancer, in part, by showing that dietary**

antioxidants act as cancer-preventive agents. Although results are promising, the research on this topic is still controversial. Thus, the aim of this study was to investigate whether **vitamins C, E and pequi oil** can, individually, provide prevention and/or be used afterward as an adjuvant in cancer therapy. Ehrlich solid tumor-bearing mice received antioxidant as follows: before tumor inoculation, before and after tumor inoculation (continuous administration), and after tumor inoculation; morphometric analyses of tumor, genotoxicity and hematology were then carried out. **Antioxidant administrations before tumor inoculation effectively inhibited its growth in the three experimental protocols**, but *administrations after the tumor's appearance accelerated tumor growth and favored metastases.* **Continuous administration of pequi oil inhibited the tumor's growth, while the same protocol with** *vitamins E and C accelerated it (tumor growth), favoring metastasis and increasing oxidative stress on erythrocytes.* Except for continuous administration with vitamin E, the development of ascites tumor metastases was linked with increased inflammation. Results suggest that the efficiency and applicability of antioxidants in the medical clinic can depend not only on the nature of the antioxidant, the type and stage of cancer being treated and the prevailing oxygen partial pressure in the tissues, but also on the type of antioxidant therapy chosen (Miranda-Vilela et al, 2011).

Prenatal exposure to flavonoids: Implication for cancer risk (Vanhees et al, 2011)

Flavonoids are potent antioxidants, freely available as high-dose dietary supplements. However, **they can induce DNA double-strand breaks (DSB) and rearrangements in the mixed-lineage leukemia (MLL) gene, which are frequently observed in childhood leukemia.** We hypothesize that a deficient DSB repair, as a result of an Atm mutation, may reinforce the clastogenic effect of dietary flavonoids and increase the frequency of Mll rearrangements. Therefore, we examined the effects of in vitro and transplacental exposure to high, but biological amounts of flavonoids in mice with different genetic capacities for DSB repair (homozygous/heterozygous knock-in for human Atm mutation [Atm-ΔSRI] vs. wild type [wt]). *In vitro exposure to genistein/quercetin induced higher numbers of Mll rearrangements in bone marrow cells of Atm-ΔSRI mutant mice compared with wt mice.* Subsequently, heterozygous Atm-ΔSRI mice were placed on either a flavonoid-poor or a genistein-enriched (270 mg/kg) or quercetin-enriched (302 mg/kg) feed throughout pregnancy. *Prenatal exposure to flavonoids associated with higher frequencies of Mll rearrangements and a slight increase in the incidence of malignancies in DNA repair-deficient mice.* These data suggest that *prenatal exposure to both genistein and quercetin supplements could increase the risk on Mll rearrangements especially in the presence of* *compromised DNA repair* (Vanhees et al, 2011). **I had posed the question some time ago, "Can antioxidants given during pregnancy (prenatal) cause the diseases associated with an EMOD insufficiency?" The answer may be "yes."**

Peroxiredoxin 6 overexpression attenuates cisplatin-induced apoptosis in human ovarian cancer cells. (Pak et al, 2011)

Investigators examined the involvement of peroxiredoxin 6 (Prdx 6) in providing chemoprotection against cisplatin cytotoxicity in **SKOV-3 ovarian cancer cells. Treatment of SKOV-3 cells with cisplatin-induced cytotoxicity that was associated with increased accumulation of intracellular reactive oxygen species (ROS) and apoptosis mediated by proteolytically activated caspase 3 and 9. Overexpression of Prdx 6 protein or exposure to N-acetylcysteine (NAC) reversed the apoptotic effect of cisplatin by reducing ROS levels and suppressing the caspase signaling pathway.** These results indicate that targeting Prdx 6 may sensitize cancer cells to ROS-producing therapeutic treatments, such as anticancer drugs and radiation (Pak et al, 2011).

Dietary phytocompounds and risk of lymphoid malignancies in the California Teachers Study cohort. 000 (Chang et al, 2010) (#110,215)

Investigators examined whether dietary intake of **isoflavones, lignans, isothiocyanates, antioxidants, or specific foods rich in these compounds** is associated with reduced risk of B-cell non-Hodgkin lymphoma (NHL), multiple myeloma (MM), or Hodgkin lymphoma (HL) in a **large, prospective cohort of women.**

METHODS: Between 1995-1996 and 31 December 2007, among **110,215 eligible members of the California Teachers Study cohort,** 536 women developed incident B-cell NHL, 104 developed MM, and 34 developed HL. Cox proportional hazards regression, with age as the time scale, was used to estimate adjusted rate ratios (RRs) with 95% confidence intervals (CIs) for risk of lymphoid malignancies.

RESULTS: Weak inverse associations with risk of diffuse large B-cell lymphoma were observed for isothiocyanates and an antioxidant index measuring hydroxyl radical absorbance capacity. **Risk of other NHL subtypes, overall B-cell NHL, MM, or HL was not generally associated with dietary intake of isoflavones, lignans, isothiocyanates, antioxidants, or major food sources of these compounds.**

CONCLUSIONS: Isoflavones, lignans, isothiocyanates, and antioxidant compounds are not associated with risk of most B-cell malignancies, but some phytocompounds may decrease the risk of selected subtypes (Chang et al, 2010). 000

Total number of participants for the above studies is approximately **11,127,347**. Some studies did not have the number of participants available.

Total 118 studies above on cancer only.

26 studies showing that antioxidants increased the risk of cancer

39 STUDIES SHOWING HARMFUL EFFECTS

REFERENCES

(approximately 631)

Abner et al, 2011) (Abner EL, et al. Vitamin E and All-cause Mortality: A Meta-Analysis. Curr Aging Sci. 2011 Jan 14).

(Adedayo and Ganiyu, 2008) (Ademiluyi Adedayo Oluwaseun and Oboh Ganiyu. Antioxidant properties of methanolic extracts of mistletoes (*Viscum album*) from cocoa and cashew trees in Nigeria. African Journal of Biotechnology Vol. 7 (17), pp. 3138-3142, 3 September, 2008).

(Agarwal et al, 1991) (Agarwal, M.L., Clay, M.E., Harvey, E.J., Evans, H.H., Antunez, A.R. and Oleinick, N.L. Photodynamic therapy induces rapid cell death by apoptosis in L5178Y mouse lymphoma cells. Cancer Res 1991; 51: 5993-5996).

(Agus et al, 1999) (Agus DB, Vera JC, Golde DW. Stromal cell oxidation: a mechanism by which tumors obtain vitamin C. Cancer Res (1999) 59(18):4555–4558).

(Ahmad et al, 1997) (Ahmad N, Feyes DK, Nieminen AL, Agarwal R, Mukhtar H. Green tea constituent epigallocatechin-3-gallate and induction of apoptosis and cell cycle arrest in human carcinoma cells. J Natl Cancer Inst 1997;89:1881–6).

(Ahmad et al, 2000) (Ahmad N, Gupta S, Mukhtar H. Green tea polyphenol epigallocatechin-3-gallate differentially modulates nuclear factor kB in cancer cells versus normal cells. Arch Biochem Biophys 2000;376:338–46).

(Ahmad et al, 2003) (K.A. Ahmad, M-V. Clement and S. Pervaiz. Pro-oxidant activity of low doses of resveratrol inhibits hydrogen peroxide - induced apoptosis. Ann. N.Y. Acad. Sci. 1010: 365–373 (2003).

(Ahmad et al, 2005) (Ahmad IM, et al. Mitochondrial O_2^*- and H_2O_2 mediate glucose deprivation-induced stress in human cancer cells. J Biol Chem. 2005 Feb 11;280(6):4254-63).

(Albanes et al, 1996) (Albanes D. et al. Alpha-Tocopherol and beta-carotene supplements and lung cancer incidence in the alpha-tocopherol, beta-carotene cancer prevention study: effects of base-line characteristics and study compliance. J Natl Cancer Inst. 1996 Nov 6;88(21):1560-70 (Albright et al, 2003) (Albright, C. D., Salganik, R. I., Craciunescu, C. N., Mar, M. H. & Zeisel, S. H. (2003) Mitochondrial and microsomal derived reactive oxygen species mediate apoptosis induced by transforming growth factor-beta1 in immortalized rat hepatocytes. J. Cell Biochem. 89:254-261).

(Albright et al, 2004) (Albright, C. D., Salganik, R. I. & Van Dyke, T. (2004) Dietary depletion of vitamin E and vitamin A inhibits mammary tumor growth and metastasis in transgenic mice. J. Nutr. 134:1139-1144).

(Alkhenizan and Hafez, 2007) (Alkhenizan A, Hafez K. The role of vitamin E in the prevention of cancer: a meta-analysis of randomized controlled trials. Ann Saudi Med. 2007 Nov-Dec;27(6):409-14).

(Al-Waili et al, 2006) (Al-Waili, NS and Butler, GJ. Phototherapy and malignancy: Possible enhancement by iron administration and hyperbaric oxygen. Med Hypotheses. 2006;67(5):1148-58).

(Andersson et al. 1996) (Andersson SO, Wolk A, Bergström R, Giovannucci E, Lindgren C, Baron J, Adami HO. Energy, nutrient intake and prostate cancer risk: a population-based case-control study in Sweden. Int J Cancer. 1996 Dec 11;68(6):716-22).

(Andoh et al, 2003) (Andoh T, Chiueh CC, Chock PB. Cyclic GMP-dependent protein kinase regulates the expression of thioredoxin and thioredoxin peroxidase-1 during hormesis in response to oxidative stress-induced apoptosis. J Biol Chem. 2003; 278: 885–890).

(Andrieu-Abadie et al, 2001) (Nathalie Andrieu-Abadie et al. Ceramide in apoptosis signaling: relationship with oxidative stress. Free Radical Biology and Medicine. Volume 31, Issue 6, 15 September 2001, Pages 717-728).

(Aoe et al, 1995) (Aoe, T., Y. Okamoto, T. Saito. 1995. Activated macrophages induce structural abnormalities of the T cell receptor-CD3 complex. J. Exp. Med. 181: 1881-1886).

(Arends et al, 1990) (Arends, M. J., Morris, R. G. & Wyllie, A. H. (1990) Apoptosis. The role of the endonuclease. Am. J. Pathol. 136:593-608).

(Arrowsmith et al, 1989) (Morbidity and mortality among low birth weight infants exposed to an intravenous vitamin E product, E-Ferol. JB Arrowsmith et al. Pediatrics. 1989 Feb;83(2):244-9).

(Asgari et al, 2009) (Maryam M. Asgari, Sonia S. Maruti, Lawrence H. Kushi, Emily White. Antioxidant Supplementation and Risk of Incident Melanomas. *Arch Dermatol.* 2009;145(8):879-882)

(Ashino et al, 2003) (Ashino H, Shimamura M, NaKajima H, Dombou M, Kawanaka S, Oikawa T, Iwaguchi T, Kawashima S. Novel function of ascorbic acid as an angiostatic factor. *Angiogenesis.* 2003;6:259–269).

(Aw, 1999) (Aw TY., 1999. Molecular and cellular responses to oxidative stress and changes in oxidation–reduction imbalance in the intestine. Am. J. Clin. Nutr. 70, 557–565).

(Aykin-Burns et al, 2009) (Aykin-Burns N, Ahmad IM, Zhu Y, Oberley LW, Spitz DR. Increased levels of superoxide and H2O2 mediate the differential susceptibility of cancer cells versus normal cells to glucose deprivation. Biochem J. 2009 Feb 15;418(1):29-37).

(Baader et al, Anticancer Res. 1994) (Baader, S. L., Bruchelt, G., Trautner, M. C., Boschert, H., and Niethammer, D. Uptake and cytotoxicity of ascorbic acid and dehydroascorbic acid in neuroblastoma (SK-N-SH) and neuroectodermal (SK-N-LO) cells. Anticancer Res., 14: 221–227, 1994).

(Baader et al, 1994) (Baader, S. L., Bruchelt, G., Trautner, M. C., Boschert, H., and Niethammer, D. Uptake and cytotoxicity of ascorbic acid and dehydroascorbic acid in neuroblastoma (SK-N-SH) and neuroectodermal (SK-N-LO) cells). Anticancer Res., 14: 221–227, 1994).

(Bachur et al, 1978) (Nicholas R. Bachur, Sandra L. Gordon, and Malcolm V. Gee. A General Mechanism for Microsomal Activation of Quinone Anticancer Agents to Free Radicals. CANCER RESEARCH 38, 1745-1750, June 1978).

(Bardia et al, 2008) (Bardia A, Tleyjeh IM, Cerhan JR, Sood AK, Limburg PJ, Montori VM. "Efficacy of antioxidant supplementation in reducing primary cancer incidence and mortality: systematic review and meta-analysis." Mayo Clin Proc. 2008 83(1):23-34).

(Bairati et al, 2005 Apr 6) (Bairati I, Meyer F, Gélinas M, Fortin A, Nabid A, Brochet F, Mercier JP, Têtu B, Harel F, Mâsse B, Vigneault E, Vass S, del Vecchio P, Roy J. A randomized trial of antioxidant vitamins to prevent second primary cancers in head and neck cancer patients. J Natl Cancer Inst. 2005 Apr 6;97(7):481-8)

(Bairati et al, 2005 Aug 20) (Bairati I, Meyer F, Gélinas M, Fortin A, Nabid A, Brochet F, Mercier JP, Têtu B, Harel F, Abdous B, Vigneault E, Vass S, Del Vecchio P, Roy J. Randomized trial of antioxidant vitamins to prevent acute adverse effects of radiation therapy in head and neck cancer patients. J Clin Oncol. 2005 Aug 20;23(24):5805-13)

(Bairati et al, J Clin Oncol. 2005) (Bairati I, Meyer F, Gelinas M, et al. Randomized trial of antioxidant vitamins to prevent acute adverse effects of radiation therapy in head and neck cancer patients. J Clin Oncol (2005) 23(24):5805–5813).

(Bairati et al, 2006) (Bairati I, Meyer F, Jobin E, et al. Antioxidant vitamins supplementation and mortality: a randomized trial in head and neck cancer patients. Int J Cancer (2006) 119(9):2221–2224).

(Baker et al, 2007) (A. F. Baker, T. Landowski, R. Dorr, W. R. Tate, J. M.C. Gard, B. E. Tavenner, T. Dragovich, A. Coon, and G. Powis. The Antitumor Agent Imexon Activates Antioxidant Gene Expression: Evidence for an Oxidative Stress Response. Clin. Cancer Res., June 1, 2007; 13(11): 3388 – 3394).

(Barbior, 1974) (Babior, B.M. Oxygen dependent microbial killing by phagocytes. N Engl J Med 1974; 298: 659-668, 721-726).

(Bareggi SR et al. 2009) (Bareggi SR et al. Effects of clioquinol on memory impairment and the neurochemical modifications induced by scrapie infection in golden hamsters. Brain Res. 2009 Jul 14;1280:195-200). Department of Pharmacology, Chemotherapy and Medical Toxicology, School of Medicine, Milano, Italy.

(Baron et al, 2003) (John A. Baron, Bernard F. Cole, Leila Mott, Robert Haile, Maria Grau, Timothy R. Church, Gerald J. Beck, E. Robert Greenberg. Neoplastic and Antineoplastic Effects of Beta Carotene on Colorectal Adenoma Recurrence: Results of a Randomized Trial. JNCI Journal of the National Cancer Institute 2003 95(10):717-722).

(Barthleman et al, 1998) (Barthelman M, Bair WB III, Stickland KK, et al. (–)-Epigallocatechin-3-gallate inhibition of ultraviolet B-induced AP-1 activity. Carcinogenesis 1998;19:2201–4).

(Beckman, Ames, 1998) (Beckman K.B., Ames, B.N., 1998. The free radical theory of aging matures. Physiol. Rev. 78, 547–581) (Finkel T, Holbrook N.J., 2000. Oxidants, oxidative stress and the biology of ageing. Nature 408, 239–247).

(Begin, 1987) (Begin ME. Effects of polyunsaturated fatty acids and of their oxidation products on cell survival. Chem Phys Lipids 1987;45:269–313).

(Begin, 1988) (Begin ME, Ells G, Horrobin DF. Polyunsaturated fatty acid induced cytotoxicity against tumor cells and its relationship to lipid peroxidation. J Natl Cancer Inst 1988;80:188–94).

(Bekhit et al, 2004) (Bekhit, A.; Geesink, G.; Ilian, M.; Morton, J.; Sedcole, J.; Bickerstaffe, R. Pro-oxidant activities of carnosine, rutin and quercetin in a beef model system and their effects on the metmyoglobin-reducing activity. European Food Research and Technology A, Volume 218, Number 6, May 2004 , pp. 507-514).

(Berg et al, 1992) (Berg, K., Steen, H.B., Windelman, J.W. and Moan, J. Synergistic effects of photo activated tetra(4-sulfonatophenyl)porphine and nocodazole on microtubule assembly, accumulation of cells in mitosis and cell survival. J Photochem Photobiol B 1992; 13: 59-70).

(Berk et al, 2007) (Berk L, Berkey B, Rich T, et al. Randomized phase II trial of high-dose melatonin and radiation therapy for RPA class 2 patients with brain metastases (RTOG 0119). Int J Radiat Oncol Biol Phys (2007) 68(3):852–857).

(Bernards, Sung, 2003) (Rene Bernards, Ph.D., Max Sung, M.D., Sept. 18, 2003, *Nature*).

(Betten et al, 2001) (Betten, A., J. Bylund, T. Cristophe, F. Boulay, A. Romero, K. Hellstrand, C. Dahlgren. 2001. A proinflammatory peptide from *Helicobacter pylori* activates monocytes to induce lymphocyte dysfunction and apoptosis. *J. Clin. Invest.* 108: 1221-1228).

(Bhalla et al, 2009) (Savita Bhalla, Sriram Balasubramanian, Kevin David, Mint Sirisawad, Joseph Buggy, Lauren Mauro, Sheila Prachand, Richard Miller, Leo I. Gordon and Andrew M. Evens. PCI-24781 Induces Caspase and Reactive Oxygen

Species–Dependent Apoptosis Through NF-kB Mechanisms and Is Synergistic with Bortezomib in Lymphoma Cells. *Clinical Cancer Research* 15, 3354, May 15, 2009).

(Biaglow et al, 1989) (Biaglow J. E., Varnes M. E., Epp E. R., Clark E. P., Tuttle S. W., Held K. D. Role of glutathione in the aerobic radiation response. Int. J. Radiat. Oncol. Biol. Phys., *16:* 1311-1314, 1989).

(Biaglow et al, 1992) (Biaglow J. E., Mitchell J. B., Held K. The importance of peroxide and superoxide in the X-ray response. Int. J. Radiat. Oncol. Biol. Phys., 22: 665-669, 1992).

(Biswas et al, 2010) (Biswas S, et al. Arsenic trioxide and ascorbic acid demonstrate promising activity against primary human CLL cells in vitro. Leuk Res. 2010 Jul;34(7):925-31).

(Bize et al, 1980) (Bize IB, Oberley LW, Morris HP. Superoxide dismutase and superoxide radical in Morris hepatomas. Cancer Res. 1980 Oct;40(10):3638-93).

(Bjelakovic et al. 2004) (Bjelakovic G, Nikolova D, Simonetti RG, Gluud C. Antioxidant supplements for preventing gastrointestinal cancers. *Cochrane Database Syst Rev.* doi: 10.1002/14651858.CD004183.pub2. 2004;(4):CD004183).

(Bjelakovic et al, Lancet 2004) (Bjelakovic G, Nikolova D, Simonetti RG, Gluud C. Antioxidant supplements for prevention of gastrointestinal cancers: a systematic review and meta-analysis. *Lancet.* 2004;364:1219-1228).

(Bjelakovic et al, 2006) (Bjelakovic G, Nagorni A, Nikolova D, Simonetti RG, Bjelakovic M, Gluud C. Meta-analysis: antioxidant supplements for primary and secondary prevention of colorectal adenoma. *Aliment Pharmacol Ther.* 2006;24:281-291).

(Bjelakovic et al, 2007) (Bjelakovic G, Nikolova D, Gluud LL, Simonetti RG, and Gluud C. "Mortality in Randomized Trials of Antioxidant Supplements for Primary and Secondary Prevention; Systematic Review and Meta-analysis." JAMA 2007;297:842-857. Vol. 297 No. 8, February 28, 2007).

(Bjelakovic, Nikolova, Simonette and Gludd, 2008 Sept) (Bjelakovic G, Nikolova D, Simonetti RG, Gluud C. Systematic review: primary and secondary prevention of gastrointestinal cancers with antioxidant supplements. Aliment Pharmacol Ther. 2008 Sep 15;28(6):689-703).

(Black and Livingston, I, 1990) (Black DJ, Livingston RB. Antineoplastic drugs in 1990: A review (part I). Drugs 39:489-501, 1990).

(Black and Livingston, II, 1990) (Black DJ, Livingston RB. Antineoplastic drugs in 1990: A review (part II). Drugs 39:652-673, 1990).

(Block et al, 2007) (Block KI, Koch AC, Mead MN, Tothy PK, Newman RA, Gyllenhaal C. Impact of antioxidant supplementation on chemotherapeutic efficacy:

a systematic review of the evidence from randomized controlled trials. Cancer Treat Rev. (2007) 33(5):407–418).

(Blot et al, 1993) (Blot WJ, Li JY, Taylor PR, Guo W, Dawsey S, Wang GQ, et al. Nutrition intervention trials in Linxian, China: supplementation with specific vitamin/mineral combinations, cancer incidence, and disease-specific mortality in the general population. J Natl Cancer Inst. 1993;85:1483-92).

(Blumenthal et al, 2000) (Blumenthal, R. D., Lew, W., Reising, A., Soyne, D., Osorio, L., Ying, Z. & Goldenberg, D. M. (2000) Anti-oxidant vitamins reduce normal tissue toxicity induced by radio-immunotherapy. Int. J. Cancer 86:276-280).

(Bocci et al, 2005) (Bocci V, Larini A, Micheli V. April 2005. "Restoration of normoxia by ozone therapy may control neoplastic growth: a review and a working hypothesis". J Altern Complement Med 11 (2): 257–65).

(Boehm et al, 2009) (Boehm et al. Green tea (Camellia sinensis) for the prevention of cancer. Chochrane Database Syst Rev. 2009 Jul 8;(3):CD005004).

(Bohlke et al, 1999) (K Bohlke, D Spiegelman, A Trichopoulou, K Katsouyanni and D Trichopoulos. Vitamins A, C and E and the risk of breast cancer: results from a case-control study in Greece. British Journal of Cancer (1999) 79, 23–29).

(Bonuccelli et al, 2010) (Bonuccelli G, et al. Ketones and lactate "fuel" tumor growth and metastasis: Evidence that epithelial cancer cells use oxidative mitochondrial metabolism. Cell Cycle. 2010 Sep;9(17):3506-14).

(Borek, 2004) (Carmia Borek. Antioxidants and Radiation Therapy. J. Nutr. 134:3207S-3209S, November 2004).

(Borek, Pardo, 2002) (Borek, C. & Pardo, F. (2002) Vitamin E and apoptosis: a dual role. Pasquier, C. eds. Biennial Meeting of the Society for Free Radicals Research International 2002:327-331 Monduzzi Editore Bologna, Italy).

(Borrego et al, 2004) (Borrego A, Zamora ZB, González R, et al. (February 2004). "Protection by ozone preconditioning is mediated by the antioxidant system in cisplatin-induced nephrotoxicity in rats". Mediators Inflamm. 13 (1): 13–9).

(Borrego et al, 2006) (Borrego A, Zamora ZB, González R, et al. (August 2006). "Ozone/oxygen mixture modifies the subcellular redistribution of Bax protein in renal tissue from rats treated with cisplatin". Arch. Med. Res. 37 (6): 717–22).

451

(Bove et al, 1985) (Vasculopathic hepatotoxicity associated with E-Ferol syndrome in low-birth-weight infants. K. E. Bove, N. Kosmetatos, K. E. Wedig, D. J. Frank, S. Whitlatch, V. Saldivar, J. Haas, C. Bodenstein and W. F. Balistreri. JAMA. Vol. 254. No. 17. November 1, 1985).

(Bracke et al, 1999) (Bracke ME, et al. Influence of tangeretin on tamoxifen's therapeutic benefit in mammary cancer. J Natl Cancer Inst 91:354-359, 1999).

(Branda et al, 2004) (Branda RF, Naud SJ, Brooks EM, Chen Z, Muss H. Effect of vitamin B12, folate, and dietary supplements on breast carcinoma chemotherapy—induced mucositis and neutropenia. Cancer (2004) 101(5):1058–1064).

(Brennan, O'Neill, 1995) (Brennan P, O'Neill LA: Effects of oxidants and anti-

oxidants on nuclear factor kB activation in three different cell lines: evidence against a universal hypothesis involving oxygen radicals. *Biochim Biophys Acta* 1995, 1260:167-175).

(Brewer, 2010) (Gregory J. Brewer. Epigenetic oxidative redox shift (EORS) theory of aging unifies the free radical and insulin signaling theories. Experimental Gerontology. Volume 45, Issue 3, March 2010, Pages 173-179).

(Brophy PM, Prichard DI 1992. Immunity to helminthes: Ready to tip the biochemical balance? *Parasitol Today 8*: 419-422).

(Buettner et al, 2006) (Buettner Garry R; Ng Chin F; Wang Min; Rodgers V G J; Schafer Freya Q. A new paradigm: manganese superoxide dismutase influences the production of H_2O_2 in cells and thereby their biological state. Free radical biology & medicine 2006;41(8):1338-50).

(Buettner et al, 1992) (Buettner G. R., Moseley P. L. Ascorbate both activates and inactivates bleomycin by free radical generation. Biochemistry, *31*: 9784-9788, 1992).

(Buettner, Jurkiewicz, 1996) (Buettner GR. & Jurkiewicz BA. (1996) Catalytic metals, ascorbate and free radicals: combinations to avoid. Radiat. Res. 145, 532-541).

(Burger, 1998) (Burger R. M. Cleavage of nucleic acids by bleomycin. Chem. Rev., 98: 1153-1169, 1998).

(Buring and Hennekens, 1992) (Buring JE, Hennekens CH. The women's health study: summary of the design. *J Myocardial Ischemia* 1992;4:27-9).

(Burlacu et al, 2001) (Burlacu A, Jinga V, Gafencu AV, et al. Severity of oxidative stress generates different mechanisms of endothelial cell death. Cell Tissue Res 2001;306:409–16).

(Byfield et al, 1976) (Byfield J. E., Lee Y. C., Tu L., Kullhanian F. Molecular interactions of the combined effects of bleomycin and X-rays on mammalian cell survival. Cancer Res., 36: 1138-1143, 1976).

(CA Cancer J Clin, 1993) ("Questionable methods of cancer management: hydrogen peroxide and other 'hyperoxygenation' therapies". CA Cancer J Clin 43 (1): 47–56. 1993).

(CA Cancer J Clin, 1994) ("Questionable methods of cancer management: electronic devices". CA Cancer J Clin 44 (2): 115–27. 1994).

Callahan et al, 1988) (Callahan HL, Crouch RK, James ER 1988. Helminth antioxidant enzymes: A protective mechanism against host oxidants? Parasitol Today 4: 218-225).

(Callahan et al, 1990) (Callahan, H. L. et al. Hydrogen peroxide is the most toxic oxygen species for Onchocerca cervicalis microfilariae. Parasitology. 1990 Jun;100 Pt 3:407-15).

(Campbell et al, 2006) (KJ Campbell, JM O'Shea and ND Perkins. Differential regulation of NF-kB activation and function by topoisomerase II inhibitors. BMC Cancer 2006, 6:101).

(Caraballoso et al, 2003) (Caraballoso M, Sacristan M, Serra C, Bonfill X. Drugs for preventing lung cancer in healthy people. Cochrane Database Syst Rev. doi: 10.1002/14651858.CD002141. 2003;(2):CD002141).

(Carr, Frei, 1999) (A Carr and B Frei. Does vitamin C act as a pro-oxidant under physiological conditions? The FASEB Journal. 1999;13:1007-1024).

(Cascinu et al, 1995) (Cascinu S, Cordella L, Del Ferro E, et al. Neuroprotective effect of reduced glutathione on cisplatin-based chemotherapy in advanced gastric cancer: a randomized double-blind placebo-controlled trial. J Clin Oncol 1995;13:26–32).

(Chabner et al, 1990) (Chabner BA, Collins JM: Cancer Chemotherapy: Principles and Practice, pp 276-297, 314-333. Philadelphia, JB Lippincott, 1990).

(Chandra et al, 2003) (Chandra J, Hackbarth J, Le S, et al. Involvement of reactive oxygen species in adaphostin-induced cytotoxicity in human leukemia cells. Blood. 2003;102: 4512-4519).

(Chang et al, 2007) (Chang ET, et al. Diet and risk of ovarian cancer in the California Teachers Study cohort. Am J Epidemiol. 2007 Apr1;165(7):802-13).

(Chang et al, 2010) (Chang ET, et al. Dietary phytocompounds and risk of lymphoid malignancies in the California Teachers Study cohort. Cancer Causes Control. 2011 Feb;22(2):237-49).

(Chapman et al, 1991) (Chapman, J.D., Stobbe, C.C., Arnfield, M.R., Santus, R., Lee, L. and McPhee, M.S. Oxygen dependency of tumor cell killing in vitro by light-activated Photofrin II. Radiat Res 1991; 126: 73-79).

(Chapmann, 1979) (William Chapmann, "A Japanese Tragedy, Dirodohydroxyquinoline," *Washington Post* 18 March1979.).

(Chen et al, 2002) (Chen Q, et al. Improvement of tumor response by manipulation of tumor oxygenation during photodynamic therapy. Photochem Photobiol, 2002 Aug;76(2):197-203).

(Chen et al, 2004) (Chen YC, et al. Flavone inhibition of tumor growth via apoptosis in vitro and in vivo. Int J Oncol, 2004 Sep;25(3):661-70).

(Chen et al, 2005) (Chen Q, Espey MG, Krishna MC, Mitchell JB, Corpe CP, Buettner GR, Shacter E, and Levine L. Pharmacologic ascorbic acid concentrations selectively kill cancer cells: Action as a pro-drug to deliver hydrogen peroxide to tissues. PNAS. September 20, 2005. Vol. 102. No. 38. pp. 13604-13609).

(Chen et al, 2007) (Chen Q, Espey MG, Sun AY, Lee J, Krishna MC, Shacter E, Choyke P, Pooput C, Kirk KL, Buettner GR, and Levine M. Ascorbate in pharmacologic concentrations selectively generates ascorbate radical and hydrogen peroxide in extracellular fluid in vivo. PNAS. May 22, 2007. Vol. 104. No. 21. pp. 8749-8754).

(Chen et al, 2008) (Chen Q, Espey MG, Sun AY, Pooput C, Kirk KL, Krishna MC, Khosh DB, Drisko J, Levine M. Pharmacologic doses of ascorbate act as a prooxidant and decrease growth of aggressive tumor xenografts in mice. PNAS. August 12, 2008. Vol. 105. No. 32. pp. 11105-11109).

(Chen J et al, 2008) (Jiping Chen, Ingo Ruczinski, Timothy J. Jorgensen, Gayane Yenokyan, Yin Yao, Rhoda Alani, Nanette J. Liégeois, Sandra C. Hoffman, Judith Hoffman-Bolton, Paul T. Strickland, Kathy J. Helzlsouer, and Anthony J. Alberg. Nonmelanoma Skin Cancer and Risk for Subsequent Malignancy. *Journal of the National Cancer Institute* Advance Access published on August 26, 2008).

(Chen et al. PLoS 2009) (Chen Y, Cairns R, Papandreou I, et al. Oxygen consumption can regulate the growth of tumors, a new perspective on the Warburg effect. PLoS One. 2009 Sep 15;4(9):e7033).

(Cheng et al, 1993) (Cheng, K.C. and Loeb, L.A. Genomic instability and tumor progression: Mechanistic considerations. Adv Cancer Res 1993; 60: 121-156).

(Chiang et al, 1994) (Chiang CD, et al. Ascorbic acid increases drug accumulation and reverses vincristine resistance of human, non-small-cell lung cancer cells. Biochem J, 301:759-764, 1994).

(Chinery et al, 1997) (Chinery R, et al. Antioxidants enhance the cytotoxicity of chemotherapeutic agents in colorectal cancer: a p53-independent induction of p21WAFI/CIPI via C/EBPbeta. Nature Medicine 3(11):1233-41, 1997).

(Cho et al, 2005) (Cho SD, et al. Involvement of c-Jun N-terminal kinase in G2/M arrest and caspase-mediated apoptosis induced by sulforaphane in DU145 prostate cancer cells. Nutr Cancer. 2005;52(2):213-24).

(Cho et al, 2006) (Cho E. et al. Intakes of vitamins A, C and E and folate and multivitamins and lung cancer: a pooled analysis of 8 prospective studies. Int J Cancer. 2006 Feb 15;118(4):970-8).

(Christen et al. 2010) (Christen WG, et al. Age-related cataract in a randomized trial of vitamins E and C in men. Arch Ophthalmol. 2010 Nov;128(11):1397-405).

(Clark et al. 1996) (Clark et al. Effects of selenium supplementation for cancer prevention in patients with carcinoma of the skin. A randomized controlled trial. Nutritional Prevention of Cancer Study Group. JAMA. 1996 Dec 25;276(24):1957-63).

(Clavo et al, 2004) (Clavo B, Pérez JL, López L, et al. June 2004. "Ozone Therapy for Tumor Oxygenation: a Pilot Study". Evid Based Complement Alternat Med 1 (1): 93–98).

(Clavo, Ruiz et al, 2004) (Clavo B, Ruiz A, Lloret M, et al. December 2004. "Adjuvant Ozonetherapy in Advanced Head and Neck Tumors: A Comparative Study". Evid Based Complement Alternat Med 1 (3): 321–325).

(Clavo et al, 2005) (Clavo B, Gutiérrez D, Martín D, Suárez G, Hernández MA, Robaina F (June 2005). "Intravesical ozone therapy for progressive radiation-induced hematuria". J Altern Complement Med 11 (3): 539–41).

(Clement et al, 1998) (Clement MV, Ponton A, Pervaiz S. Apoptosis induced by hydrogen peroxide is mediated by decreased superoxide anion concentration and reduction of intracellular milieu. FEBS Lett 1998; 440:13-18).

(Conklin, 2000) (Conklin KA. Dietary antioxidants during cancer chemotherapy: Impact on chemotherapeutic effectiveness and development of side effects. *Nutrition and Cancer.* 2000;37(1):1-18).

(Conklin, 2004) (Conklin KA. Supplement: Free Radicals: The Pros and Cons of Antioxidants. Cancer Chemotherapy and Antioxidants. The American Society for Nutritional Sciences J. Nutr. 134:3201S-3204S, November 2004).

(Conklin, 2005) (Conklin KA. Coenzyme q10 for prevention of anthracycline-induced cardiotoxicity. Integr Cancer Ther (2005) 4(2):110–130).

(Connelly et al, 2003) (Connelly, A.E., Satia-Abouta, J., Martin, C.F., Keku, T.O., Woosley, J.T., Lund, P.K. and Sandler, R.S. (2003) Vitamin C intake and apoptosis in normal rectal epithelium. Cancer Epidemiol. Biomarkers Prev., 12, 559–565).

(Cook et al, 2004) (Cook JA, Gius D, Wink DA, Krishna MC, Russo A, Mitchell JB: Oxidative stress, redox, and the tumor microenvironment. *Semin Radiat Oncol 14:* 259-266, 2004).

(Cosse et al, 2008) (Cosse, Jean-Philippe; Michiels, Carine. Tumour Hypoxia Affects the Responsiveness of Cancer Cells to Chemotherapy and Promotes Cancer Progression. Anti-Cancer Agents in Medicinal Chemistry [Formerly Current Medicinal Chemistry], Volume 8, Number 7, October 2008, pp. 790-797(8).

(Coulter et al, 2006) (Antioxidants Vitamin C and Vitamin E for the Prevention and Treatment of Cancer. Coulter, Ian D.; Hardy, Mary L.; Morton, Sally C.; Hilton, Lara G.; Tu, Wenli; Valentine, Di; Shekelle, Paul G. Journal of General Internal Medicine, Volume 21, Number 7, July 2006, pp. 735-744(10).

(Coursin et al, 1996) (Coursin, D. B., Cihla, H. P., Sempf, J., Oberley, T. D. & Oberley, L. W. (1996) An immunohistochemical analysis of antioxidant and gluta-thione S-transferase enzyme levels in normal and neoplastic human lung. Histol. Histopathol. 11:851-860).

(Creagan et al, 1979) (Creagan ET, Moertel CG, O'Fallon JR, et al. Failure of high-dose vitamin C (ascorbic acid) therapy to benefit patients with advanced cancer. A controlled trial. N Engl J Med. 1979 Sep 27;301(13):687-90).

(Cullen et al, 2003) (Cullen, J. J., Hinkhouse, M. M., Grady, M., Gaut, A. W., Liu, J., Zhang, Y., Weydert, C. J. D., Domann, F. E., and Oberley, L. W. (2003) Cancer Res. 63, 5513-5520).

(D'Andrea, 2005) (D'Andrea GM. Use of antioxidants during chemotherapy and ra-diotherapy should be avoided. CA 2005;55:319–21).

(D'Incalci et al, 2007) (D'Incalci M, Steward W, Gescher A "Modulation of Response to Cancer Chemotherapeutic Agents by Diet Constituents - Is the Available Evidence Sufficiently Robust for Advice to Patients?", Cancer Treatment Review, May 2007, pp 223-229).

(Dai et al, 1999) (Dai J, Weinberg RS, Waxman S, Jing Y. Malignant cells can be sen-sitized to undergo growth inhibition and apoptosis by arsenic trioxide through modulation of the glutathione redox system. Blood 1999;93:268–77).

(Daly et al, 2009) (Daly TJ, et al. Lack of genoprotective effect of phytosterols and conjugated linoleic acids on Caco-2 cells. Food and Chemical toxicology Vol. 47. Issue 8. August 2009. pp. 1791-1796).

(Das et al, 1987) (Das UN, Begin ME, Ells G, Huang YS, Horrobin DF. Polyunsaturated fatty acids augment free radical generation in tumor cells in vitro. Biochem Biophys Res Commun 1987;145:15–24).

(Das, 2002) (U. Das. A radical approach to cancer. Med Sci Monit. 2002 Apr;8(4):RA79-92).

(Davies, Doroshow, 1986) (Davies KJ, Doroshow JH: Redox cycling of anthracy-clines by cardiac mitochondria. I. Anthracycline radical formation by NADH dehy-drogenase. J Biol Chem 1986, 261:3060-3076).

(Davies, 1999) (Davies KJ. The broad spectrum of responses to oxidants in prolifer-ating cells: a new paradigm for oxidative stress. IUBMB Life. 1999 Jul; 48(1):41-7).

(Davies et al, 2006) (Davies AA, Davey Smith G, Harbord R, et al. Nutritional in-terventions and outcome in patients with cancer or preinvasive lesions: systematic review. J Natl Cancer Inst. 2006;98:961-973).

(DeChatelet, 1975) (DeChatelet, L.R. Oxidative bactericidal mechanisms of poly-morphonuclear leukocytes. J Infect Dis 1975; 131: 295-303).

(de Gast et al, 2000) (de Gast GC, Klümpen HJ, Vyth-Dreese FA; et al. Phase I trial of combined immunotherapy with subcutaneous granulocyte macrophage colony-stimulating factor, low-dose interleukin 2, and interferon alpha in progressive meta-static melanoma and renal cell carcinoma. Clin Cancer Res. 2000;6(4):1267-1272).

(DeLorenze et al. 2010) (DeLorenze GN, McCoy L, Tsai AL, Quesenberry CP Jr, Rice T, Il'yasova D, Wrensch M. Daily intake of antioxidants in relation to survival among adult patients diagnosed with malignant glioma. BMC Cancer. 2010 May 19;10:215).

(DeLuca et al, 1996) (De Luca, L. M. & Ross, S. A. (1996) Beta-carotene increases lung cancer incidence in cigarette smokers. Nutr. Rev. 54:178-180).

(De Maria et al, 1992) (De Maria D, Falchi AM, Venturino P. Adjuvant radiotherapy of the pelvis with or without reduced glutathione: a randomized trial in patients oper-ated on for endometrial cancer. Tumori. 78(6):374-6, 1992).

(Deneke, 2000) (Deneke S. M. Thiol-based antioxidants. Curr. Top. Cell Regul., 36: 151-180, 2000).

(Dennert, Horneber, 2006) (Dennert G, Horneber M. Selenium for alleviating the side effects of chemotherapy, radiotherapy and surgery in cancer patients. Cochrane Database Syst Rev (2006) 3. CD005037).

(Dharamainder et al, 1997) (Dharamainder Choudhary, Dhyan Chandra and Raosaheb K. Kale. Influence of methylglyoxal on antioxidant enzymes and oxidative damage. Toxicology Letters. Volume 93, Issues 2-3, 1 December 1997, Pages 141-152).

(Dharmarahan et al, 1999) (A.M. Dharmarahan et al. Antioxidants mimic the ability of chorionic gonadotropin to suppress apoptosis in the rabbit corpus luteum in vitro: a novel role for superoxide dismutase in regulating bax expression. Endocrinology. 1999 Jun;140(6):2555-61).

(Diplock, 1994) (Diplock AT. Antioxidants and disease prevention. Mol Aspects Med. 1994;15:293-376).

(Diplock et al, 1998) (Diplock AT, Charleux JL, Crozier-Willi G, et al. Functional food science and defence against reactive oxidative species. Br J Nutr. 1998;80 (suppl 1):S77-S112).

(Djavaheri-Mergny et al, 2003) (Djavaheri-Mergny, M., Wietzerbin, J. and Besancon, F. (2003) 2-Methoxyestradiol induces apoptosis in Ewing sarcoma cells through mitochondrial hydrogen peroxide production. Oncogene, 22, 2558–2567).

(Dockrek, Playfair, 1984) (Dockrek H. M. and Playfair, JH. Killing of Plasmodium yoelii by enzyme-induced products of the oxidative burst. Infect Immun. 1984 Feb;43(2):451-6).

(Donnelly et al, Mutagenesis. 1999) (Donnelly ET, McClure N, Lewis SE. The effect of ascorbate and alpha-tocopherol supplementation in vitro on DNA integrity and hydrogen peroxide-induced DNA damage in human spermatozoa. Mutagenesis. 1999 Sep;14(5):505-12).

(Dorgan et al, 1998) (Dorgan JF, Sowell A, Swanson CA, et al. Relationships of serum carotenoids, retinol, alpha-tocopherol, and selenium with breast cancer risk: results from a prospective study in Columbia, Missouri (United States). Cancer Causes Control. 1998;9(1):89-97).

(Doroshenko et al, 2004) (Doroshenko N, Doroshenko P: The glutathione reductase inhibitor carmustine induces an influx of Ca2+ in PC12 cells. Eur J Pharmacol 497: 17-24, 2004).

(Doroshow, 1986) (Doroshow JH. Prevention of doxorubicin-induced killing of MCF-7 human breast cancer cells by oxygen radical scavengers and iron chelating agents. Biochemical & Biophysical Research 135(1):330-5, 1986).

(Doroshow, Davies, 1986) (Doroshow JH, Davies KJ: Redox cycling of anthracy-clines by cardiac mitochondria. II. Formation of superoxide anion, hydrogen perox-ide, and hydroxyl radical. J Biol Chem 1986, 261:3068-3074).

(Doyle et al, 1989) (Doyle LA, et al. Differentiation of human variant small cell can-cer cell lines to a classic morphology by retinoic acid. Cancer Res 49:6745-6751, 1989).

(Drisko et al, 2003) (Drisko JA, Chapman J, Hunter VJ. The use of antioxidants with first-line chemotherapy in two cases of ovarian cancer. J Am Coll Nutr 2003;22:118–23).

(Du et al, 2006) (Du J, Daniela DH, Asbury C, et al. Mitochondrial production of re-active oxygen species mediate dicumarol-induced cytotoxicity in cancer cells. J Biol Chem, 2006 Dec 8;281(49):37416-26).

(Du et , 2010) (Du J, Martin SM, Levine M. et al. Mechanisms of ascorbate-induced cytotoxicity in pancreatic cancer. Clin Cancer Res, 2010 Jan 15;16(2):509-20).

(Duarte, Lunec, 2005) (Duarte TL, Lunec J. When is an antioxidant not an an-tioxidant? a review of novel actions and reactions of vitamin C. Free Radic Res. 2005;39:671-686).

(Duffield-Lillico, 2003) (Duffueld-Lillico AJ, et al, Selenium supplementation and secondary prevention of nonmelanoma skin cancer in a randomized trial. J Natl Cancer Inst, 2003 Oct 1;95(19):1477-81).

(Dunn, 1997) (Dunn T. 1997. "Oxygen and cancer". N C Med J 58 (2): 140–3).

(Duranteau et al, 1998) (Duranteau J, Chandel NS, Kulisz A, Shao Z, Schumacker PT, 1998. Intracellular signaling by reactive oxygen species during hypoxia in cardio-myocytes. J. Biol. Chem. 273, 11619–11624).

(Dussan et al, 2008) (Dussan C, Zubor P, Fernandez M, Yabar A, Szunyogh N, Visnovsky J. Spontaneous regression of a breast carcinoma: a case report. Gynecol Obstet Invest. 2008;65(3):206-211).

(Eisenberg et al, 1993) (Eisenberg DM, Kessler RC, Foster C, et al: Unconventional medicine in the United States: Prevalence, costs, and patterns of use. N Engl J Med 328(4):246-252, 1993).

(Enger et al, 1995) (Enger SM, Longnecker MP, Shikany JM, et al: Questionnaire assessment of intake of specific carotenoids. Cancer Epidemiol Biomarkers Prev 4(3):201-205, 1995).

(Epplein, 2009) (Meira Epplein et al. Plasma carotenoids, retinol, and tocopherols and postmenopausal breast cancer risk in the Multiethnic Cohort Study: a nested case-control study. *Breast Cancer Research.* 2009, 11:R49).

(Erhola et al, 1996) (Erhola M, Kellokumpu-Lehtinen P, Metsa-Ketela T, et al: Effect of anthracycline-based chemotherapy on total plasma antioxidant capacity in small-cell lung cancer patients. Free Radic Biol Med 21(3):383-390, 1996).

(Ernst, 2001) (Ernst E (January 2001). "A primer of complementary and alternative medicine commonly used by cancer patients". Med. J. Aust. 174 (2): 88–92).

(Esposti et al, 1999) (Esposti M. D., Hatzinisiriou I., McLennan H., Ralph S. Bcl-2 and mitochondrial oxygen radicals. New approaches with reactive oxygen species-sensitive probes. J. Biol. Chem., 274: 29831-29837, 1999).

(Evens et al, 2005) (Andrew M. Evens, Philip Lecane, Darren Magda, Sheila Prachand, Seema Singhal, Jeff Nelson, Richard A. Miller, Ronald B. Gartenhaus, and Leo I. Gordon. Motexafin gadolinium generates reactive oxygen species and induces apoptosis in sensitive and highly resistant multiple myeloma cells. Blood, 1 February 2005, Vol. 105, No. 3, pp. 1265-1273).

(Fairfield et al, 2001) (Fairfield KM, Hankinson SE, Rosner BA, Hunter DJ, Colditz GA, Willett WC. Risk of ovarian carcinoma and consumption of vitamins A, C, and E and specific carotenoids: a prospective analysis. Cancer. 2001 Nov 1;92(9):2318-26).

(Fang et al, 2002) (Fang J, Sawa T, Akaike T and Maeda H. Tumor-targeted Delivery of Polyethylene Glycol-conjugated D-Amino Acid Oxidase for Antitumor Therapy via Enzymatic Generation of Hydrogen Peroxide. *Cancer Research* 62, 3138-3143, June 1, 2002).

(Fang et al, 2007) (Fang J, Nakamura H, Iyer AK. Tumor-targeted induction of oxystress for cancer therapy. J Drug Target. 2007 Aug-Sep;15(7-8):475-86).

(Fang, Nakamura, Iyer, 2007) (Fang J, Nakamura H, Iyer AK. Tumor-targeted induction of oxystress for cancer therapy. J Drug Target. 2007 Aug-Sep;15(7-8):475-86).

(Fang et al, 2008) (Fang J, Deng D, Nakamura H, et al. Oxystress inducing antitumor therapeutics via tumor-targeted delivery of PEG-conjugated D-amino acid oxidase. Int J Cancer. 2008 Mar 1;122(5):1135-44).

(Fantappie et al, 2004) (Fantappie O, Lodovici M, Fabrizio P, et al. Vitamin E protects DNA from oxidative damage in human hepatocellular carcinoma cell lines. Free Radic Res (2004) 38(7):751–759).

(Farah and Begum, 2003) (I. O. Farah and R. A. Begum. Effect of Nigella sativa and oxidative stress on the survival pattern of MCF-7 breast cancer cells. Biomedical Sciences Instrumentation. 39. 2003: 359-64).

(Fath et al, 2009) (Fath MA, Diers AR, Aykin-Burns N, Simons AL, Hua L, Spitz. DR. Mitochondrial electron transport chain blockers enhance 2-deoxy-D-glucose induced oxidative stress and cell killing in human colon carcinoma cells. Cancer Biol Ther. 2009 Jul;8(13):1228-36).

(Feng et al, 2007) (Feng R., Ni H., Wang S.Y., Tourkova I. L., Shurin M. R., Harada H. and Yin X. Cyanidin-3-rutinoside, a Natural Polyphenol Antioxidant, Selectively Kills Leukemic Cells by Induction of Oxidative Stress. The Journal of Biological Chemistry. 2007; 282(18): 13468–13476).

(Ferlat et al, 1993) (Ferlat S; Favier A. C R Seances. Tumor necrosis factor (TNF) and oxygen free radicals: potential effects for immunity. Soc Biol Fil. 1993;187(3):296-307).

(Ferlini et al, 1999) (Ferlini C, Scambia G, Marone M, Distefano M, Gaggini C, Ferrandina G, Fattorossi A, Isola G, Benedetti Panici P, Mancuso S. Tamoxifen induces oxidative stress and apoptosis in estrogen receptor-negative human cancer cell lines. Br J Cancer 1999;**79**:257–263).

(Ferreira et al, 2004) (Ferreira PR, Fleck JF, Diehl A, et al. Protective effect of alpha-tocopherol in head and neck cancer radiation-induced mucositis: a double-blind randomized trial. Head Neck (2004) 26(4):313–321).

(Fiers, et al, 1999) (Fiers W, Beyaert R, Declercq W, Vandenabeele P. More than one way to die: apoptosis, necrosis and reactive oxygen damage. Oncogene (1999) 18: 7719-30).

(Figueiredo et al, 2009) (Figueiredo JC et al. Folic acid and risk of prostate cancer: results from a randomized clinical trial. J Natl Cancer Inst. 2009 Mar 18;101(6):432-5).

(Finkel, Holbrook, 2000) (Finkel T, Holbrook N.J., 2000. Oxidants, oxidative stress and the biology of ageing. Nature 408, 239–247).

(Finney et al, 1961) (Finney, J.W., Collier, R.E., Balla, G.A., Tomme, J.W., Wakley, J., Race, G.J., Urschel, H.C., D'Errico, A.D. and Mallams, J.T. The preferential localization of radioisotopes in malignant tissue by regional oxygenation. Nature 1961; 202: 1172).

(Finney et al, 1965) (Finney, J.W., Balla, G.A., Collier, R.E., Wakely, J., Urschel, H.C. and Mallams, J.T. Differential localization of isotopes in tumors through the use of intra-arterial hydrogen peroxide: Part I: Basic science. Amer J Roentgen 1965; 94: 783).

(Fluery et al, 2002) (Fleury C, Mignotte B, Vayssiere JL. Mitochondrial reactive oxygen species in cell death signaling. Biochimie 2002; 84:131-41).

(Food and chemical toxicology, 2007) (Antioxidant and prooxidant effects of quercetin on glyceraldehyde-3-phosphate dehydrogenase. Food and chemical toxicology. 2007;45(10):1988-93).

(Franka et al, 2010) (Franca C, Nogewira C, Ramalho A, et al. Serum levels of selenium in patients with breast cancer before and after treatment of external beam radiotherapy. Ann Oncol 2010. doi: 10.1093/annonc/mdq547. First published online: Oct 5, 2010).

(Fredrik et al, 2006) (*Fredrik B. Thorén, Ana I. Romero and Kristoffer Hellstrand*. Oxygen Radicals Induce Poly(ADP-Ribose) Polymerase-Dependent Cell Death in Cytotoxic Lymphocytes. *The Journal of Immunology,* 2006, 176: 7301-7307).

(Frieling et al, 2000) (Frieling UM, et al. A randomized, 12-year primary-prevention trial of beta carotene supplementation for nonmelanoma skin cancer in the physician's health study. Arch Dermatol. 2000 Feb;136(2):179-84).

(Frommel et al, 1995) (Frommel TO, Sohrab M, Doria M, et al: Effect of beta-carotene supplementation on indices of colonic cell proliferation. J Natl Cancer Inst 87(23):1781-1787, 1995).

(Gali-Muhtasib et al, 2008) (Hala Gali-Muhtasib et al. Thymoquinone Triggers Inactivation of the Stress Response Pathway Sensor *CHEK1* and Contributes to Apoptosis in Colorectal Cancer Cells. Cancer Res 2008;68(14):5609–18).

(Galleano et al, 2002) (Galleano M, Aimo L, Puntarulo S. Ascorbyl radical/ascorbate ratio in plasma from iron overloaded rats as oxidative stress indicator. *Toxical Lett.* 2002;133:193–201).

(Gallicchio et al, 2008) (Gallicchio L. et al. Carotenoids and the risk of developing lung cancer: a systematic review. Am J Clin Nutr. 2008 Aug;88(2):372-83).

(Gaziano et al, 2009) (Vitamins E and C in the prevention of prostate and total cancer in men: the Physicians' Health Study II randomized controlled trial. Gaziano, JM., JAMA. 2009 Jan 7;301(1):52-62. Epub 2008 Dec 9).

(Gandara et al, 1995) (Gandara DR, et al. A randomized placebo-controlled multi-center evaluation of diethyldithiocarbamate for chemoprotection against cisplatin-induced toxicities. J Clin Oncol 13:490-496, 1995).

(Garewal, 1997) (Garewal HS: Antioxidants and Disease Prevention, pp 19-26. New York, CRC Press, 1997).

(Garland et al, 1995) (Garland M, Morris S, Meir J. et al. Prospective study of toenail seleniumlevels and cancer among women. JNCI J Natl Cancer Inst (1995) 87 (7): 497-505).

(Genkinger et al. 2004) (Genkinger JM, Platz EA, Hoffman SC, Comstock GW, Helzlsouer KJ. Fruit, vegetable, and antioxidant intake and all-cause, cancer, and cardiovascular disease mortality in a community-dwelling population in Washington County, Maryland. Am J Epidemiol. 2004 Dec 15;160(12):1223-33).

(Gerwirtz, 1999) (Gewirtz DA: A critical evaluation of the mechanisms of action proposed for the antitumor effects of the anthracycline antibiotics Adriamycin and daunorubicin. Biochem Pharmacol 1999, 57:727-741).

(Gianfranco et al, 2004) (C. Gianfranco et al. The Journal of biological chemistry. 2004, vol. 279, pp. 13738-13745).

(Giovannucci, et al., 1998) (Giovannucci, E., M.J. Stampfer, G.A. Colditz, D.J. Hunter, C. Fuchs, B.A. Rosner, F.E. Speizer & W.C. Willett. 1998. Multivitamin use, folate, and colon cancer in women in the Nurses' Health Study. Ann. Intern. Med. 129(7):517-524)

(Giovannucce, Chan, 2010) (Giovannucce E, Chan AT. Role of vitamin and mineral supplementation and aspirin use in cancer survivors. J Clin Oncol. 2010 Sep 10;28(26):4081-5).

(Gleave et al, 1998) (Gleave ME, Elhilali M, Fradet Y; et al, Canadian Urologic Oncology Group. Interferon gamma-1b compared with placebo in metastatic renal-cell carcinoma. *N Engl J Med.* 1998;338(18):1265-1271).

(Gogvadze et al, 2009) (Gogvadze V, Orrenius S, Zhivotovsky B. Mitochondria as targets for cancer chemotherapy. <u>Semin Cancer Biol.</u> 2009 Feb;19(1):57-66).

(Gonzalez et al, 2004) (González R, Borrego A, Zamora Z, et al. (December 2004). "<u>Reversion by ozone treatment of acute nephrotoxicity induced by cisplatin in rats</u>". Mediators Inflamm. 13 (5-6): 307–12).

(Goodman et al, 2004) (Goodman GE, Thornquist MD, Balmes J, Cullen MR, Meyskens Jr. FL, Omenn GS, et al. The Beta-Carotene and Retinol Efficacy Trial: Incidence of Lung Cancer and Cardiovascular Disease Mortality During 6-Year Follow-up After Stopping Beta-Carotene and Retinol Supplements. J Natl Cancer Inst 2004;96:1743-50).

(Gottlieb, 1999) (Gottlieb, N. (1999) Cancer treatment and vitamin C: the debate lingers. J. Natl. Cancer Inst. 24:2073-2075).

(Grad et al, 2001) (<u>Grad</u> JM, <u>Bahlis</u> NJ, <u>Reis</u> I, <u>Oshiro</u> MM, <u>Dalton</u> WS, <u>Boise</u> LH. Ascorbic acid enhances arsenic trioxide-induced cytotoxicity in multiple myeloma cells. Blood (2001) 98: 805-13).

(Graham et al, 1992) (Graham S, Sielezny M, Marshall J, Priore R, Freudenheim J, Brasure J, Haughey B, Nasca P, Zdeb M. Diet in the epidemiology of Postmenopausal Breast Cancer in the New York State Cohort. Am J Epidemiol 1992;136:3127-37).

(Gray et al, 1953) (Gray LH, Conger AD, Ebert M, Hornsey S, Scott OC (December 1953). "The concentration of oxygen dissolved in tissues at the time of irradiation as a factor in radiotherapy". Br J Radiol 26 (312): 638–48).

(Green, Reed, 1998) (Green DR, Reed JC. Mitochondria and apoptosis. Science 1998;281:1309–12).

(Green et al, 1999) (Green A, Williams G, Neale R, et al.: Daily sunscreen application and beta carotene supplementation in prevention of basal-cell and squamous-cell carcinomas of the skin: a randomised controlled trial. Lancet 354 (9180): 723-9, 1999)

(Greenberg et al, 1994) (Greenberg ER, Baron JA, Tosteson TD, Freeman DH Jr, Beck GJ, Bond JH, Colacchio TA, Coller JA, Frankl HD, Haile RW, et al. A clinical trial of antioxidant vitamins to prevent colorectal adenoma. Polyp Prevention Study Group. N Engl J Med. 1994 Jul 21;331(3):141-7).

(Greenberg et al, 1996) (Greenberg ER, Baron JA, Karagas MR, Stukel TA, Nierenberg DW, Stevens MM, Mandel JS, Haile RW. Mortality associated with low plasma concentration of beta carotene and the effect of oral supplementation. JAMA. 1996; 275: 699-703).

(Greenlee et al, 2009) (Greenlee H, Gammon MD, Abrahamson PE, et al. Prevalence and predictors of antioxidant supplement use during breast cancer treatment: the Long Island Breast Cancer Study Project. Cancer. 2009 Jul 15;115(14):3271-82).

(Greenlee, Hershman et al, 2009) (Greenlee H, Hershman DL, Jacobson JS. Use of antioxidant supplements during breast cancer treatment: a comprehensive review. Breast Cancer Res Treat. 2009 Jun;115(3):437-52).

(Grechkanev et al, 2002) (Gretchkanev et al., Role of Ozone Therapy in Prevention and Treatment of Complications of Drug Therapy for Ovarian Cancer. Akusherstvo Ginekologiya No 4, 57-58, 2002).

(Grimm et al, 2011) (Grimm S, Mvondo d, Grune T, Bruesing N. The outcome of 5-ALA-mediated photodynamic treatment inmelamomacells is influenced by vitamin C and heme oxygenase-1. Biofactors. 2011 Jan;37(1):17-24).

(Guaiquil et al, 1997) (Guaiquil VH, Farber CM, Golde DW, Vera JC. Efficient transport and accumulation of vitamin C in HL-60 cells depleted of glutathione. J Biol Chem. 1997;272:9915–9921).

(Guaiquil et al, 2001) (Guaiquil VH, Vera JC, Golde DW. Mechanism of vitamin C inhibition of cell death induced by oxidative stress in glutathione- depleted HL-60 cells. J Biol Chem. 2001;276:40955–40961).

(Gundimeda et al 1996) (Gundimeda U, Chen Z-H and Gopalakrishna R. Tamoxifen Modulates Protein Kinase C via Oxidative Stress in Estrogen Receptor-negative Breast Cancer Cells. J. Biol. Chem. Volume 271, Number 23, Issue of June 7, 1996 pp. 13504-13514).

(Gupta et al, 2000) (Gupta S, Ahmad N, Nieminen AL, Mulhtar H. Growth inhibition, cell-cycle dysregulation, and induction of apoptosis by green tea constituent (–)-epigallocatechin-3-gallate in androgen-sensitive and androgen-insensitive human prostate carcinoma cells. Toxicol Appl Pharmacol 2000;164:82–90).

(Guzik, Harrison, 2006) (Guzik TJ, Harrison DG. Vascular NADPH oxidases as drug targets for novel antioxidant strategies. Drug Discov Today. 2006 Jun;11(11-12):524-33).

(Hadzic et al, 2010) (Hadzic T, Aykin-Burns N, Zhu Y, Coleman MC, Leick K, Jacobson GM, Spitz DR. Paclitaxel combined with inhibitors of glucose and hydroperoxide metabolism enhances breast cancer cell killing via H2O2-mediated oxidative stress. Free Radic Biol Med. 2010 Apr 15;48(8):1024-33).

(Haendeler et al, 1996) (Haendeler, J., Zeiher, A. M. & Dimmler, S. (1996) Vitamin C and vitamin E prevent lipopolysaccharide-induced apoptosis in human endothelial cells by modulating Bcl-2 and Bax. Eur. J. Pharmachol. 17:407-411).

(Hahm et al, 2007) (Hahm E, Jin DH, Kang JS, Kim YI, Hong SW, Lee SK, Kim HN, Jung da J, Kim JE, Shin DH, Hwang YI, Kim YS, Hur DY, Yang Y, Cho D, Lee MS, Lee WJ. The molecular mechanisms of vitamin C on cell cycle regulation in B16F10 murine melanoma. J Cell Biochem. 2007;102:1002–1010).

(Hail et al, 2008) (Numsen Hail Jr. Marcela Cortes, Edgar N. Drake and Julian E. Spallholz. Cancer chemoprevention: A radical Perspective. Free Radical Biology and Medicine. Volume 45, Issue 2, 15 July 2008, Pages 97-110).

(Hall, 2000) (Hall E. Repair of radiation damage and the dose-rate effect. In: In: John J-R, Sutton P, Marino D, eds. Radiobiology for the Radiologist (2000) 5th ed. Philadelphia, PA: Lippincott Williams and Wilkins. 67–90).

(Halliwell, 1989) (Halliwell B, Gutteridge JMC: Free Radicals in Biology and Medicine. Oxford University Press; 1989).

(Halliwell, 1990) (Halliwell B. (1990) "How to characterize a biological antioxidant", Free Radical Res. Commun. 9, 1-32).

(Halliwell et al, 2000) (B Halliwell et al. Hydrogen peroxide in the human body. FEBS Lett. 2000 Dec 1;486(1):10-3).

(Halliwell et al, 2007) (Halliwell B (2007). "Dietary polyphenols: good, bad, or indifferent for your health?". Cardiovasc. Res. 73 (2): 341-7).

(Halperin et al, 1993) (Halperin EC, Gaspar L, George S, et al: A double-blind, randomized, prospective trial to evaluate topical vitamin C solution for the prevention of radiation dermatitis: CNS Cancer Consortium. Int J Radiat Oncol Biol Phys 26:413-416, 1993).

(Hampton, Orrenius, 1997) (MB Hampton, S Orrenius. Dual regulation of caspase activity by hydrogen peroxide: implications for apoptosis. FEBS Lett (1997) 414: 552-6).

(Hanck, 1988) (Hanck AB. Vitamin C and cancer. Progress in Clinical & Biological Research 259:307-20, 1988).

(Hansson et al, 1996) (Hansson, M., A. Asea, U. Ersson, S. Hermodsson, K. Hellstrand. 1996. Induction of apoptosis in NK cells by monocyte-derived reactive oxygen metabolites. J. Immunol. 156: 42-47).

(Hansson et al, 1999) (Hansson, M., S. Hermodsson, M. Brune, U. H. Mellqvist, P. Naredi, A. Betten, K. R. Gehlsen, K. Hellstrand. 1999. Histamine protects T cells and natural killer cells against oxidative stress. J. Interferon Cytokine Res. 19: 1135-1144).

(Harder et al, 2006) (Simone Harder, Meike Bente, Kerstin Isermann, and Iris Bruchhaus. Expression of a Mitochondrial Peroxiredoxin Prevents Programmed Cell Death in Leishmania donovani. Eukaryotic Cell, May 2006, p. 861-870, Vol. 5, No. 5).

(Harman, 1956) (Harman D. Aging: a theory based on free radical and radiation chemistry. J Gerontol 11: 298–300, 1956).

(Harman D., 1981. The aging process. Proc. Natl Acad. Sci. USA 78, 7124–7128).

(Harman, 1961) (Harman D. 1961. Mutation, cancer and aging. Lancet 1: 200-201).

(Hasinoff, Davey, 1988) (Hasinoff B. B., Davey J. P. Adriamycin and its iron(III) and copper(III) complexes, glutathione-induced dissociation, cytochrome c oxidase inactivation and protection: binding to cardiolipin. Biochem. Pharmacol., 37: 3663-3669, 1988).

(Hawkins et al, 1998) (Hawkins, R. A., Sangster, K. & Arends, M. J. (1998) Apoptotic death of pancreatic cancer cells induced by polyunsaturated fatty acids varies with double bond number and involves an oxidative mechanism. J. Pathol. 185:61-70).

(Hayakawa et al, 2003) (Hayakawa M, Miyashita H, Sakamoto I, Kitagawa M, Tanaka H, Yasuda H, Karin M, Kikugawa K: Evidence that reactive oxygen species do not

mediate NF-kB activation. *EMBO J* 2003, 22:3356-3366).

(Healy et al, 1998) (Healy, C. G., J. W. Simons, M. A. Carducci, T. L. DeWeese, M. Bartkowski, K. P. Tong, W. E. Bolton. 1998. Impaired expression and function of signal-transducing zchains in peripheral T cells and natural killer cells in patients with prostate cancer. *Cytometry* 32: 109-119).

(Heaney et al, 2008) (Heaney ML, Gardner JR, Karasavvas N, Golde DW, Scheinberg DA, Smith EA, O'Connor OA. Vitamin C antagonizes the cytotoxic effects of antineoplastic drugs. *Cancer Res.* 2008;68:8031–8038).

(Heinonen et al, 1994) (Heinonen, O.P., J.K. Huttunen, D. Albanes & ATBC cancer prevention study group. 1994. The effect of vitamin E and beta carotene on the incidence of lung cancer and other cancers in male smokers. N. Engl. J. Med. 330:1029-1035).

(Heinonen et al, 1998) (Heinonen, O. P., Albanes, D., Virtamo, J., Taylor, P. R., Huttunen, J. K., Hartman, A. M., Haapakoski, J., Malila, N. & Rautalahti, M., et al (1998) Prostate cancer and supplementation with alpha-tocopherol and beta-carotene: incidence and mortality in a controlled trial. J. Natl. Cancer Inst. 90:440-446).

(Henderson, Dougherty, 1992) (Henderson, B.W. and Dougherty, T.J. How does photodynamic therapy work? Photochem Photobiol 1992; 55: 145-157).

(Henderson, Fingar, 1987) (Henderson, B.W. and Fingar, V.H. Relationship of tumor hypoxia and response to photodynamic treatment in an experimental mouse tumor. Cancer Res 1987; 47: 3110-3114).

(Hennekens et al, 1996) (Hennekens CH, Buring JE, Manson JE, et al. Lack of effect of long-term supplementation with beta carotene on the incidence of malignant neoplasms and cardiovascular disease. N Engl J Med. 1996;334:1145-1149).

(Herbert et al. 2006) (Herbert KE, Fletcher S, Chauhan D, Ladapo A, Nirwan J, Munson S, Mistry P. Dietary supplementation with different vitamin C doses: no effect on oxidative DNA damage in healthy people. Eur J Nutr. 2006 Mar;45(2):97-104).

(Hercberg et al, 2004) (Hercberg S, Galan P, Preziosi P, Bertrais S, Mennen L, Malvy D, Roussel A-M, Favier A, Briançon S. SU.VI.MAX Study. Arch Intern Med 2004;164:2335–42).

(Hercberg et al, 2007) (Serge Hercberg et al. Antioxidant Supplementation Increases the Risk of Skin Cancers in Women but Not in Men. <u>American Society for Nutrition</u> J. Nutr. 137:2098-2105, September 2007).

(Hileman et al, 2004) (Hileman EO, Liu J, Albitar M, Keating MJ, Huang P. Intrinsic oxidative stress in cancer cells: a biochemical basis for therapeutic selectivity. Cancer Chemother Pharmacol. 2004 Mar;53(3):209-19).

(Hirpara et al, 2001) (Hirpara JL, Clement MV, Pervaiz S. Intracellular acidification triggered by mitochondrial-derived hydrogen peroxide is an effector mechanism for drug-induced apoptosis in tumor cells. J Biol Chem 2001;276:514-521).

(Hiraoka et al, 1998) (W Hiraoka, N Vazquez, W Nieves-Neira, S J Chanock and Y Pommier. Role of oxygen radicals generated by NADPH oxidase in apoptosis induced in human leukemia cells. *J. Clin. Invest.* 102(11): 1961-1968 (1998).

(Ho et al, 2007) (Ho et al, 2007) (J. C. Ho et al. Disturbance of systemic antioxidant profile in nonsmall cell lung carcinoma. Eur Respir J 2007; 29:273-278).

(Hofstad et al, 1996) (Hofstad B, Vatn MH, Andersen SN; et al. Growth of colorectal polyps: redetection and evaluation of unresected polyps for a period of three years. *Gut.* 1996;39(3):449-456).

(Hohn, 1997) (Hohn, D.C. Oxygen and leukocyte microbial killing. Davis, J.C., Hunt, T.K. Eds. Hyperbaric Oxygen Therapy, Bethesday, Undersea Med Soc 1977; 101-110).

(Horneber et al, 2008) (Horneber et al. Mistletoe therapy in oncology. Cochrane Database Syst Rev. 2008 Apr 16;(2):CD003297).

(Hotaling et al, 2010) ((James Hotaling, Jonathan Wright, Gaia Pocobelli, Michael Porter and Emily White. Long-Term Use of supplemental vitamin C, vitamin D and vitamin E does not reduce the risk of urothelial cell carcinoma of the bladder in the VITamins and Lifestyle Study. The Journal of Urology. Vol. 183, Issue 4, Supplement 1, April 2010, Page e450).

(Hotaling et al, 2011) (JM Hotaling, et al. Long-Term Use of supplemental vitamins and minerals does not reduce the risk of urothelial cell carcinoma of the bladder in the VITamins and Lifestyle Study. In press. Available online 2-18-2011).

(Hou et al, 2005) (Hou D-X, Tong X, Terahara N, Luo D, Fujii M. Delphinidin 3-sam-bubioside (Dp3-Sam), a Hibiscus anthocyanin, induces apoptosis in human leukemia cells through reactive oxygen species-mediated mitochondrial pathway. Arch-Biochem-Biophys. 2005 Aug 1; 440(1): 101-9).

(Howes, Steele, 1971) (Howes, R. M. and Steele, R. H., Microsomal chemilumines-cence induced by NADPH and its relation to lipid peroxidation, Res. Commun. Chem. Path. Pharmacol., July-Sept. 1971, 2; 4 & 5:619-626).

(Howes, Steele, 1972) (Howes, R.M. and Steele, R.H., Microsomal chemilumines-cence induced by NADPH and its relation to aryl-hydroxylations, Res Commun. Chem. Path. Pharmacol., March 1972, 3; 2:349-357).

(Howes et al, 1976) (Howes, R. M., Allen, R.C., Su, C.T. and Hoopes, J.E., Altered polymorphonuclear leukocyte bioenergetics in patients with thermal injury, the Surgical Forum, 1976, 27:558-560).

(Howes, Steele, 1976) (Howes, R.M., Steele, R.H. and Hoopes, J.E., Peroxide induced Chemiluminescence in an in vitro proline hydroxylation system, 1976, 8; 1:77-84).

(Howes et al, 1977) (Howes, R.M., Steele, R.H. and Hoopes, J.E., The role of Electronic excitation states in collagen biosynthesis, Persp. In Biol. And Med., Summer 1977, 20; 4:539-544).

(Howes, 2004) (Howes, R. M. U.T.O.P.I.A. - Unified Theory of Oxygen Participation in Aerobiosis. © 2004. Free Radical Publishing Co. Kentwood, LA, available at www. iwillfindthecure.org.).

(Howes, 2005) (Howes, R.M. Tumoricidal Activity of An Injectable Singlet Oxygen System Generated From Physiological Agents: The Howes Singlet Oxygen Cancer Therapy System). In The Medical and Scientific Significance of Oxygen Free Radical Metabolism. © 2005. Free Radical Publishing Co. Kentwood, LA. pp. 893-912).

(Howes, Farber, 2005) (Howes, R.M. and Farber, G. Tumoricidal Activity of the Howes Singlet Oxygen Delivery System in Human Basal Cell Carcinoma. In The Medical and Scientific Significance of Oxygen Free Radical Metabolism. © 2005. Free Radical Publishing Co. Kentwood, LA. pp. 883-892).

(Howes, 2006) (Howes R.M. The Free Radical Fantasy: A Panoply of Paradoxes. Ann. N.Y. Acad. Sci. 2006;1067:22-26).

(Howes, Philica. Feb 26, 2007) (Howes M.D., PhD., R. (2007). Cancer, Apoptosis and Reactive Oxygen Species: A New Paradigm. PHILICA.COM Article number 86. Published on 26th February, 2007).

(Howes, Philica. April 5, 2007) (Howes M.D., PhD., R. (2007). Antioxidant Vitamins A, C & E; Death in Small Doses and Legal Liability? PHILICA.COM Article number 89. Published April 5, 2007).

(Howes, Am J Cos Surg. 2009) (Antioxidant Vitamins: A Review of Policy Statements and Recommendations. R.M. Howes. The American Journal of Cosmetic Surgery. Vol. 26, No. 2, pg. 63-78, 2009).

(Howes, Philica. Feb 7, 2009) (Howes M.D., PhD., R. (2009). Dangers of Antioxidants in Cancer Patients: A Review. PHILICA.COM Article number 153. Published 7th February, 2009).

(Howes, 2009) (Howes, R. M. Reactive Oxygen Species Insufficiency (ROSI) as the Basis for Disease Allowance and Coexistence. © 2009. Free Radical Publishing Co. Kentwood, LA, available at www.iwillfindthecure.org.).

(Howes R : Hydrogen Peroxide: 2010) (R. Howes : Hydrogen Peroxide: A review of a scientifically verifiable omnipresent ubiquitous essentiality of obligate, aerobic, carbon-based life forms. The Internet Journal of Plastic Surgery. 2010 Volume 7 Number 1)

(Howes, 2010) (Howes R. Death In Small Doses? Trafford Publishing. Indianapolis, USA. 2010).

(Howes R : Cancer Therapy, 2010) (Howes R : Cancer Therapy: A Review with Scientific Validation for the Role of Electronically Modified Oxygen Derivatives in Oncologic Treatment Modalities. The Internet Journal of Alternative Medicine. 2010 Volume 8 Number 1).

(Howes, 2010) (Howes R. Death In Small Doses? Trafford Publishing. Indianapolis, USA. 2010).

(Huang et al, 2000) (Huang P., Feng L., Oldham E.A., Keating M. J., Plunkett W. Superoxide dismutase as a target for the selective killing of cancer cells. Nature (Lond.), 407: 390-395, 2000).

(Huang et al, 2006) (Huang HY, Caballero B, Chang S, et al. The efficacy and safety of multivitamin and mineral supplement use to prevent cancer and chronic disease in adults: a systematic review for a National Institutes of Health state-of-the-science conference. *Ann Intern Med.* 2006;145:372-385).

(Huang et al, 2006 May) (Huang HY, Caballero B, Chang S, Alberg A, Semba R, Schneyer C, Wilson RF, Cheng TY, Prokopowicz G, Barnes GJ 2nd, Vassy J, Bass EB. Multivitamin/mineral supplements and prevention of chronic disease. Evid Rep Technol Assess (Full Rep). 2006 May;(139):1-117).

(Huang et al, 2006 Sept) (H. Huang et al. The Efficacy and Safety of Multivitamin and Mineral Supplement Use To Prevent Cancer and Chronic Disease in Adults: A Systematic Review for a National Institutes of Health State-of-the-Science Conference. September 5, 2006, Vol. 145. Issue 5. Pages 372-385).

(Hughes et al, 1998) (Hughes CM, Lewis SE, McKelvey-Martin VJ, Thompson W. The effects of antioxidant supplementation during Percoll preparation on human sperm DNA integrity. Hum Reprod. 1998 May;13(5):1240-7).

(Hulten, 2001) (Hulten K, Van Kappel AL, Winkvist A, et al. Carotenoids, alpha-to-copherols, and retinol in plasma and breast cancer risk in northern Sweden. Cancer Causes Control. 2001;12(6):529-537).

(Hunter et al, 1993) (A Prospective Study of the Intake of Vitamins C, E, and A and the Risk of Breast Cancer. David J. Hunter, JoAnn E. Manson, Graham A. Colditz, Meir J. Stampfer, Bernard Rosner, Charles H. Hennekens, Frank E. Speizer, and Walter C. Willett. The New England Journal of Medicine. Vol. 329:234-240. No. 4. July 22, 1993).

(Il'yasova et al. 2009) (Il'yasova D, Marcello JE, McCoy L, Rice T, Wrensch M. Total dietary antioxidant index and survival in patients with glioblastoma multiforme. Cancer Causes Control. 2009 Oct;20(8):1255-60)

(Inoue et al, 2009) (Inoue et al. Green tea consumption and gastric cancer in Japanese: a pooled analysis of six cohort studies. Gut. 2009 Oct;58(10):1323-32).

(Institute of Medicine, 2000) (Institute of Medicine. *Dietary Reference Intakes for Vitamin C, Vitamin E, Selenium, and Carotenoids.* Washington, DC: National Academy Press; 2000).

(Isham et al, 2007) (C. R. Isham, J. D. Tibodeau, W. Jin, R. Xu, M. M. Timm, and K. C. Bible. Chaetocin: a promising new antimyeloma agent with in vitro and in vivo activity mediated via imposition of oxidative stress. Blood, March 15, 2007; 109(6): 2579 - 2588).

(Israel et al, 1985) (Israel L, et al. Augmentation par la vitamin A des effets de la chimiotherapie dans le cancer du sein metastases apres la menopause. Ann Med Interne 136:551-554, 1985).

(Ishikawa et al, 2006) (Ishikawa et al. Smoking, alcohol drinking, green tea consumption and the risk of esophageal cancer in Japanese men. J Epidemiol. 2006 Sep;16(5):185-92).

(Iwasaki et al, 2010) (Motoki Iwasaki; Manami Inoue; Shizuka Sasazuki; Norie Sawada; Taiki Yamaji; Taichi Shimazu; Walter C Willett; Shoichiro Tsugane. Green Tea Drinking and Subsequent Risk of Breast Cancer in a Population to Based Cohort of Japanese Women. Breast Cancer Research. 2010;12(5:R88).

(J. Nutr. 134, 2004) (FREE RADICALS: THE PROS AND CONS OF ANTIOXIDANTS. Division of Cancer Prevention National Cancer Institute. Division of Cancer Treatment and Diagnosis, National Cancer Institute. National Cancer Institute. National Center for Complementary and Alternative Medicine National Institutes of Health. Office of Dietary Supplements National Institutes of Health. (at http://www.nutrition.org, References to the published, final version of this manuscript should include the following citation: Seifried HE, Anderson EE, Sorkin BC, Costello RB. J. Nutr. 134:3143S-3163S, 2004).

(Jaakkola et al, 1992) (Jaakkola K, Lahteenmaki P, Laakso J, et al. Treatment with antioxidant and other nutrients in combination with chemotherapy and irradiation in patients with small-cell lung cancer. Anticancer Res 1992;12:599-606).

(Jacobs, 2001) (Jacobs EJ, Connell CJ, Patel AV, Chao A, Rodriguez C, Seymour J, McCullough ML, Calle EE, Thun MJ. Vitamin C and vitamin E supplement use and colorectal cancer mortality in a large American Cancer Society cohort. Cancer Epidemiol Biomarkers Prev, 2001 Jan;10(1):17-23).

(Jacobs et al., 2002) (Jacobs EJ, Henion AK, Briggs PJ, Connell CJ, McCullough ML, Jonas CR, Rodriguez C, Calle EE, Thun MJ. Vitamin C and vitamin E supplement use and bladder cancer mortality in a large cohort of US men and women. American Journal of Epidemiology 2002;156: 1002-10).

(Jacobs et al. Jan. 2002) (Jacobs EJ, Connell CJ, McCullough ML, Chao A, Jonas CR, Rodriguez C, Calle EE, Thun MJ. Vitamin C, vitamin E, and multivitamin supplement use and stomach cancer mortality in the Cancer Prevention Study II cohort. Cancer Epidemiol Biomarkers Prev, 2002 Jan;11(1):35-41).

(Jaganjac et al, 2008) (M. Jaganjac, M. Poljak-Blazi, K. Zarkovic, R. Schaur, N. Zarkovic. The involvement of granulocytes in spontaneous regression of Walker 256 carcinoma. *Cancer Letters*, Volume 260, Issue 1, 18 February 2008, Pages 180-186).

(James, 1994) (James ER 1994. Superoxide dismutase. Parasitol Today 10:481-484).

(Jang, Surh, 2001) (Jang JH, Surh YJ. Protective effects of resveratrol on hydrogen peroxide-induced apoptosis in rat pheochromocytoma (PC12) cells. Mutat Res (2001) 496: 181-90).

(Jarvinen, 1995) (Jarvinen R: Carotenoids, retinoids, tocopherols, and tocotrienols in the diet—the Finnish mobile clinic health examination survey. Int J Vitam Nutr Res 65(1):24-30, 1995).

(Jiang et al, 2009) (Jiang YY, et al. The protective effect of silibinin against mitomycin C-induced intrinsic apoptosis in human melanoma A375-S2 cells. J Pharmacol Sci. 2009 Oct;111(2):137-46).

(Johnson et al, 1996) (Johnson, T. M., Yu, Z. X., Ferrans, V. J., Lowenstein, R. A. & Finkel, T. (1996) Reactive oxygen species are downstream mediators of p53-dependent apoptosis. Proc. Natl. Acad. Sci. U.S.A. 93:11848-11852).

(Jonas et al, 2000) (Jonas CR, Puckett AB, Jones DP, et al. Plasma antioxidant status after high-dose chemotherapy: a randomized trial of parenteral nutrition in bone marrow transplantation patients. Am J Clin Nutr (2000) 72(1):181–189).

(Judy et al, 1984) (Judy WV, Hall JH, Dugan W, et al. Coenzyme Q10 reduction of adriamycin cardiotoxicity. In: Folkers K, Yamamura Y, eds. Biomedical and Clinical Aspects of Coenzyme Q, Vol. 4, Elsevier, 1984:231–41).

(Kagreud, Peterson, 1981) (Kagreud A, Peterson HI. Tocopherol in irradiation of experimental neoplasms. Acta Radiol Oncol 1981;20:97-100).

(Kang et al, 2003) (Kang JS, Cho D, Kim YI, Hahm E, Yang Y, Kim D, Hur D, Park H, Bang S, Hwang YI, Lee WJ. L-ascorbic acid (vitamin C) induces the apoptotic of B16 murine melanoma cells via a caspase-8-independent pathway. *Cancer Immunol Immunother.* 2003;52:693–698).

(Kay, 2006) (Kay NE. ROS: double-edged sword for leukemic cells. Blood, 15 March 2006, Vol. 107, No. 6, pp. 2212-2213).

(Kemp et al, 1996) (Kemp G, et al. Amifostine pre-treatment for protection against cyclo-phosphamide-induced and cisplatin-induced toxicities: results of a randomized controlled trial in patients with advanced ovarian cancer. J Clin Oncol 14:2101-2112, 1996) (Venturini M, et al, 1996).

(Key, 2011) (Key TJ. Fruit and vegetables and cancer risk. *British Journal of Cancer* (2011) 104, 6–11).

(Kim et al, 2008) (Kim JE, Jin DH, Lee SD, Hong SW, Shin JS, Lee SK, Jun DJ, Kang JS, Lee WJ. Vitamin C inhibits p53-induced replicative senescence through suppression of ROS production and p38 MAPK activity. *Int J Mol Med.* 2008;22:651–655).

(Kirsh et al, 2006) (Kirsh VA, Hayes RB, Mayne ST, Chatterjee N, Subar AF, Dixon LB, et al. Supplemental and Dietary Vitamin E, Beta-Carotene, and Vitamin C Intakes and Prostate Cancer Risk. PCLO. J Natl Cancer Inst 2006;98:245-254).

(Kirshner et al, 2008) (Kirshner JR, He S, Balasubramanyam V, Kepros J, Yang C-Y, Zhang M, Du Z, Barsoum J and Bertin J. Elesclomol [STA-4783] induces cancer cell apoptosis through oxidative stress. *Molecular Cancer Therapeutics* 7, 2319-2327, August 1, 2008).

(Kochevar et al, 2000) (Kochevar IE, Lynch MC, Zhuang S, Lambert CR. Singlet oxygen, but not oxidizing radicals, induces apoptosis in HL-60 cells. Photochem Photobiol. 2000 Oct;72(4):548-53).

(Kockar MC, et al. N-acetylcysteine modulates doxorubicin-induced oxidative stress and antioxidant vitamin concentrations in liver or rats. Cell Biochem Funct. 2010 Dec 2;28(8):673-7).

(Kokileva, 1994) (Kokileva, L. (1994) Multi-step chromatin degradation in apoptosis. Int. Arch. Allergy Immunol. 105:339-343).

(Kono et al, 1996) (Kono, K., F. Salazar-Onfray, M. Petersson, J. Hansson, G. Masucci, K. Wasserman, T. Nakazawa, P. Anderson, R. Kiessling. 1996. Hydrogen peroxide secreted by tumor-derived macrophages down-modulates signal-transducing zeta molecules and inhibits tumor-specific T cell-and natural killer cell-mediated cyto-toxicity. *Eur. J. Immunol.* 26: 1308-1313).

(Konogaya et al.) (Konogaya M, et al. Clinical analysis of longstanding subacute myelo-optico-neuropathy: sequelae of clioquinol at 32 years after its ban. Journal of the Neurological Sciences. <u>Volume 218, Issue 1</u> , Pages 85-90, 15 March 2004).

(Kontorschikova et al, 2001) (Kontorschikova et al., Ozonetherapy In A Complex Treatment Of Breast Cancer. In Proceedings of the 15th Ozone World Congress, 11-15th Sept 2001, Medical Therapy Conference (IOA 2001, Ed.), Speedprint Macmedia Ltd, Ealing, London, UK, 2001).

(Korbelik, 1996) (Korbelik, M. Induction of tumor immunity by photodynamic therapy. J Clin Laser Med Surg 1996; 14: 315-334).

(Korebelic, Dougherty, 1999) (Korbelik, M. and Dougherty, G.J. Photodynamic therapy-mediated immune response against subcutaneous mouse tumors. Cancer Research 1999; 59: 1441-1446).

(Koushik et al, 2005) (Koushik A, et al. Fruits and vegetables and ovarian cancer risk in a pooled analysis of 12 cohort studies. <u>Cancer Epidemiol Biomarkers Prev.</u> 2005 Sep;14(9):2160-7).

(Koushik et al, 2006) (Koushik A, et al. Intake of major carotenoids and the risl of epithelial ovarian cancer in a pooled analysis of 10 cohort studies. Int J Cancer. 2006 Nov 1;119(9):2148-54).

(Krutchik et al, 1978) (Krutchik AN, Buzdar AU, Blumenschein GR, Lukeman JM. Spontaneous regression of breast carcinoma. *Arch Intern Med.* 1978;138(11):1734-1735).

(Kuipers, Lafleur, 1998) (Kuipers, G. K. & Lafleur, M.V. (1998) Characterization of DNA damage induced by gamma-radiation-derived water radicals, using DNA repair enzymes. Int. J. Radiat. Biol. 74:511-519).

(Kwon et al, 2003) (Kwon YW, Masutani H., Nakamura H, Ishii Y, Yodoi J, 2003. Redox regulation of cell growth and cell death. Biol. Chem. 384, 991–996).

(Kuninaka et al, 2000) (Kuninaka S., Ichinose Y., Koja K., Toh Y. Suppression of manganese superoxide dismutase augments sensitivity to radiation, hyperthermia, and doxorubicin in colon cancer cell lines by inducing apoptosis. Br. J. Cancer, 83: 928-934, 2000).

(Kurbacher, 1996) (Kurbacher CM. Ascorbic acid improves the antineoplastic activity of doxorubicin, cispaltin, and paclitaxil in human breast carcinoma cells in vitro. Cancer letters 103:183-189, 1996).

(Kwok, Richardson, 2002) (Kwok JC, Richardson DR: The iron metabolism of neoplastic cells: alterations that facilitate proliferation? *Crit Rev Oncol Hematol 42*: 65-78, 2002)

(Labriola, 1999) (Dan Labriola. Possible interactions between dietary antioxidants and chemotherapy. Oncology 13(7):1003-1008, 1999).

(Labriola and Livingston, 1999) (Labriola D, Livingston R. Possible interactions between dietary antioxidants and chemotherapy. Oncology 13:1003-12, 1999).

(Ladas et al, 2004) (Ladas EJ, Jacobson JS, Kennedy DD, Teel K, Fleischauer A, Kelly KM. Antioxidants and cancer therapy: a systematic review. J Clin Oncol (2004) 22(3):517–528).

(Lamson, Brignall, 1999) (Lamson DW, Brignall MS. Antioxidants in cancer therapy; their actions and interactions with oncologic therapies. Altern Med Rev 1999;4(5):304-29).

(Lamson et al, 2010) (Lamson DW et al, The vitamin C: vitamin K3 system - enhancers and inhibitors of the anticancer effect. Altern Med Rev. 2010 Dec;15(4):345-51).

(Langemann et al, 1989) (Langemann, H., Torhorst, J., Kabiersch, A., Krenger, W., and Honegger, C. G. Quantitative determination of water- and lipid-soluble antioxidants in neoplastic and non-neoplastic human breast tissue. Int. J. Cancer, 43: 1169–1173, 1989).

(Larsson et al, 2010) (Susanna C Larsson, Agneta Åkesson, Leif Bergkvist, and Alicja Wolk. Multivitamin use and breast cancer incidence in a prospective cohort of Swedish women. Am J Clin Nutr Published online 24 March 2010. Am J Clin Nutr Vol. 91, No. 5, 1268-1272, May 2010).

(Lawson et al, 2007) (Lawson KA, Wright ME, Subar A, Mouw T, Schatzkin A, Leitzmann MF. Multivitamin use and risk of prostate cancer in the National Institutes of Health–AARP Diet and Health Study. J Natl Cancer Inst (2007) 99:754–64).

(Laurent et al, 2005) (Alexis Laurent et al. Controlling Tumor Growth by Modulating Endogenous Production of Reactive Oxygen Species. *Cancer Research* 65, 948-956, February 1, 2005).

(Lawenda et al, 2007) (Lawenda BD, Smith DE, Xu L, et al. Do the dietary supplements epigallocatechin gallate or vitamin e cause a radiomodifying response on tumors in vivo? A pilot study with murine breast carcinoma. J Soc Integr Oncol (2007) 5(1):11–17).

(Lawenda et al, 2008) (Lawenda BD, Kelly KM, Ladas EJ, Sagar SM, Vickers A, Blumberg J. 2008. Should supplemental antioxidant administration be avoided during chemotherapy and radiation therapy?. Journal of the National Cancer Institute. May 27, 2008. 100(11)773-783).

(Lecane et al, 2005) (P. S. Lecane, M. W. Karaman, M. Sirisawad, L. Naumovski, R. A. Miller, J. G. Hacia, and D. Magda. Motexafin Gadolinium and Zinc Induce Oxidative Stress Responses and Apoptosis in B-Cell Lymphoma Lines. Cancer Res., December 15, 2005; 65(24): 11676 – 11688).

(Lee et al, 2001) (Lee SH, Oe T, Blair IA. Vitamin C-induced decomposition of lipid hydroperoxides to endogenous genotoxins. *Science.* 2001;292:2083–2086).

(Lee et al, 2004) (Lee HC, Kim DW, Jung KY, Park IC, Park MJ, Kim MS, et al: Increased expression of antioxidant enzymes in radioresistant variant from U251 human glioblastoma cell line. *Int J Mol Med 13*: 883-887, 2004).

(Levine et al, PNAS 2001) (Levine M, Wang Y, Padayatty SJ, Morrow J. A new recommended dietary allowance of vitamin C for healthy young women. *Proc Natl Acad Sci U S A.* 2001;98:9842–9846).

(Lee et al., 1999) (Lee IM, Cook NR, Manson JE, Buring JE, Hennekens CH. Beta-carotene supplementation and incidence of cancer and cardiovascular disease: the Women's Health Study. J Natl Cancer Inst. 1999 Dec 15;91(24):2102-6).

(Lee et al, 2003) (Lee KW, Lee HJ, Surh YJ, Lee CY. Vitamin C and cancer chemoprevention: reappraisal. *Am J Clin Nutr.* 2003;78:1074–1078).

(Lee J, et al, 2003) (Lee J.-C.; Kim J.; Park J.-K.; Chung G.-H.; Jang Y.-S. Experimental Cell Research, Volume 291, Number 2, 10 December 2003 , pp. 386-397).

(Lee et al, 2004) (Lee HC, Kim DW, Jung KY, Park IC, Park MJ, Kim MS, et al: Increased expression of antioxidant enzymes in radioresistant variant from U251 human glioblastoma cell line. Int J Mol Med 13: 883-887, 2004).

(Lee et al, 2005) (Vitamin E in the primary prevention of cardiovascular disease and cancer: the Women's Health Study: a randomized controlled trial. Lee IM, Cook NR, Gaziano JM, Gordon D, Ridker PM, Manson JE, et al. JAMA. 2005;294:56–65).

(Lee et al, 2008) (Lee SK, Kang JS, Jung da J, Hur DY, Kim JE, Hahm E, Bae S, Kim HW, Kim D, Cho BJ, Cho D, Shin DH, Hwang YI, Lee WJ. Vitamin C suppresses proliferation of the human melanoma cell SK-MEL-2 through the inhibition of cyclooxygenase (COX-2) expression and the modulation of insulin- like growth factor (IGF-II) production. J Cell Physiol. 2008;216:180–188).

(Lee W, 2009) (Wang-jae Lee. The prospects of vitamin C in cancer therapy. Immune Netw. 2009 October; 9(5): 147-152).

(Lepley et al, 1996) (Lepley DM, Li B, Birt DF, Pelling JC. The chemopreventive flavonoid apigenin induces G_2/M arrest in keratinocytes. Carcinogenesis 1996;17:2367–75).

(Lesperance et al, 2002) (Lesperance ML, Olivotto IA, Forde N, et al. Mega-dose vitamins and minerals in the treatment of non-metastatic breast cancer: an historical cohort study. Breast Cancer Res Treat (2002) 76(2):137–143).

(Levine, 1986) (Levine M. (1986) New concepts in the biology and biochemistry of ascorbic acid. New Engl. J. Med. 314,892-902).

(Levine et al, 2008) (Levine M, Espey MG, and Chen Q. Losing and finding a way at C: New promise for pharmacologic ascorbate in cancer treatment. Free Radical Biology & Medicine. 47 (2008) pp. 27-29).

(Lhuillery et al, 1997) (Lhuillery C, Cognault S, Germain E, Jourdan ML, Bougnoux P. Suppression of the promoter effect of polyunsaturated fatty acids by the absence of dietary vitamin E in experimental mammary carcinoma. Cancer Lett 1997;114:233–4).

(Li et al, 2008) (L. Li, E. Abdel Fattah, G. Cao, C. Ren, G. Yang, A. A. Goltsov, A. C. Chinault, W.-W. Cai, T. L. Timme, and T. C. Thompson. Glioma Pathogenesis-Related

Protein I Exerts Tumor Suppressor Activities through Proapoptotic Reactive Oxygen Species c-Jun NH2 Kinase Signaling. Cancer Res 2008;68(2):434–43).

(Liede et la, 1998) (Liede KE, Alfthan G, Hietanen JH, Haukka JK, Saxen LM, Heinonen OP. Beta-carotene concentration in buccal mucosal cells with and without dysplastic oral leukoplakia after long-term beta-carotene supplementation in male smokers. Eur J Clin Nutr (1998) 52(12):872–876).

(Lin et al, 2005) (Lin C, Kang J, Zheng R. Vitamin K3 triggers human leukemia cell death through hydrogen peroxide generation and histone hyperacetylation. Pharmazie. 2005 Oct;60(10):765-71).

(Lin et al, 2009) (Lin J, Cook N, Albert C. et al. Vitamins C and E and Beta Carotene Supplementation and Cancer Risk: A Randomized Controlled Trial JNCI J Natl Cancer Inst 2009 101: 14-23).

(Ling et al, 2003) (Ling Y-H, Liebes L, Zou Y and Perez-Soler R. Reactive Oxygen Species Generation and Mitochondrial Dysfunction in the Apoptotic Response to Bortezomib, a Novel Proteasome Inhibitor, in Human H460 Non-small Cell Lung Cancer Cells. J. Biol. Chem., Vol. 278, Issue 36, 33714-33723, September 5, 2003).

(Lippman et al, 2009) (Effect of selenium and vitamin E on risk of prostate cancer and other cancers: the Selenium and Vitamin E Cancer Prevention Trial (SELECT). Lippman, SM. JAMA. 2009 Jan 7;301(1):39-51. Epub 2008 Dec 9).

(Lissoni et al, 1996) (Lissoni P, Meregalli S, Nosetto L, Barni S, Tancini G, Fossati V, Maestroni G. Increased survival time in brain glioblastomas by a radioneuroendocrine strategy with radiotherapy plus melatonin compared to radiotherapy alone. Oncology. 53(1):43-6, 1996).

(Little et al, 1993) (Little JB. Cellular, molecular, and carcinogenic effects of radiation. Hematol Oncol Clin N Am 7:337–352, 1993).

(Liu et al, 2003) (Liu, L., Trimarchi, J.R., Navarro, P., Blasco, M.A. and Keefe, D.L. (2003) Oxidative stress contributes to arsenic-induced telomere attrition, chromosome instability and apoptosis. J. Biol. Chem., 278, 31998–32004).

(Liu et al, 2008) (Qing Liu et al. NADPH oxidase-mediated generation of reactive oxygen species: A new mechanism for X-ray-induced HeLa cell death. Biochemical and Biophysical Research Communications Volume 377, Issue 3, 19 December 2008, Pages 775-779).

(Llobet et al, 2008) (Llobet D, et al. Antioxidants block proteasome inhibitor function in endometrial carcinoma cells. Anti-Cancer Drugs. 19(2):115-124, February 2008).

(Loeve et al, 2004) (Loeve F, Boer R, Zauber AG; et al. National Polyp Study data: evidence for regression of adenomas. *Int J Cancer.* 2004;111(4):633-639).

(Longnecker, 1997) (Longnecker MP, Newcomb PA, Mittendorf R, Greenberg ER, Willett WC. Intake of carrots, spinach, and supplements containing vitamin A in relation to risk of breast cancer. Cancer Epidemiol Biomarkers Prev. 1997;6(11):887-892).

(Lonn et al, 2005) (Effects of long-term vitamin E supplementation on cardiovascular events and cancer: a randomized controlled trial. E. Lonn et al. JAMA. 2005 Mar 16;293(11):1338-47).

(Lowe et al, 1993) (Lowe, S.W., Ruley, H. E., Jacks, T. & Housman, D. E. (1993) p53-Dependent apoptosis modulates the cytotoxicity of anticancer agents. Cell 34:957-967) (Thompson, 1995).

(Luna et al, 1994) (Luna, M.C., Wong, S. and Gomer, C.J. Photodynamic therapy mediated induction or early response genes. Cancer Res 1994; 14: 315-321).

(Machlin, Bendich, 1987) (Machlin LJ, Bendich A. Free radical tissue damage: protective role of antioxidant nutrients. *FASEB J.* 1987).

(Maehara et al, 2004) (Maehara S, et al. Selenoprotein P, as a predictor for evaluating gemcitabine resistance in human pancreatic cancer cells. Int J Cancer. 2004 Nov 1;112(2):184-9).

(Maier et al, 2000) (Maier A et al. Combined photodynamic therapy and hyperbaric oxygenation in carcinoma of the esophagus and the esophago-gastric junction. Eur J Cardiothorac Surg. 2000 Dec;18(6):649-54).

(Malik et al, 2003) (Minnie Malik, Cuiwei Zhao, Norberta Schoene, M Monica Guisti, Mary P Moyer, Bernadene A Magnuson. **Anthocyanin-Rich Extract From Aronia meloncarpa E. Induces a Cell Cycle Block in Colon Cancer but Not Normal Colonic Cells.** Nutr Cancer. 2003 ;46 (2):186-96).

(Mallams et al, 1965) (Mallams, J.T., Balla, G.A. and Finney, J.W. Regional oxygenation and irradiation in the treatment of malignant tumors. Prog Clin Cancer 1965; 1: 137).

(Manakata et al, 1985) (Manakata T, Semba U, Shibuya Y, et al. Induction of interferon-gamma production by human natural killer cells stimulated by hydrogen peroxide. J Immunol 1985;134(4):2449-2455).

(Mannisto et al, 2004) (Mannisto S, et al. Dietary carotenoids and risk of lung cancer in a pooled analysis of seven cohort studies. Cancer Epidemiol Biomarkers Prev. 2004 Jan;13(1):40-8).

(Mannisto et al, 2007) (Mannisto S, et al. Dietary carotenoids and risk of colorectal cancer in a pooled analysis of 11 cohort studies. Am J Epidemiol. 2007 Feb 1;165(3):246-55).

(Mansat-De Mas et al, 1999) (Ve´ Ronique Mansat-De Mas et al. Implication of Radical Oxygen Species in Ceramide Generation, c-Jun N-Terminal Kinase Activation and Apoptosis Induced by Daunorubicin. Molecular Pharmacology, 56:867–874 (1999).

(Mantovani et al, 2002) (Mantovani G, Maccio A, Madeddu L, et al. Reactive oxygen species, antioxidant mechanisms and serum cytokine levels in cancer patients: impact of an antioxidant treatment. J Cellular and Mol Med. Oct. 2002. Vol. 6, Issue 4, pp. 570-82).

(Marcin et al, 2005) (Marcin O, Wojciech W, Ewa S, Andrzej M, Jacek B. A novel mechanism of action of the fumagillin analog, TNP-470, in the B16F10 murine melanoma cell line. Anti-Cancer Drugs. 16(8):817-823, September 2005).

(Maserejian et al, 2007) (Maserejian NW, Giovanncci E, Rosner B, Joshipura K. Prospective Study of Vitamins C, E, A, and Carotenoids and Risk of Oral Premalignant Lesions in Men. International J of Cancer. 120(5):970-7; 2006).

(Mates et al, 2000) (José M. Matés and Francisca M. Sánchez-Jiménez. Role of reactive oxygen species in apoptosis: implications for cancer therapy. The International Journal of Biochemistry & Cell Biology. Volume 32, Issue 2, February 2000, Pages 157-170).

(Mattson et al, 2009) (Mattson DM, et al. Cisplatin combined with zidovudine enhances cytotoxicity and oxidative stress in human head and neck cancer cells via a thiol-dependent mechanism. Free Radical biology and Medicine. 46 (2009): 232-237).

(Mayne et al, 2001) (Susan T. Mayne et al. Randomized Trial of Supplemental ß-Carotene to Prevent Second Head and Neck Cancer. *Cancer Research* 61, 1457-1463, February 15, 2001).

(McGough et al, 2004) (McGough C, Baldwin C, Frost G, Andreyev HJ. Role of nutritional intervention in patients treated with radiotherapy for pelvic malignancy. Br J Cancer. 2004 Jun 14;90(12):2278-87).

(McKallip et al, 2006) (McKallip RJ, et al. Cannabidiol-Induced Apoptosis in Human Leukemia Cells: A Novel Role of Cannabidiol in the Regulation of p22^{phox} and Nox4 Expression. *Mol Pharmacol* 70:897-908, 2006).

(Mei et al, 1995) (Mei H, LoVerde PT 1995. Schistosoma mansoni: cloning the gene encoding glutathione peroxidase. Exp Parasitol 80:319-322).

(Mell et al, 2007) (Mell LK, Malik R, Komaki R, et al. Effect of amifostine on response rates in locally advanced non-small cell lung cancer patients treated on randomized controlled trials: a meta-analysis. Int J Radiat Oncol Biol Phys (2007) 68(1):111–118).

(Mercer et al, 2011) (Mercer AE. et al. The role of heme and the mitochondrion in the chemical and molecular mechanisms of mammalian cell death induced by the artemisinin antimalarials. J Biol. Chem. 2011 Jan 14;286(2):987-96).

(Metz et al, 2004) (Metz JM, Smith D, Mick R, et al: A phase I study of topical Tempol for the prevention of alopecia induced by whole brain radiotherapy. Clin Cancer Res 10:6411-6417, 2004).

(Meyer et al, 2007) (Meyer F, Bairati I, Jobin E, Gélinas M, Fortin A, Nabid A, Têtu B. Acute adverse effects of radiation therapy and local recurrence in relation to dietary and plasma beta carotene and alpha tocopherol in head and neck cancer patients. Nutr Cancer. 2007;59(1):29-35).

(Meyer et al, 2008) (Meyer F, Bairati I, Fortin A, et al. Interaction between antioxidant vitamin supplementation and cigarette smoking during radiation therapy in relation to long-term effects on recurrence and mortality: a randomized trial among head and neck cancer patients. Int J Cancer (2008) 122(7):1679–1683).

(Meyers et al, 1996) (Meyers DG, Maloley PA, Weeks D. Safety of antioxidant vitamins. *Arch Intern Med.* 1996;156:925-35).

(Michels et al, 2001) (Michels KB, et al, Dietary antioxidant vitamins, retinol, and breast cancer incidence in a cohort of Swedish women. Int J Cancer. 2001 Feb 15;91(4):563-7).

(Milanesa et al, 2000) (Dan M. Milanesa, Muhammad S. Choudhury, Camille Mallouh, Hiroshi Tazaki, Sensuke Konno. Methylglyoxal-Induced Apoptosis in Human Prostate Carcinoma: Potential Modality for Prostate Cancer Treatment. *Eur Urol* 2000;37:728-734).

(Miller et al, 2002) (Miller WH, Jr., Schipper HM, Lee JS, Singer J, Waxman S. Mechanism of action of arsenic trioxide. Cancer Res 2002;62:3893–903).

(Miller et al, 2005) (Miller ER III, Pastor-Barriuso R, Dalal D, Riemersma RA, Appel LJ, Guallar E. Meta-analysis: high-dosage vitamin E supplementation may increase all-cause mortality. *Ann Intern Med.* 2005;142:37-46).

(Miller et al, 2009) (Miller PE, Vasey JJ, Short PF et al. Dietary supplement use in adult cancer survivors. Oncol Nurs Forum. 2009 Jan;36(1):61-8).

(Mills, 1988) (Mills EE: The modifying effect of beta-carotene on radiation and chemotherapy induced oral mucositis. Br J Cancer 57:416-417, 1988).

(Miranda-Vilela et al, 2011) (Miranda-Vilela AL, et al. The protective effects of nutritional antioxidant therapy on Ehrlich solid tumor-bearing mice depend on the type of antioxidant therapy chosen: histology, genotoxicity and hematology evaluations. J Nutr Biochem. 2011 Jan 25. [Epub ahead of print]).

(Mishra et al, 2007) (Mishra V, et al. Effect of selenium supplementation on biochemical markers and out come in critically ill patients. Clin Nutr. 2007 Feb;26(1):41-50).

(Misirlioglu et al, 2006) (Misirlioglu CH, Erkal H, Elgin Y, Ugur I, Altundag K. Effect of concomitant use of pentoxifylline and alpha-tocopherol with radiotherapy on the clinical outcome of patients with stage IIIB non-small cell lung cancer: a randomized prospective clinical trial. Med Oncol (2006) 23(2):185–189).

(Mitchell et al, 1989) (Mitchell JB, et al, Glutahtione modulation in cancer treatment: will it work? Int J Radiat Oncol Biol Phys. 1989 May;16(5):1289-95).

(Miyajima et al, 1999 - human bladder cancer KU-1 cell line) (Miyajima A, et al. N-acetylcysteine modifies cis-dichlorodiamineplatinum induced effects in bladder cancer cells. Jap J Cancer Res 90:565-570, 1999).

(Mkoji et al, 1988a) (Mkoji GM, Smith JM, Prichard RK 1988a. Antioxidant systems in Schistosoma mansoni. Correlation between susceptibility to oxidant killing and the levels of scavengers of hydrogen peroxide and oxygen free radicals. Int J Parasitol. 18: 661-666).

(Mkoji et al, 1988b) (Mkoji GM, Smith JM, Prichard RK 1988b. Antioxidant systems in Schistosoma mansoni: Evidence for their role in protection of the adult worms against oxidant killing. Int J Parasitol 18: 667-673).

(Moertel et al, 1985) (Moertel CG, Fleming TR, Creagan ET, Rubin J, O'Connell MJ, Ames MM. High-dose vitamin C versus placebo in the treatment of patients with advanced cancer who have had no prior chemotherapy. A randomized double-blind comparison. N Engl J Med, 1985 Jan 17;312(3):137-41)

(Moertel, Creagan, 1980) (Moertel CG, Creagan ET. Vitamin C therapy and advanced cancer (letter). New England Journal of Medicine 302:694-695, 1980).

(Moscicki et al, 2004) (Moscicki AB, Shiboski S, Hills NK; et al. Regression of low-grade squamous intra-epithelial lesions in young women. *Lancet.* 2004;364(9446):1678-1683).

(Mosienko et al, 1990) (Mosienko VS, et al. Effectiveness of combined action of vitamins A, E, and C and Cyclophosphane or Adriamycin on growth of transpslanted tumors in mice. Eksperimentalaia Oncologiia. 12:55-7, 1990).

(Moss, 2006) (Moss RW. Should patients undergoing chemotherapy and radiotherapy be prescribed antioxidants? Integr Cancer Ther. 2006 Mar;5(1):63-82).

(Moss, Sept 2007) (Moss, R.W. Do antioxidants interfere with radiation therapy for cancer? Integr Cancer Ther Sept. 2007. Vol.6, No. 3. pp. 281-292).

(Mothersill et al, 1986) (Mothersill C, Moriarty MJ, Seymour CB. Radiobiologic response of CHO-KI cells treated with vitamin A. Acta Radiol Oncol (1986) 25(4–6):275–280).

(Movsas. 2009) (Benjamin Movsas. "Hypoxic Prostate/Muscle pO2 (P/M pO2) Ratio Predicts for Biochemical Failure in Patients with Localized Prostate Cancer: Long-term Result." Abstract # 5136. ASCO 2009).

(Mow et al, 2002) (Mow BM, Chandra J, Svingen PA, et al. Effects of the Bcr/abl kinase inhibitors STI5 71 and adaphostin (NSC 680410) on chronic myelogenous leukemia cells in vitro. Blood. 2002;99: 664-671).

(Moyad et al. 2002) (Moyad MA. Selenium and vitamin E supplements for prostate cancer: evidence or embellishment? Urology. 2002 Apr;59(4 Suppl 1):9-19).

(Murphy et al, 1992) (Murphy PG, Myers DS, Davies MJ, et al. The antioxidant potential of propofol (2,6-diisopropylphenol). Br J Anaesth 1992;68:613–8).

(Murry et al, 1998) (Murry CE, Richard VJ, Jennings RB, Reimer KA. Preconditioning with ischemia: is the protective effect meditated by free radical induced myocardial stunning? Circulation 1988;78 (Suppl. II):77).

(Myung et al, 2009) (Myung, S.-K., Kim, Y., Ju, W., Choi, H. J., Bae, W. K. (2010). Effects of antioxidant supplements on cancer prevention: meta-analysis of randomized controlled trials. Ann Oncol 21: 166-179).

(Myung, Int J Cancer. et al, 2009) (Myung et al, Green tea consumption and risk of stomach cancer: a meta-analysis of epidemiologic studies. Int J Cancer. 2009 Feb1;124(3):670-7).

(Nakazato et al, 2005) (Nakazato T, Ito K, Kizaki YI and M. Green Tea Component, Catechin, Induces Apoptosis of Human Malignant B Cells via Production of Reactive Oxygen Species. Clinical Cancer Research Vol. 11, 6040-6049, August 15, 2005).

(Nam et al, 2001) (Nam S, Smith DM, Dou QP. Ester bound-containing tea polyphenols potently inhibit proteasome activity in vitro and in vivo. J Biol Chem 2001;276:13322–30).

(Nare et al, 1990) (Nare B, Smith JM, Prichard RK 1990. Schistosoma mansoni: levels of antioxidants and resistance to oxidants increase during development. Exp Parasitol 70: 389-397).

(Nathan et al, 1979) (C. F. Nathan et al. Extracellular cytolysis by activated macrophages and granulocytes, Journal of Experimental Medicine. January 1979. 149(1): 84-99).

(Nathan et al, vol 153, 1981) (Nathan CF et al. Tumor cell anti-oxidant defenses. Inhibition of the glutathione redox cycle enhances macrophage-mediated cytolysis. J Exp Med 1981 Apr 1;153(4): 766-82).

(Nathan, Cohn, 1981) (CF Nathan and ZA Cohn. Antitumor effects of hydrogen peroxide in vivo. Journal of Experimental Medicine, November 1981. Vol 154, 1539-1553).

(Nelson, 2004) (Nelson, W. G. (2004) Prostate cancer prevention. J. Nutr. 134:3211S-3212S).

(Nechuta et al, 2010) (Nechuta S, Lu W, Chen Z. et el. Vitamin supplement use during breast cancer treatment and survival: a prospective cohort study. Cancer Epidemiol Biomarkers Prev. 2010 Dec 21. [Epub ahead of print])

(Neuhouser et al, 2009) (Neuhouser ML, barnett MJ, Kristal, et al. Dietary supplement use and prostate cancer risk in the Carotene and Retinol Efficacy Trial. Cancer Epidemiol Biomarkers Prev. 2009 Aug;18(8):2202-6).

(Nicholson, 297–301. 1996) (Nicholson, D.W. (1996) ICE/CED3-like proteases as therapeutic targets for the control of inappropriate apoptosis. Nature Biotechnol., 14, 297–301).

(Nicholson, 810-816. 1996) (Nicholson, D.W. (1996) From bench to clinic with apoptosis-based therapeutic agents. Nature, 407, 810–816).

(Nicholson et al, 1998) (N. C. Nicholson et al., Hydrogen peroxide inhibits giant cell tumor and osteoblast metabolism in vitro. Clinical Orthopedics and Related Research 347. February 1998: 250-60).

(NIH State-of-the Science Panel. 2007). (National Institutes of Health State-of-the-Science Conference Statement: Multivitamin/Mineral Supplements and Chronic Disease Prevention. NIH State-of-the-Science Panel. ANN INTERN MED 2006;145:364-371).

(Nishikawa et al, 2004) (Takeshi Nishikawa, Satoshi Nishikawa, Nobuko Akiyama and Shunji Natori. Correlation between the Catalase Level in Tumor Cells and Their Sensitivity to N-ß-Alanyl-5-S-Glutathionyl-3,4-Dihydroxyphenylalanine (5-S-GAD). J. Biochem, 2004, Vol. 135, No. 4 465-469).

(Noguchi et al, 2002) (Noguchi, N., Nakad, A., Itoh, Y., Watanabe, A. and Niki, E. Formation of active oxygen species and lipid peroxidation induced by hypochlorite. 2002, Arch Biochem Biophys. 397; 2:440-447).

(Oberley et al, 1996) (Oberley, T. D., Sempf, J. M. & Oberley, L. W. (1996) Immunogold analysis of antioxidant enzymes in common renal cancers. Histol. Histopathol. 11:153-160).

(Oberley, Oberley, 1997) (Oberley, T. D. & Oberley, L. W. (1997) Antioxidant enzyme levels in cancer. Histol. Histopathol. 12:525-535).

(Obrenovich et al, 2011) (Obrenovich ME et al. Antioxidants in health, disease and aging. CNS Neurol Disord Drug Targets. 2011 Mar;10(2):192-207).

(O'Brien, 1991) (O'Brien PJ. Molecular mechanism of quinone cytotoxicity. Chem Biol Interact 80:1–41, 1991).

(Ogunleye et al, 2010) (Ogunleye AA, Xue F, Michels KB: Green tea consumption and breast cancer risk or recurrence: a meta-analysis. *Breast Cancer Res Treat* 2010, 119:477–484).

(Okroj et al, 2005) (*Okroj, Marcin; Kamysz, Wojciech; Slominska, Ewa M.; Mysliwski, Andrzej; Bigda, Jacek.* A novel mechanism of action of the fumagillin analog, TNP-470, in the B16F10 murine melanoma cell line. Anti-Cancer Drugs. 16(8):817-823, September 2005).

(Okroj et al, 2006) (Okrój M, Stawikowska D, Słomińska EM, Myśliwski A, Bigda J. The atypical pattern of cell death in B16F10 melanoma cells treated with TNP-470. Cell Mol Biol Lett. 2006;11(3):384-95).

(O'Leary et al, 1991) (O'Leary KA, Tracy JW 1991. Schistosoma mansoni: glutathione S-transferase-catalyzed detoxication of dichlorvos. Exp Parasitol 72: 355-361).
(O'Leary et al, 1992) (O'Leary KA, Hathaway KM, Tracy JW 1992. Schistosoma mansoni: Single-step purification and characterization of gutathione 5-transferase isoenzyme 4. Exp Parasitol 75:47-55).

(Olson et al, 1983) (Olson RD, Stroo WE, Boerth RC. Influence of N-acetylcysteine on the antitumor activity of doxorubicin. Semin Oncol 1983;10:S29-S34).

(Omenn et al, 1996) (Omenn GS, Goodman GE, Thornquist MD, et al: Risk factors for lung cancer and for intervention effects in CARET, the Beta-Carotene and Retinol Efficacy Trial. J Natl Cancer Inst 88:1550-1559, 1996).

(Otsuji et al, 1996) (Otsuji, M., Y. Kimura, T. Aoe, Y. Okamoto, T. Saito. 1996. Oxidative stress by tumor-derived macrophages suppresses the expression of CD3 zeta chain of T-cell receptor complex and antigen-specific T-cell responses. *Proc. Natl. Acad. Sci. USA* 93: 13119-13124).

(Pace et al, 2003) (Pace A, Savarese A, Picardo M, et al. Neuroprotective effect of vitamin E supplementation in patients treated with cisplatin chemotherapy. J Clin Oncol (2003) 21(5):927–931).

(Padayatty et al, 2004) (Padayatty SJ, Sun H, Wang Y, et al. Vitamin C pharmacokinetics: implications for oral and intravenous use. Ann Intern Med (2004) 140(7):533–537).

(Padayatty et al, 2010) (Padayatty SJ, Sun AY, Chen Q, Espey MG, Drisko J, Levine M. Vitamin C: intravenous use by complementary and alternative medicine practitioners and adverse effects. PLoS One. 2010 Jul 7;5(7):e11414).

(Pak et al, 2011) (Pak JH et al. Peroxiredoxin 6 overexpression attenuates cisplatin-induced apoptosis in human ovarian cancer cells. Cancer Invest. 2011 Jan;29(1):21-8).

(Palazzo et al, 2003) (Palozza P, Serini S, Di Nicuolo F, et al: Prooxidant effects of beta-carotene in cultured cells. Mol Aspects Med 24:353-362, 2003).

(Papas et al, 1999) (Papas AM. Antioxidant Status, Diet, Nutrition, and Health (1999) Boca Raton, FL: CRC Press).

(Park et al, 1998) (Park TK, et al. Interferon alpha 2a, 13-cis-retinoic acid and radiotherapy for locally advanced carcinoma of the cervix: a pilot study. Eur J Gynaecol Oncol. 19:35-38, 1998).

(Park et al, 2008) (Park S, et al. vitamin and mineral supplements: barriers and challenges for older adults. J Nutr Eldeer. 2008;27(3-4):297-317).

(Parker-Pope, 2005) (Parker-Pope T. Cancer and Vitamins: Patients Urged to Avoid Supplements During Treatment; The Wall Street Journal 2005 Sep 20 Sect. D:1).

(Pathak et al, 2005) (Pathak AK, Bhutani M, Guleria R, et al. Chemotherapy alone vs. chemotherapy plus high dose multiple antioxidants in patients with advanced non small cell lung cancer. J Am Coll Nutr (2005) 24(1):16–21).

(Pelicano et al, 2003) (Hélène Pelicano et al. Inhibition of Mitochondrial Respiration. A Novel Strategy to Enhance Drug-induced apoptosis in human leukemia cells by a reactive oxygen species-mediated mechanism. J. Biol. Chem., 2003. Vol. 278, Issue 39, 37832-37839).

(Peralta et al, 2006) (Peralta EA, Viegas ML, Louis S, Engle DL and Dunnington GL. Effect of vitamin E on tamoxifen-treated breast cancer cells. Surgery. Volume 140, Issue 4, October 2006, Pages 607-615).

(Perez Ripoll et al, 1986) (Perez Ripoll EA, Rama BN, Webber MM. Vitamin E enhances the chemotherapeutic effects of adriamycin on human prostatic carcinoma cells in vitro. J Urol 1986;136:529-531).

(Peters et al, 2008) (U. Peters et al. Vitamin E and selenium supplementation and risk of prostate cancer in the Vitamins and lifestyle (VITAL) study cohort. Cancer Causes Control. 2008 Feb;19(1):75-87).

(Picardo et al, 1996) (Picardo M, Grammatico P, Roccella F, et al. Imbalance in the antioxidant pool in melanoma cells and normal melanocytes from patients with melanoma. J Invest Dermatol (1996) 107(3):322–326).

(Pietrangeli, Mondovi, 2008) (Paola Pietrangeli and Bruno Mondovì. On the Biochemical Basis of Tumour Damage by Hypothermia. Book: Hyperthermia in Cancer Treatment: A Primer. Springer Link May 8, 2008).

(Piyathilake et al, 2000) (Piyathilake CJ, Bell WC, Johanning GL, Cornwell PE, Heimburger DC, Grizzle WE. The accumulation of ascorbic acid by squamous cell carcinomas of the lung and larynx is associated with global methylation of DNA. Cancer (2000) 89(1):171–176).

(Podmore et al, 1998) (Podmore ID, Griffiths HR, Herbert KE, Mistry N, Mistry P, Lunec J. Vitamin C exhibits pro-oxidant properties. Nature. 1998;392:559).

(Potanin et al, 2000) (Potanin et al., Ozonotherapy In The Early Postoperative Period In The Surgical Treatment Of The Lung Cancer. [Written in Russian] Kazanskij Medicinskij Zurnal No. 4, 263-265, 2000).

(Prasad KN, et al, 1979) (Prasad KN, et al. Sodium ascorbate potentiates the growth inhibitory effects of certain agents on neuroblastoma cells and culture. Int J Vitam Nutr Res 19: 155-166, 1979).

(Prasad et al, PNAS. 1979) (Prasad, KN et al. Sodium ascorbate potentiates the growth inhibitory effect of certain agents on neuroblastoma cells in culture. Proc Natl Acad Sci USA. 76(2):829-832, 1979).

(Prasad et al, 1994) (Prasad KN, et al. Modification of the effect of tamoxifen, cisplatin, DTIC, and interferon-alpha 2B on human melanoma cells in culture by a mixture of vitamins. Nutr Cancer 22:233-245, 1994).

(Prasad, Kumar, 1996) (Prasad KN, Kumar R. Effect of individual and multiple antioxidant vitamins on growth and morphology of human nontumorigenic and tumorigenic parotid acinar cells in culture. Nutr Cancer (1996) 26(1):11–19).

(Prasad et al, 1999) (Prasad KN, Kumar A, Kochupillai V, Cole WC. High doses of multiple antioxidant vitamins: essential ingredients in improving the efficacy of standard cancer therapy. J Am Coll Nutr 1999;18(1):13-25).

(Prasad et al, 2001) (Prasad KN, Cole WC, Kumar B, Prasad KC. Scientific rationale for using high-dose multiple micronutrients as an adjunct to standard and experimental cancer therapies. J Am Coll Nutr (2001) 20(5 suppl):450S–463S. discussion 473S–475S).

(Pradad, 2004) (Prasad KN. Multiple dietary antioxidants enhance the efficacy of standard and experimental cancer therapies and decrease their toxicity. Integrative Cancer Therapies. 2004;3(4):310-322).

(Priemé et al. 1997) (Priemé H, Loft S, Nyyssönen K, Salonen JT, Poulsen HE. No effect of supplementation with vitamin E, ascorbic acid, or coenzyme Q10 on oxidative DNA damage estimated by 8-oxo-7,8-dihydro-2'-deoxyguanosine excretion in smokers. Am J Clin Nutr. 1997 Feb;65(2):503-7).

(Printz 2001) (Printz C. Spontaneous regression of melanoma may offer insight into cancer immunology. J Natl Cancer Inst. 2001;93(14):1047-1048).

(Qiao et al, 2009) (Y.-L. Qiao, S. M. Dawsey, F. Kamangar, J.-H. Fan, C. C. Abnet, X.-D. Sun, L. L. Johnson, M. H. Gail, Z.-W. Dong, B. Yu, et al. Total and Cancer Mortality After Supplementation With Vitamins and Minerals: Follow-up of the Linxian

General Population Nutrition Intervention Trial. J Natl Cancer Inst, April 1, 2009; 101(7): 507 - 518).

(Qu et al, 2007) (Chen-Xu Qu et al, Chemoprevention of Primary Liver Cancer: A Randomized, Double-Blind Trial in Linxian, China. Journal of the National Cancer Institute. Vol 99, Issue 16. August 15, 2007. pp. 1240-1247).

(Rabinowich et al, 1996) (Rabinowich, H., M. Banks, T. E. Reichert, T. F. Logan, J. M. Kirkwood, T. L. Whiteside. 1996. Expression and activity of signaling molecules in T lymphocytes obtained from patients with metastatic melanoma before and after interleukin 2 therapy. *Clin. Cancer Res.* 2: 1263-1274).

(Ratnam et al, 2006) (Ratnam DV, Ankola DD, Bhardwaj V, Sahana DK, Kumar MN. Role of antioxidants in prophylaxis and therapy: a pharmaceutical perspective. J Control Release (2006) 20(113):189–207).

(Ristow, 2006) (Ristow M. Oxidative metabolism in cancer growth. Curr Opin Clin Nutr Metab Care. 2006 Jul;9(4):339-45).

(Rock et al, 2004) (Rock, C. L., Newman, V. A., Neuhouser, M. L., Major, J. & Barnett, M. J. (2004) Antioxidant supplement use in cancer survivors and the general population. J. Nutr. 134:3194S-3195S).

(Rohan et al. 1995) (Rohan TE, Howe GR, Burch JD, Jain M. Cancer Causes Control, Dietary factors and risk of prostate cancer: a case-control study in Ontario, Canada. 1995 Mar;6(2):145-54).

(Roller, Weller, 1998) (Roller A, Weller M. Antioxidants specifically inhibit cisplatin cytotoxicity of human malignant glioma cells. Anticancer Res 1998;18:4493-4497).

(Russo, Mitchell, 1985) (Russo A, Mitchell JB. Potentiation and protection of doxorubicin cytotoxicity by cellular glutathione modulation. Cancer Treat Rep. 1985 Nov;69(11):1293-6).

(Sagar, 2005) (Sagar S. Should patients take or avoid antioxidant supplements during anticancer therapy? An evidence-based review. Curr Oncol (2005) 12:44–54).

(Sakamoto, Sakka, 1973) (Sakamoto K, Sakka M. Reduced effect of irradiation on normal and malignant cells irradiated in vivo in mice pretreated with vitamin E. Br J Radiol (1973) 46(547):538–540).

(Sakhi et al, 2009) (Sakhi AK et al, Pre-radiotherapy plasma carotenoids and markers of oxidative stress are associated with survival in head and neck squamous cell carcinoma patients: a prospective study. BMC Cancer. 2009 Dec 21;9:458).

(Saldew et al, 1990) (Saldew GS, et al. Selective reduction of cis-diamminedichloroplatinim nephrotoxicity by ebselen. Cancer Res 50: 7031-7036. 1990).

(Salganik et al, 2000) (Salganik, R. I., Albright, C. D., Rodgers, J., Kim, J., Zeisel, S. H., Sivashinskiy, M. S. & Van Dyke, T. A. (2000) Dietary antioxidant depletion: enhancement of tumor apoptosis and inhibition of brain tumor growth in transgenic mice. Carcinogenesis 21:909-914).

(Salganik, 2001) (Salganik RI. The benefits and hazards of antioxidants: controlling apoptosis and other protective mechanisms in cancer patients and the human population. J Am Coll Nutr. 2001;20(suppl):464S-472S).

(Samoszuk et al, 1989) (M. K. Samoszuk et al., In vitro sensitivity of Hodgkin's disease to hydrogen peroxide toxicity. Cancer 63 (1989): 2114).

(Sanchiz et al, 1996) (Sanchiz F, Milla A, Artola N, et al: Prevention of radioinduced cystitis by orgotein: A randomized study. Anticancer Res 16:2025-2028, 1996).

(Sasaki et al, 1967) (H. Sasaki et al, "Application of hydrogen peroxide to maxillary cancer," Yango Acta Medica 11, no. 3 (1967): 149).

(Sastre et al, 2000) (Sastre J., Pallardo F.V., Garcia de la Asucion J., Vian J. Mitochondria, oxidative stress and aging. Free Radical Res., 32: 189-198, 2000).

(Satia et al, 2009) (Satia JA, Littman A, Slatore CG, Galanko JA, White E. Long-term use of beta-carotene, retinol, lycopene, and lutein supplements and lung cancer risk: results from the VITamins And Lifestyle (VITAL) study. Am J Epidemiol. 2009 Apr 1;169(7):815-28).

(Sato et al, 2002) (Sato R, et al, Prospective study of carotenoids, tocopherols, and retinoid concentrations and the risk of breast cancer. Cancer Epidemiol Biomarkers Prev. 2002 May;11(5):451-7).

(Satoh et al, 1992) (Satoh M, et al. Effect of the co-administration of selenite on the toxicity and antitumor activity of cisdiamminedichloroplatinum given repeatedly to mice. Cancer Chemother Pharmacol. 30: 439-443, 1992).

(Scarabelli et al, 2001) (Scarabelli T, Stephanou A, Rayment N, et al. Apoptosis of endothelial cells precedes myocyte cell apoptosis in ischemia/reperfusion injury. Circulation 2001;104:253–6).

(Schlecht et al, 2003) (Schlecht NF, Platt RW, Duarte-Franco E; et al. Human papillomavirus infection and time to progression and regression of cervical intraepithelial neoplasia. *J Natl Cancer Inst.* 2003;95(17):1336-1343).

(Schilling et al, 2002) (Schilling FH, Spix C, Berthold F; et al. Neuroblastoma screening at one year of age. *N Engl J Med.* 2002;346(14):1047-1053).

(Schmitt-Graff and Schuelen, 1986) (Schmitt-Graff A, Schuelen ME. Prevention of adriamycin cardiotoxicity by niacin, isocitrate, or N-acetylcysteine in mice. Path Res Pract 181: 168-174, 1986).

(Schoonbroodt et al, 2000) (Schoonbroodt S, Piette J: Oxidative stress interference with the nuclear factor-kB activation pathways. *Biochem Pharmacol* 2000, 60:1075-1083).

(Schreiner, 1974) (Schreiner, A. Hyperbaric oxygen therapy in bactericides infections. Acta Chir Scand 1974; 140: 73-76).

(Schulz et al, 2006) (Schulz TJ, Thierbach R, Voight A, et al. Induction of oxidative metabolism by mitochondrial frataxin inhibits cancer growth: Otto Warburg revisited. J Biol Chem. 2006 Jan 13;281(2):977-81).

(Schreck et al, 1991) (Schreck R, Rieber P, Baeuerle PA: Reactive oxygen intermediates as apparently widely used messengers in the activation of the NF-kB transcription factor and HIV-1. *EMBO J* 1991, 10:2247-2258).

(Seifried et al, 2003) (Seifried, H. E., McDonald, S. S., Anderson, D. E., Greenwald, P. & Milner, J. A. (2003) The antioxidant conundrum in cancer. Cancer Res 63:4295-4298).

(Seifter et al, 1984) (Seifter E, et al. Vitamin A and beta-carotene as adjunctive therapy to tumor excision radiation therapy and chemotherapy. In Prasad K ed., Vitamins, Nutrition and Cancer. New York, Karger Press: 2-19, 1984).

(Seija et al, 2004) (Sieja K, Talerczk M. Selenium as an element in the treatment of ovarian cancer in women receiving chemotherapy. *Gynecol Oncol* 2004;93:320-27).

(Selbo et al, 2002) (Selbo, P.K., Hogset, A., Prasmickaite, L. and Berg, K. Photochemical internalization: A novel drug delivery system. Tumour Bio 2002; 23(2): 103-112).

(Senturker et al, 2002) (Sentürker, S., Tschirret-Guth, R, Morrow, JD, Levine, RL, and Shacter, E. (2002) Induction of apoptosis by chemotherapeutic drugs without generation of reactive oxygen species. *Arch. Biochem. Biophys.* 397, 262-272).

(Sergediene et al, 1999) (Sergediene E, Jönsson K, Szymusiak H, Tyrakowska B, Rietjens IMCM, Cenas N. Prooxidant toxicity of polyphenolic antioxidants to HL-60 cells: description of quantitative structure-activity relationship. FEBS Lett 1999;462:392–6).

(Shacter et al, 2000) (Shacter, E., Williams, J.A., Hinson, R.M., Sentürker, S., and Lee, Y.J. (2000) Oxidative stress reduces the efficacy of cancer chemotherapy drugs. Inhibition of lymphoma cell apoptosis and phagocytosis. *BLOOD* 96, 307-313).

(Shanafelt et al, 2005) (Shanafelt TD, Lee YK, Bone ND, et al. Adaphostin-induced apoptosis in CLL B cells is associated with induction of oxidative stress and exhibits synergy with fludarabine. Blood. 2005;105: 2099-2106).

(Shenkin, 2006) (Shenkin A. The key role of micronutrients. Clin Nutr. 2006;25(1):1-13).

(Shi et al, 2009) (Shi R, et al. N-acetylcysteine amide decreases oxidative stress but not cell death induced by doxorubicin in H9c2 cardiomyocytes. BMC Pharmacol. 2009 Apr 15;7).

(Shimoda et al, 2003) (Shimoda R, et al. Human hepatocellular liver carcinoma), 24 h pretreatment with cadmium resulted in concentration-dependent increases in MT levels and marked decreases in etoposide-induced apoptosis. (Metallothionein Is a Potential Negative Regulator of Apoptosis. Toxicological Sciences 73, 294-300 (2003).

(Shimoda et al, 2003) (Ryuya Shimoda et al. Metallothionein Is a Potential Negative Regulator of Apoptosis. Toxicological Sciences 73, 294-300 (2003).

(Shimpo et al, 1991) (Shimpo K, et al. Ascorbic acid and adriamycin toxicity. Am. J Clin Nutr. 54: 1298SS-1301S, 1991).

(Shimizu et al, 1995) (Shimizu, S., Eguchi, Y., Kosaka, H., Kamiike, W., Matsuda, H. and Tsujimoto, Y. Prevention of hypoxia-induced cell death by Bel-2 and Bel-xL. Nature 1995; 374: 811-813).

(Sieja, 2000) (Sieja K. Protective role of selenium against the toxicity of multi-drug chemotherapy in patients with ovarian cancer. Pharmazie (2000) 55(12):958–959)

(Sieja, Talerczyk, 2004) (Sieja K, Talerczyk M. Selenium as an element in the treatment of ovarian cancer in women receiving chemotherapy. Gynecol Oncol 2004;93:320–27).

(Sigounas et al, 1997) (Sigounas, G., Anagnostu, A. & Steiner, M. (1997) Dl-alpha tocopherol induces apoptosis in erythroleukemia, prostate and breast cancer cells. Nutr. Cancer 28:30-35).

(Simone et al, 2007) (Simone CB 2nd, Simone NL, Simone V, Simone CB. Antioxidants and other nutrients do not interfere with radiation or chemotherapy. Altern Ther Health Med. 2007 Mar-Apr;13(2):40-7).

(Simone, Simone, Simone, 2007) (Simone CB 2nd, Simone NL, Simone V, Simone CB. Antioxidants and other nutrients do not interfere with chemotherapy or radiation therapy and can increase kill and increase survival, part 1. Altern Ther Health Med (2007) 13(1):22–28).

(Simons et al, 2007) (Simons AL, Ahmad IM, Mattson DM, Dornfeld KH, Spitz DR. 2-Deoxy-D-glucose combined with cisplatin enhances cytotoxicity via metabolic oxidative stress in human head and neck cancer cells. Cancer Res. 2007 Apr 1;67(7):3364-70).

(Simons et al, 2009) (Simons AL, Mattson DM, Dornfeld K, Spitz, DR. Glucose deprivation-induced metabolic oxidative stress and cancer therapy. J Cancer Res Ther. 2009 Sep;5 Suppl 1:S2-6).

(Simizu et al, 1998) (Simizu S, Umezawa K, Takada M, Arber N, Imoto M. Induction of hydrogen peroxide production and Bax expression by caspase-3(-like) proteases in tyrosine kinase inhibitor-induced apoptosis in human small cell lung carcinoma cells. Exp Cell Res 1998;238:197-203).

(Singh et al, 2005) (Singh SV, et al. Sulforaphane-induced Cell Death in Human Prostate Cancer Cells Is Initiated by Reactive Oxygen Species. J. Biol. Chem., Vol. 280, Issue 20, 19911-19924, May 20, 2005).

(Siveski-Iliskovic et al, 1995) (Siveski-Iliskovic N, et al. Probucol protects against adriamycin cardiotoxicity without interfering with its antitumor effect. Circulation 91: 10-15, 1995).

(Skibsted et al, 2006) (Skibsted LH, Dragsted LO, Dyerberg J, Hansen HS, Kiens B, Ovesen LF, Tjonneland AM. Antioxidants and Health. JAMA. 2006 Aug 21;168(34):2787-9).

(Slater et al, 1995) (Slater, A. F., Nobel, C. S. & Orrenius, S. (1995) The role of intra-cellular oxidants in apoptosis. Biochim. Biophys. Acta 1271:59-62).

(Slatore et al, 2008) (Christopher G. Slatore, Alyson J. Littman, David H. Au, Jessie A. Satia, and Emily White Long-Term Use of Supplemental Multivitamins, Vitamin C, Vitamin E, and Folate Does Not Reduce the Risk of Lung Cancer. Am. J. Respir. Crit. Care Med. 2008 Mar. 1;177(5): 524-530).

(Soengas et al, 1999) (Soengas, M.S., Alarcon, R.M., Yoshida, H., Giaccia, A.J., Hakem, R. and Mak, T.W., et al. Apaf-1 and caspace-9 in p53-dependent apoptosis and tu-mor inhibition. Science 1999; 284: 156-159).

(Sonnevald, 1976) (Sonnevald P. Effect of alpha-tocopherol on cardiotoxicity of adriamycin in the rat. Cancer Treatment Rep 62:961-962, 1976).

(Spielholz et al, 1997) (Spielholz, C., Golde, D. W., Houghton, A. N., Nualart, F., and Vera, J. C. Increased facilitated transport of dehydroascorbic acid without changes in sodium-dependent ascorbate transport in human melanoma cells. Cancer Res., 57: 2529–2537, 1997).

(Stanner et al, 2004) (Stanner SA, Hughes J, Kelly CN, Buttriss J (2004). "A review of the epidemiological evidence for the 'antioxidant hypothesis'". Public Health Nutr 7 (3): 407–22).

(Stevens et al, 2005) (Stevens VL, McCullough ML, Diver WR, Rodriguez C, Jacobs EJ, Thun MJ, Calle EE. Use of multivitamins and prostate cancer mortality in a large co-hort of US men. Cancer Causes Control. 2005 Aug; 16(6):643-50).

(Stratton, Godwin, 2011) (Stratton J, Godwin M. The effect of supplemental vitamins and minerals on the development of prostate cancer: a systematic review and
meta-analysis. Fam Pract. 2011. Jan 27. [Epub ahead of print]).

(Sue et al, 1998) (Sue K, et al. Combined effects of Vitamin E and cisplatin on the
growth of murine neuroblastoma in vivo. Eur J Cancer Clin Oncol 24: 1751-1758,
1988).

(Sugiyama et al, 1996) (Sugiyama, H., Kashihara, N., Makino, H., Yamasaki, Y. & Ota, Z.
(1996) Reactive oxygen species induce apoptosis in cultured human mesangial cells.
J. Amer. Soc. Nephrol. 7:2357-2363).

(Suhail et al, 2011) (Suhail N et al. Effect of vitamins C and E on antioxidant status
of breast-cancer patients undergoing chemotherapy. J Clin Pharm Ther. 2011 Jan 4).

(Sunday, Willett, 1992) (Mary E. Sunday and Christopher G. Willett. Induction
and Spontaneous Regression of Intense Pulmonary Neuroendocrine Cell
Differentiation in a Model of Preneoplastic Lung Injury. (CANCER RESEARCH
(SUPPL.) 52. 2677s-2686s. May 1. 1992).

(Sweet et al, 1980) (Sweet F, Kao MS, Lee SC, Hagar WL, Sweet WE (August 1980).
"Ozone selectively inhibits growth of human cancer cells". Science (journal) 209
(4459): 931–3).

(Symonds et al, 2001) (M. C. Symonds et al., Hydrogen peroxide: A potent cytotoxic
agent effect in causing cellular damage and used in the possible treatment for certain tumors. Medical Hypothesis 57. July 2001: 56-58).

(Sztarovski et al, 1991) (Sztarovski, T. R. & Nathan, C. F. (1991) Production of large
amounts of hydrogen peroxide by human tumor cells. Cancer Res 51:794-798).

(Takahashi et al, 1998) (Takahashi, H., Kosaka, N. & Nakagawa, S. (1998) Alpha-
tocopherol protects PC12 cells from hyperoxia-induced apoptosis. J. Neurosci. Res.
52:184-191).

(Takeuchi et al, 1997) (Takeuchi T, Matsugo S and Morimoto K. (1997) Mutagenicity
of oxidative DNA damage in Chinese hamster V79 cells. Carcinogenesis, 18,
2051–2055).

(Tang et al, 2009) (Tang et al, Green tea, black tea consumption and risk of lung
cancer: a meta-analysis. Lung Cancer. 2009 Sep;65(3):274-83).

(Tangrea et al, 1992) (Tangrea JA, Edwards BK, Taylor PR, et al.: Long-term therapy with low-dose isotretinoin for prevention of basal cell carcinoma: a multicenter clinical trial. Isotretinoin-Basal Cell Carcinoma Study Group. J Natl Cancer Inst 84 (5): 328-32, 1992).

(Taper et al, 1996) (Taper HS, et al. Potentiation of radiotherapy by nontoxic pre-treatment with combined vitamins C and K3 in mice bearing solid transplantable tumor. Anticancer Res 16: 499-504. 1996).

(Taylor et al, 1995) (Taylor PR, Wang GQ, Sanford MD, et al: Effect of nutrition in-tervention on intermediate end points in esophageal and gastric carcinogenesis. Am J Clin Nutr 62(suppl):1420S-1423S, 1995).

(Teicher et al, 1990) (Teicher, B.A, Holden, S.A., Al-Achi, A. and Herman, T.S. Classification of antineoplastic treatments by their differential toxicity toward pu-tative oxygenated and hypoxic tumor subpopulations in vivo in the FSaII murine fibrosarcoma. Cancer Res 1990; 50: 3339-3344).

(Teicher et al, 1994) (Teicher BA, et al. In vivo modulation of several anticancer agents by beta-carotene. Cancer Chemother Pharmacol 34:235-241, 1994).

(Teramoto et al, 2000) (Teramoto S, Suzuki M, Matsuse T, Ishii T, Fukuchi Y, Ouchi Y. Effects of angiotensin-converting enzyme inhibitors on spontaneous or stimu-lated generation of reactive oxygen species by bronchoalveolar lavage cells har-vested from patients with or without chronic obstructive pulmonary disease. Jpn J Pharmacol. 2000 May;83(1):56-62).

(The ATBC Cancer Prevention Study Group, 1994) (The alpha-tocopherol, beta-carotene lung cancer prevention study: Design, methods, participant characteristics, and compliance—The ATBC Cancer Prevention Study Group. Ann Epidemiol 4:1-10, 1994).

(Thompson, 1995) (Thompson, C. B. (1995) Apoptosis in the pathogenesis and treatment of disease. Science 267:1456-1462).

(Tome et al, 2001) (Margaret E. Tome, Amanda F. Baker, Garth Powis, Claire M. Payne and Margaret M. Briehl. Catalase-overexpressing Thymocytes Are Resistant to Glucocorticoid-induced Apoptosis and Exhibit Increased Net Tumor Growth. *Cancer Research* 61, 2766-2773, March 15, 2001).

(Tomiselli et al, 2001) (Tomaselli F, et al. Photodynamic therapy enhanced by hyperbaric oxygen in acute endoluminal palliation of malignant bronchial stenosis. Eur J Cardiothorac Surg. 2001 May;19(5):549-54).

(Tomaselli et al, Lasers Surg Med. 2001) (Tomaselli F, et al. Acute effects of combined photodynamic therapy and hyperbaric oxygenation in lung cancer. Lasers Surg Med. 2001;28(5):399-403).

(Tomlison, Bodmer, 1995) (Tomlinson, I.P.M. & Bodmer, W. F. (1995) Failure of programmed cell death and differentiation as causes of tumors: Some simple mathematical models. Proc. Natl. Acad. Sci. U.S.A. 92:11130-11134).

(Tomko et al, 2006) (Robert J. Tomko, Jr., Pallavi Bansal and John S. Lazo. Airing Out an Antioxidant Role for the Tumor Suppressor p53. *Molecular Interventions* 6:23-25, (2006).

(Toyokune et al, 1995) (Toyokuni, S., Okamoto, K., Yodoi, J. & Hiai, H. (1995) Hypothesis: persistent oxidative stress in cancer. FEBS Lett 358:1-3).

(Troyano et al, 2001) (Troyano A, Fernandez C, Sancho P, de Blas E, Aller P. Effect of glutathione depletion on antitumor drug toxicity (apoptosis and necrosis) in U937 human promyelocytic cells. J Biol Chem 2001;276:47107–15).

(Tsang et al, 2003) (Tsang, W.P., Chau, S.P., Kong, S.K., Fung, K.P. and Kwok, T.T. (2003) Reactive oxygen species mediate doxorubicin induced p53-independent apoptosis. Life Sci., 73, 2047–2058).

(Umegaku et al, 1995) (Umegaku, K., Aoki, S. & Esashi, T. (1995) Whole body irradiation to mice decrease ascorbic acid concentrations in bone marrow: comparison with vitamin E. Free Radic. Biol. Med. 19:493-497).

(Ungvari, 2007) (Zoltan Ungvari. Resveratrol increases vascular oxidative stress resistance. Am J Physiol Heart Circ Physiol 292: H2417-H2424, 2007).

(van Poppel, vanden Berg, 1997) (van Poppel G, van den Berg H. Vitamins and cancer. *Cancer Lett.* 1997;114:195-202).

(Vanden Hoek et al, 2000) (Vanden Hoek TL, Becker LB, Shao Z, Li C, Schumacker PT. Preconditioning in cardiomyocytes protects by attenuating oxidant stress at reperfusion. Circ Res 2000;86:534–40).

(Vanhees et al, 2011) (Vanhees K, et al. Prenatal exposure to flavonoids: Implication for cancer risk. Toxicol Sci. 2011 Mar;120(1):59-67).

(Valko et al, 2006) (Valko M, et al. Free radicals and antioxidants in normal physiological functions and human disease. Int J Biochem Cell Biol. 2007;39(1):44-84. Epub 2006 Aug 4).

(Varro, 1974) (J. Varro, "Die Krebsbehandlung mit Ozon," Erfahungsheilkunde 23, 1974: 178-181).

(Vasquez et al., 1998) (The SUVIMAX (France) study: the role of antioxidants in the prevention of cancer and cardiovascular disease. Vasquez, Martínez C, Galán P, Preziosi P, Ribas L, Serra LL, Hercberg S. Rev Esp Salud Publica. 1998 May-Jun;72(3):173-83).

(Vaupel, Harrison, 2004) (Vaupel P and Harrison L. Tumor Hypoxia: Causative Factors, Compensatory Mechanisms, and Cellular Response. Oncologist, November 1, 2004; 9(suppl_5): 4 – 9).

(Venkataraman et al, 2004) (Venkataraman Sujatha; Wagner Brett A; Jiang Xiaohong; Wang Hong P; Schafer Freya Q; Ritchie Justine M; Patrick Burns C; Oberley Larry W; Buettner Garry R. Overexpression of manganese superoxide dismutase promotes the survival of prostate cancer cells exposed to hyperthermia. Free radical research 2004;38(10):1119-32).

(Venkataraman et al, 2005) (Venkataraman Sujatha; Jiang Xiaohong; Weydert Christine; Zhang Yuping; Zhang Hannah J; Goswami Prabhat C; Ritchie Justine M; Oberley Larry W; Buettner Garry R. Manganese superoxide dismutase over-expression inhibits the growth of androgen-independent prostate cancer cells. Oncogene 2005;24(1):77-89).

(Venturini et al, 1996) (Venturini M, et al., Multicenter randomized controlled clinical trial to evaluate cardioprotection of dexrazoxane vs. no cardioprotection in women receiving epirubicin chemotherapy for advanced breast cancer. J Clin Oncol 14:3112-3120, 1996).

(Vera et al, 1993) (Vera JC, Rivas CI, Fischbarg J, Golde DW. Mammalian facilitative hexose transports mediate the transport of dehydroascorbic acid. *Nature.* 1993;364:79–82).

(Vera et al, 1994) (Vera JC, Rivas CI, Zhang RH, Farber CM, Golde DW. Human HL-60 myeloid leukemia cells transport dehydroascorbic acid via the glucose transporters and accumulate reduced ascorbic acid. *Blood.* 1994;84:1628–1634).

(Verrier et al, 1996) (Verrier ED, Boyle EM Jr. Endothelial cell injury in cardiovascular surgery. Ann Thorac Surg 1996;62:915–22).

(Virtamo et al, 2003) (Virtamo J, et al. Incidence of cancer and mortality following alpha-tocopherol and beta-carotene supplementation: a post intervention follow-up. JAMA, 2003 Jul 23;290(4):476-85).

(Vivekanagthan et al, 2003) (Vivekananthan DP, Penn MS, Sapp SK, Hsu A, Topol EJ. Use of antioxidant vitamins for the prevention of cardiovascular disease: meta-analysis of randomised trials. *Lancet.* 2003;361:2017-2023).

(Vivekananthan et al., 2003) (Vivekananthan DP, Penn MS, Sapp SK, Hsu A, Topol EJ. Use of antioxidant vitamins for the prevention of cardiovascular disease: meta-analysis of randomised trials 2003 *Lancet* 2003 June 14; 361: 2017–23).

(Vrablic et al, 2001) (Vrablic, A. S., Albright, C. D., Craciunescu, C. N., Salganik, R. I. & Zeisel, S. H. (2001) Altered mitochondrial function and over generation of reactive oxygen species precede the induction of apoptosis by 1-O-octadecyl-2-methyl-rac-glycero-3-phosphocholine in p53-defective hepatocytes. FASEB J 15:1739-1744).

(Wagner et al, 2000) (Wagner B A; Buettner G R; Oberley L W; Darby C J; Burns C P. Myeloperoxidase is involved in H_2O_2-induced apoptosis of HL-60 human leukemia cells. The Journal of biological chemistry 2000;275(29):22461-9).

(Wagner et al, 1996) (Wagner B A; Buettner G R; Burns C P. Vitamin E slows the rate of free radical-mediated lipid peroxidation in cells. Archives of biochemistry and biophysics 1996;334(2):261-7).

(Warburg, 1996) (Otto Warburg, *The Prime Cause and Prevention of Cancer,* Wurzburg, Germany: K. Tritsch, 1996)

(Watters et al. 2009) (Watters JL, Gail MH, Weinstein SJ, Virtamo J, Albanes D. Associations between alpha-tocopherol, beta-carotene, and retinol and prostate cancer survival. Cancer Res. 2009 May 1;69(9):3833-41).

(Weijl, et al, 1997) (Weijl, N. I., Cleton, F. J. & Osanto, S. (1997) Free radicals and antioxidants in chemotherapy-induced toxicity. Cancer Treat. Rev. 23:209-240).

(Weijl et al, 2004) (Weijl NI, Elsendoorn TJ, Moison RM, Lentjes EG, Brand R, Berger R, et al: Non-protein bound iron release during chemotherapy in cancer patients. *Clin Sci (Lond) 106:* 475-484, 2004).

(Wells et al, 1995) (Wells WW, et al. Ascorbic acid and cell survival of adriamycin resistant and sensitive MCF-7 breast tumor cells. Free Rad Biol Med 18:699-708, 1995).

(Wentworth et al, 2001) (Wentworth P Jr, Jones LH, Wentworth AD, Zhu X, Larsen NA, Wilson IA, Xu X, Goddard WA 3rd, Janda KD, Eschenmoser A, Lerner RA. Antibody catalysis of the oxidation of water. Science. 2001 Sep 7;293(5536):1806-11).

(Wentworth et al, 2002) (Wentworth P Jr, McDunn JE, Wentworth AD, Takeuchi C, Nieva J, Jones T, Bautista C, Ruedi JM, Gutierrez A, Janda KD, Babior BM, Eschenmoser A, Lerner RA. Evidence for antibody-catalyzed ozone formation in bacterial killing and inflammation. Science. 2002 Dec 13;298(5601):2195-9).

(Wenzel et al, 2003) (Wenzel, U., Kuntz, S., Jambor de Sousa, U. and Daniel, H. (2003) Nitric oxide suppresses apoptosis in human colon cancer cells by scavenging mitochondrial superoxide anions. Int. J. Cancer, 106, 666–675).

(Wenzel et al, 2004) (Wenzel U, Nickel A, Kuntz S and Daniel H. Ascorbic acid suppresses drug-induced apoptosis in human colon cancer cells by scavenging mitochondrial superoxide anions. Carcinogenesis, Vol. 25, No. 5, 703-712, May 2004).

(Wenzel et al, 2005) (Wenzel U, Nickel A and Daniel H. Alpha-lipoic acid induces apoptosis in human colon cancer cells by increasing mitochondrial respiration with a concomitant O_2^- generation. Apoptosis. Volume 10, Number 2 / March, 2005. pp. 359-368).

(Weydert et al, 2003) (Weydert CJD, Smith BB, Xu L, Kregel KC, Ritchie JM, Davis CS, Oberley LW. Inhibition of oral cancer cell growth by adenovirus *MnSOD* plus BCNU treatment. Free Radic Biol Med 2003;34:316–29).

(White, McCubrey, 2001) (White MK. and McCubrey JA. (2001) Suppression of apoptosis: role in cell growth and neoplasia. Leukemia, 15, 1011–10121).

(Wiernik et al, 1992) (Wiernik PH, Yeap B, Vogl SE, et al. Hexamethylmelamine and low or moderate dose cisplatin with or without pyridoxine for treatment of advanced ovarian carcinoma: a study of the Eastern Cooperative Oncology Group. Cancer Invest (1992) 10(1):1–9).

(Williams, Fisher, 2005) (Williams, K.J. and Fisher, E.A. Oxidation, lipoproteins, and atherosclerosis: which is wrong, the antioxidants or the theory? Current Opinion in Clinical Nutrition & Metabolic Care. 8(2):139-146, March 2005).

(Winkler et al, 1999) (Winkler BS, Boulton ME, Gottsch JD, Sternberg P. Oxidative damage and age-related macular degeneration. Mole Vis. 1999;5:32).

(Witenberg et al, 1999) (Witenberg B, Kletter Y, Kalir HH, et al. Ascorbic acid inhibits apoptosis induced by X irradiation in HL60 myeloid leukemia cells. Radiat Res (1999) 152(5):468–478).

(Wu et al, 2002) (Wu K, Willett WC, Chan JM, Fuchs CS, Colditz GA, Rimm EB, Giovannucci EL. A prospective study on supplemental vitamin E intake and risk of colon cancer in women and men. Cancer Epidemiol Biomarkers Prev 2002;11:1298-304).

(Wu et al, 2004) (Wu SJ, et al. Effects of vitamin E on the cinnamaldehyde-induced apoptotic mechanism in human PLC/PRF/5 cells. Clin Exp Pharmacol Physiol. 2004 Nov;31(11):770-6).

(Wu, Ng, Lin, 2004) (Wu. S-J, Ng L-T and Lin C-C. Effects of vitamin E on the cinnamaldehyde-induced apoptotic mechanism in human PLC/PRF/5 cells. Clinical and Experimental Pharmacology and Physiology, Volume 31, Number 11, November 2004 , pp. 770-776(7).

(Wu et al, 2005) (Wu SJ, et al. Effects of antioxidants and caspase-3 inhibitor on the phenylethyl isothiocyanate-induced apoptotic signaling pathways in human PLC/PRF/5 cells. Eur J Pharmacol. 2005 Aug 22;518(2-3):96-106).

(Wu et al, 2006) (Xin-jiang Wu et al. The Production of Reactive Oxygen Species and the Mitochondrial Membrane Potential Are Modulated during Onion Oil–Induced Cell Cycle Arrest and Apoptosis in A549 Cells. American Society for Nutrition J. Nutr. 136:608-613, March 2006).

(Wu, Hua, 2007) (XJ Wu, X Hua. Targeting ROS: Selective Killing of Cancer Cells by a Cruciferous Vegetable Derived Pro-Ox . Cancer Biol Ther (2007) 6(1):5).

(Wyllie, 1987) (Wyllie, A. H. (1987) Cell death. Int. Rev. Cytol. 17(suppl.):755-785)

(Xiao et al, 2006) (Xiao D, et al. Phenethyl isothiocyanate-induced apoptosis in PC-3 human prostate cancer cells is mediated by reactive oxygen species-dependent disruption of the mitochondrial membrane potential. Carcinogenesis 2006 27(11):2223-2234).

(Xiao et al, Mol Cancer Ther. 2006) (Xiao et al. Benzyl isothiocyanate–induced apoptosis in human breast cancer cells is initiated by reactive oxygen species and regulated by Bax and Bak. D, Mol Cancer Ther. 2006;5:2931-2945).

(Xu et al,) (Minqi Xu, James E. Scott, Kan-Zhi Liu, Hannah R. Bishop, Diane E. Renaud, Richard M. Palmer, Abdel Soussi-Gounni, and David A. Scott. The influence of nicotine on granulocytic differentiation - inhibition of the oxidative burst and bacterial killing and increased matrix metalloproteinase-9 release. *BMC Cell Biology*, Apr 2008, 15;9:19).

(Yamamoto et al, 1998) (Yamamoto K, Hanada R, Kikuchi A; et al. Spontaneous regression of localized neuroblastoma detected by mass screening. *J Clin Oncol.* 1998;16(4):1265-1269).

(Yang et al, 1993) (Yang CS, Wang ZY. Tea and cancer (review). J Natl Cancer Inst 1993;85:1038–49).

(Yang et al, 2996) (Yang JY, Della-Fera MA, Nelson-Dooley C, Baile CA. Molecular Mechanisms of Apoptosis Induced by Ajoene in 3T3-L1 Adipocytes. Obesity (Silver Spring). 2006 Mar;14(3):388-97).

(Yasui et al, 2002) (Yasui, H., Deo, K., Ogura, Y., Yoshida, H., Shiraga, T., Kagayama, A. and Sakurai, H., Evidence for singlet oxygen involvement in rat and human cytochrome P450-dependent substrate oxidations, Drug Metab. Pharmacokin. 2002, 17 (5): 416-426).

(Yedjou et al, 2008) (Yedjou CG, Rogers C, Brown e, Tchounwou PB. Differential effect of ascorbic acid and n-acetyl-L-cysteine on arsenic trioxide-mediated oxidative stress in human leukemia (HL-60) cells. J Biochem Mol Toxicol. 2008;22(2):85-92).

(Yokomizo et al, 1995) (Yokomizo A, Ono M, Nanri H, Makino Y, Ohga T, Wada M, Okamoto T, Yodoi J, Kuwano M, Kohno K. Cellular levels of thioredoxin associated with drug sensitivity to cisplatin, mitomycin C, doxorubicin, and etoposide. Cancer Res 1995;**55**:4293–4296).

(Young et al, 2001) (Young, A. J. & Lowe, G. M. (2001) Antioxidant and prooxidant properties of carotenoids. Arch. Biochem. Biophys. 385:20-27).

(Yu et al, 2006) (Li Yu et al. Autophagic programmed cell death by selective catalase degradation. PNAS, March 28, 2006; 103(13): 4952 - 4957).

(Zanker, Kroczek, 1990) (Zänker KS, Kroczek R (1990). "In vitro synergistic activity of 5-fluorouracil with low-dose ozone against a chemoresistant tumor cell line and fresh human tumor cells". Chemotherapy 36 (2): 147–54).

(Zeisel, 2004) (Zeisel SH. Antioxidants suppress apoptosis. J. Nutr. Nov 1, 2004. Vol. 134. No. 11. pp. 21795-31805).

(Zeisel (2), 2004) (Zeisel, S.H. (2004) Antioxidants suppress apoptosis. J. Nutr. 134:319S-3180S).

(Zhang et al. 2009) (Zhang Y, Coogan P, Palmer JR, Strom BL, Rosenberg L. Vitamin and mineral use and risk of prostate cancer: the case-control surveillance study. Cancer Causes Control. 2009 Jul;20(5):691-8).

(Zhivotovsky et al, 1994) (Zhivotovsky, B., Wade, D., Nicotera, P. & Orrenius, S. (1994) Role of nucleases in apoptosis. Int. Arch. Allergy Immunol. 105:333-338).

(Zhong et al, 1995) (Zhong W, Oberley LW, Oberley TD, Yan T, Domann FE, St. Clair DK. Inhibition of cell growth and sensitization to oxidative damage by over-expression of manganese superoxide dismutase in rat glioma cells. Cell Growth Differentiation 1995;7:1175–86).

(Zilberstein et al, 1997) (Zilberstein, J., Bromberg, A., Frantz, A., Rosenbach-Belkin, V., Kritzman, A. and Pfefermann, R., et al. Light-dependent oxygen consumption in bacterio-chlorophyll-serine-treated melanoma tumors: On-line determination using a tissue-inserted oxygen microsensor. Photochem Photobiol 1997; 65: 1012-1019).

(Zimmerman et al, 2001) (Zimmermann, K. C., Bonzon, C. & Green, D. R. (2001) The machinery of programmed cell death. Pharmachol. Ther. 92:57-70).

(Zou et al, 2006) (Wei Zou et al. Vitamin C Inactivates the Proteasome Inhibitor PS-341 in Human Cancer Cells. Clinical Cancer Research Vol. 12, 273-280, January 2006).

www.ingramcontent.com/pod-product-compliance
Lightning Source LLC
Chambersburg PA
CBHW081102170526
45165CB00008B/2298